Traveling with Sugar

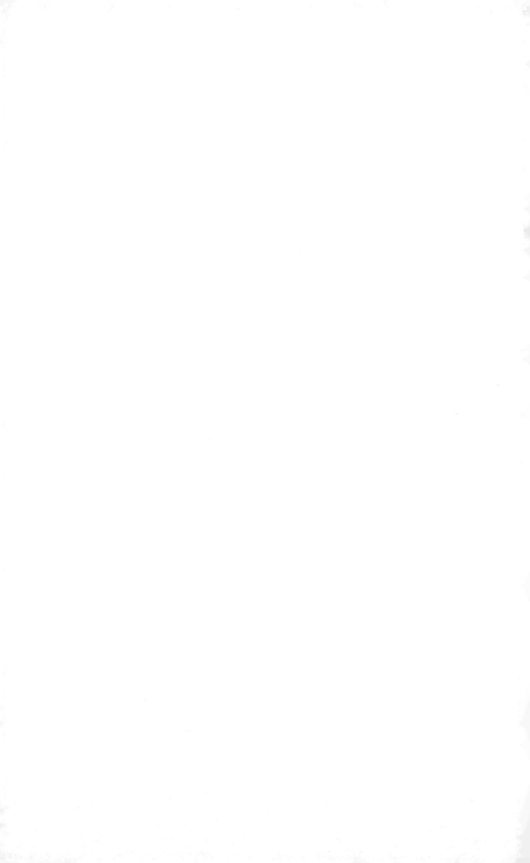

Traveling with Sugar

Chronicles of a Global Epidemic

Amy Moran-Thomas

UNIVERSITY OF CALIFORNIA PRESS

University of California Press
Oakland, California

© 2019 by Amy Moran-Thomas

Library of Congress Cataloging-in-Publication Data

Names: Moran-Thomas, Amy, author.
Title: Traveling with sugar : chronicles of a global
   epidemic / Amy Moran-Thomas.
Description: Oakland, California : University of
   California Press, [2019] | Includes bibliographical
   references and index. |
Identifiers: LCCN 2018054745 (print) | LCCN 2018056398
   (ebook) | ISBN 9780520969858 (ebook)
   | ISBN 9780520297531 (cloth : alk. paper)
   | ISBN 9780520297548 (pbk. : alk. paper)
Subjects: LCSH: Diabetes—Belize. | Diabetics—Case
   studies.
Classification: LCC RA645.D5 (ebook) | LCC RA645.D5
   M67 2019 (print) | DDC 616.4/62—dc23
LC record available at https://lccn.loc.gov/2018054745

Manufactured in the United States of America

26 25 24 23 22 21 20 19
10 9 8 7 6 5 4 3 2 1

Travel with (chravl wid): to be troubled with, suffer from; have a recurring medical problem.

Travel (chravl): euphemism for being on one's death bed.
—Belize Kriol dictionary

A lot of people, countrywide, in the whole entire world, here in Belize and Dangriga, are traveling with sugar . . .
—Anne, reflecting on diabetic sugar across three generations of her family, 2010

Contents

PART ONE

Contexts

Approach

Emergency in Slow Motion

Sugar . . . has been one of the massive demographic forces in world history.

—Sidney Mintz, *Sweetness and Power*

A lot of people, countrywide, in the whole entire world, here in Belize and Dangriga, are traveling with sugar.

Diabetic is a dangerous thing . . . It's like cancer . . . It makes you get weak, it makes you get blind, because of the sugar in your eyes and the pressure . . . It makes you get slim, especially if you don't know . . .

That is the most [serious] thing that is hampering the whole entire world. The diabetic sugar . . .

The whole of your family can get the diabetic. You have to look out [even] if you don't catch it—maybe your children later on to come . . .

—Anne, expanding on living with diabetic sugar in Belize

I have never seen a good stand-alone picture of "diabetes." If not for Mr. P's storytelling, I might never have glimpsed it at all. He was paging through a family album on the kitchen table in his home on Belize's south coast, showing me pictures of his wife. He smiled back at the old photos of her as a Garifuna teacher standing firm beside a rural schoolhouse. We watched as on the pages she became a mother, then a grandmother. The next time Mrs. P appeared in the album, she was suddenly on crutches. "Sugar," Mr. P said simply as he paged forward in time, the photographs sharpening in color and filling with grandchildren. In a family Christmas picture his wife's entire right foot was missing. At one wedding, both of Mrs. P's legs were gone below the knee. We watched her disappear a piece at a time from the pictures, until she was absent altogether.

Later, that scene kept looping in my memory: Mr. P turning the album's pages carefully so as not to crinkle its plastic sleeves, the photographic record of loss a surreal counterpoint to the stories he told about raising a family and caring for the generations to come. About the harrowing parts, he only ever repeated, "Sugar." Back then, I didn't know about the dozens of different cellular pathways and blood capillary injuries by which you can lose a limb to diabetic sugar's wears. But I could never forget how he narrated a series of slow losses that somehow had come to feel inevitable.

At the time, I thought I would be writing about another health topic altogether. Early in graduate school, I went for a preliminary visit to Belize to lay foundations for what I thought would become an anthropology project about people's perspectives on worm control programs. Mr. P had obligingly shown me the apazote leaves in his garden, which could be added to a pot of stew beans for worm treatment. But clearly, intestinal parasites seemed a minor footnote to him, in contrast to the pink housedress still floating on a hanger near their kitchen window. The more people I talked with, the more it appeared that the pressing health issue on many people's minds was not parasites, but rather the shape-shifting disease of diabetes.

The worms I had initially planned to write about are so easy to visualize. Public health campaigns focused on parasites often put cartoons of their targets on T-shirts and sponsor museum exhibits that display worms in glass bottles of formaldehyde. Fascinated viewers frequently do not read the captions; they just stare at the grotesque-looking specimens. Diabetes, in contrast, is strangely ineffable. You can't show it to anyone in a jar. It has no totem: no insect vector to put on letterhead like malaria-bearing mosquitoes, no virus to blow up under a microscope and target like Ebola, no tumor to visualize fighting like cancer, no clot to bust like a stroke. It eludes any single, self-evident image.

As Mr. P showed me, in order for most pictures of diabetic sugar to mean much at all, you need to know something about their before and after in time and place. Yet traces of diabetes were everywhere in Belize, once people taught me to pay attention to the quiet, constant presences that so many lived with. I began to glimpse the negative spaces of what was missing: Bodies that sometimes slowly stopped healing. Potent medicines and devices that sometimes slowly stopped working. Specters of lifesaving technologies that existed somewhere else in the world. Memories of former vegetable gardens and lost homelands. Loved ones changing in photograph albums. Missing limbs, failing organs. An empty dress left hanging to outline an absence.

I didn't know how to read those signs when I first walked Belize's southern coast, observing what washed up along the tideline. But like my interviews about the health of people and places, the tide arriving from the deep ocean presented a knot of entwined lives I didn't know how to untangle: the last nylon strings of "ghost nets" that now make up half of the ocean's plastic debris, long abandoned by fishermen but still catching life until they unravel; curds of broken Styrofoam in clotted algae; hunks of dying coral from the heat-bleached reef; thin gleaming strips of brown seaweed that looked as if they'd been unspooled from the reels of an old cassette tape. Odds were that most of the bright microplastic shards had once been food containers, perhaps ejected from passing cruise ships decades ago in order to be worn down to such confetti-sized slivers. I watched as local women deftly swept the day's debris from their stretch of beach, treating the sand underfoot like the floor of a well-tended kitchen.

SHORELINES

These are some of the shorelines of sugar to which the stories ahead will keep returning.[1] On a nearby wooden porch worn gray by brooms and sand, I used to sit sometimes with Cresencia and her Aunt Dee in the afternoon when it was too hot to walk anywhere. They would laugh about how I looked even whiter when sweating out beads of sunblock and invite me to stretch with them along the steps, trying to catch a little breeze from the sea. Dee liked to show me the latest foil punch card of tablets from her small bucket of "sugar pills"—an old joke that stayed funny both because they were pills for her sugar, and because she honestly could never tell whether the clinic's diabetes medications were working better than a placebo. Cresencia had stopped taking insulin injections for carefully weighed reasons after the hospital had last given her up for dead. But from the porch, you could see the tree where a meal of lavish Garifuna dishes had once been buried in the sand as part of an emergency *chugú*, offerings for the ancestral spirits who had revived her from what her physicians were certain would be an irreversible coma.

Not far from there, on a sunny overgrown highway parallel to the coast, a teenager with type 1 diabetes named Jordan used to walk in a determined half delirium, trying to reach the hospital before diabetic ketoacidosis set in. It was also along this coastline that a legendary healer with diabetes named Arreini used to send me with a tub to hang her sopping laundry after we finished at the washboard, little chores that were part of the daily test and price of being an old midwife's student. If I didn't use enough extra clothespins for her heaviest shirts to stay on the line in the stiff sea wind, she would snap at me, "*Merigan!*" (American), and I was not allowed to ask her any more questions for the night.

Somewhere far across this water lay the sugar islands from which her ancestors had come, and toward which this story will slowly wend back in trying to understand the sugar now rising in her family's bodies. It was also in Arreini's seaside kitchen where I met her daughter Guillerma when she was hoping to receive dialysis to clean her blood—even though such intricate technologies from abroad were nearly impossible to procure at that time, much less maintain. Some of these friends have thrived for many years past medical predictions. Other people I knew dealt with limbs that eroded from diabetic sugar and eventually required amputation. Many of their heaviest losses happened between my irregular trips back, although over the past decade I have also known many people whose injuries were painstakingly mended.

Most everyone in Belize had somehow witnessed the long list of strange ravages caused by diabetes: blindness, renal failure, bone disease, deadened nerves and numb limbs, pain shooting through limbs or stinging like needles, hunger that did not stop when you ate, thirst that lasted no matter how much water you drank. Whenever I thought I finally knew what diabetic injuries looked like, it seemed I would encounter some new manifestation. Like a dream or a nightmare that kept revealing more images. Once, a friend called me to come over after midnight, but there was nothing either of us could do. We stood watching her mother, Sulma, running through the house as it got harder to catch her breath or even breathe, after years of diabetes complications had contributed to organ failure. Her children had saved up to buy her an oxygen tank, but it cost one hundred dollars and had already run out. Sulma thrashed through the kitchen like someone trying to claw toward the surface, only there was no water. It looked like someone drowning in the open air.

"Far from being a disease of higher income nations, diabetes is very much a disease associated with poverty," Jean Claude Mbanya of Cameroon has argued, writing as president of the International Diabetes Federation. "The global community still has not fully appreciated the urgent need to increase funding for non-communicable diseases (NCDs), to make essential NCD medicines available for all and to include the treatment of diabetes and other NCDs into strengthened primary healthcare systems. The evidence for the need to act will soon be overwhelming."[2]

The president of the Belize Diabetes Association, Anthony Castillo, once told me how strangers often tell him he doesn't *look* like he has diabetes. He laughed about this: "Well, how are you supposed to look? Is there a look?" And it's true that if you went by the pictures that tend to show up in international papers, it would be easy to mistake globally rising diabetes for a well-understood, generally mild affliction simply linked to excess. When international media coverage of diabetes appears at all, it often implies individual misbehavior—as if people with diabetes simply cause their own conditions—like the upsettingly typical *Economist* headline "Eating Themselves to Death."[3]

These commonplace news stories and assumptions probably would not upset me so much now, if I had not once accepted some version of them myself.

A GLOBAL EPIDEMIC AS SEEN FROM BELIZE

Although it took me awhile to realize, I was one in a long line of outsiders who traveled to places like Belize assuming that infectious diseases must be the country's key health issues. Contagious conditions could be serious matters too—the Stann Creek District, where most of this book is anchored, was experiencing one of the highest HIV/AIDS rates in Belize, and Belize had the highest rate in Central America.[4] Yet as Garifuna anthropologist Joseph Palacio observed of HIV/AIDS in Belize: "It is a disease that is killing our people. But there are other diseases that are not receiving as much attention. They are diabetes, hypertension, and glaucoma. There is hardly one of us over 40 years of age, who does not have one or more of these public health problems."[5]

During my initial visit to Dangriga, I asked a prominent Garifuna physician for feedback on my proposed project. He urged me to focus on diabetes and its many chronic complications instead of parasitic worms. He also offered to mentor the project if I came back to spend a year in Belize, getting to know people who were interested in being interviewed about their experiences and trying to learn something about the ways they were making sense of what was happening.

Many doctors worldwide are also confused by the ways diabetes is now changing. Type 1 (about 5 percent of the world's cases) used to be commonly called "juvenile diabetes," while more gradually developing type 2 was labeled "adult onset diabetes" (about 95 percent of cases). They are both rising steeply. Over one million children and teenagers worldwide are now estimated to have type 1 alone.[6] But today, more children are also developing type 2, and more adults type 1. In untreated versions of either type, high or low blood sugar wears on the blood vessels carrying it. These vascular complications can accrue into severe injuries over time, including organ damage and limbs with circulation so limited that even tiny ulcers might end in amputation. Some researchers today propose to frame types of diabetes instead more like gradations on a spectrum, offering new labels: severe autoimmune diabetes; severe insulin-deficient diabetes; severe insulin-resistant diabetes; mild obesity-related diabetes; and mild age-related diabetes.[7] Many of the first people I met in Belize, though, simply called it all *sugar*. I framed this project's scope accordingly.

By the time I returned to live for a year in southern Belize in 2009–10, I had read everything I could find about diabetes. There was an odd dissonance between the tenor of U.S. public health conversations at the time, where the topic was still often assumed to be minor background noise, and statistics I could not really fathom. For instance, the International Diabetes Federation estimated that diabetes annually killed more people worldwide than HIV/AIDS and breast cancer combined.[8] Somehow, I typed abstract numbers over and over into research proposals back then without grasping the implication that a significant number of the people I was getting to know were going to face untimely deaths.

This book is set in Belize, but it also signals a global story. Diabetes takes specific shape in each life, family, and nation—but it's also spreading and causing unevenly patterned injuries and deaths in nearly all countries in the world today. Belize was dealing with the situation about as well as a very small country with limited resources initially could manage. Most health workers and policy makers I encountered in Belize cared greatly about trying to address the rising issue of diabetes. The uneasy scenes in this book show just how complicated a global problem diabetes is—even for a small country labeled "middle income" by the World Bank's relative standards, where so many community leaders and caregivers are working hard to respond. Many health officials and doctors in Belize actively encouraged critical dialogue, and were trying to expand discussions about the next steps against a growing epidemic in which their offices and many others have some role to play in future

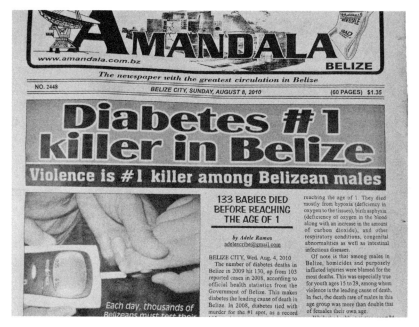

National headline, August 2010.

policies. But the fact is that the food systems and agricultural toxicities contributing to diabetes are domains far beyond the purview of any Ministry of Health alone. Even the wealthiest governments in the world have not managed to bring diabetes under control.

Belize is so beautiful that its reputation as a vacation spot for Europeans and North Americans can saturate even academic visions and distract from serious life struggles. The country's name often brings cruise ship brochures to mind. But many citizens, of course, also struggle with material constraints and social issues similar to those in neighboring countries, as much careful anthropology in Belize has shown.[9] Still, I have received enough questions over the years from audiences who have not taken social struggles in Belize seriously that it is worth reprising a thumbnail sketch of resource context: Belize is somewhere toward the lower economic range of countries in Latin America and the Caribbean. It is among the countries where the average income is more than four thousand dollars but less than five thousand dollars, according to World Bank estimates of GDP per capita in 2016. For a sense of regional reference, the other five countries listed in that income range include Jamaica, Guyana, El Salvador, Guatemala, and Paraguay.[10]

The Stann Creek District has the highest rate of diabetes in the country, nearly double the national average.[11] I talked with all kinds of people across Belize's tiny and diverse population. But as I began to be introduced to families dealing with diabetes, I ended up meeting a disproportionate number of Garifuna people (more properly, in plural, Garinagu). Both Black and Indigenous,[12] Garinagu make up some 5 percent of Belize's overall population but represent the majority of residents in Dangriga. They number among the world's surviving speakers of a Carib-Arawak Kalinago language and widely consider themselves a "nation across borders," as Joseph Palacio puts it,[13] with thriving communities across Guatemala, Honduras, Belize, Nicaragua, and U.S. cities from New York and Los Angeles to Chicago. "Certain diseases are known to have high incidence among the Garinagu relative to the wider population," the National Garifuna Council (NGC) of Belize wrote in its statement on health. "These include diabetes, hypertension, hepatitis, cataracts, and glaucoma. There is urgent need for studies to be carried out as well as the provision of treatment."[14]

Wading with patients across washed-out roads knee deep in mud to keep doctor's appointments, or traveling by canoe alongside everyone else when Tropical Storm Arthur washed out Kendall Bridge (which cut off the single road that linked southern Belize to the rest of the country and its only tertiary care hospital), I saw how realities often labeled "environmental" in the keywords of an academic journal were already part of the terrain that people with diabetes were negotiating in life. Nurse Suzanne recalled floating from rooftop to rooftop a few days after Hurricane Iris to deliver diabetic pills and insulin. The rough boat ride through floodwaters made her seasick, but she had heard how many families—on nearly every rooftop—had at least one person going into a coma or other diabetic emergency on top of their houses.

Once, I rode through the Maya Mountains in the back of a slow-moving ambulance with Paulo and his young daughter Elisa, wondering about tipping points. Elisa's pharmaceutically induced high blood sugar was a secondary concern to the fact that her skin was "coming unglued," which may also have been a side effect of the steroid medicines. We never knew for sure. There was no IV rack, so Paulo and I took turns holding the bag until our arms shook. None of us had been inside an ambulance before. We had imagined speeding to Belize City, but instead we told each other jokes about wishing bus drivers would travel this slowly along the precipitous highway.

Years later I followed behind Paulo as he chopped dense jungle plants away to clear Elisa's grave, the surrounding vegetation's growth a ruthless account of the years I had been gone. I have never felt more responsibility than when I learned that her mother, Angeline, had waited three years for me, and together we made the trip to see her daughter's grave for the first time. Afterward, Angeline handed me a photo of herself kneeling with open arms as Elisa took her first baby steps. The fact that the picture's chemical exposures had outlasted Elisa's seemed to dissolve all the words we tried to say. I gave them an image in return, an ornament engraved at a Pennsylvania Christmas shop. They cut the ribbon off and nailed it to the dash of their pickup truck.

Elisa's real name is written on that ornament, but not in this book. One difficult decision in finalizing this project was that most of its contributors requested that I use their actual names. "But then it wouldn't be true," one research contributor protested, when I asked for her input choosing a pseudonym. Others did prefer to create new names, as Belize is such a small place.[15] For this reason, I have mostly stuck with typical anthropological conventions of changing people's names unless they are public figures whose names have been previously published, changing place names except for district capitals, and at times blurring particular identifying details. Still I remain uneasy about these trade-offs, wanting to recognize people's intellectual contributions to this project.

On the other hand, most everyone I met in Belize has more than one name. When Antonia later told me to call her Beh, she said that when I first arrived at her door with a nurse asking for her by her legal name, she knew we had not been sent by friends. Her neighbor Kara had not even known her own legal name until she went to vote for the first time and discovered that in the state's eyes her name was Roseanne. Her mother had chosen to call her children by one set of names in real life and to write another name on official documents for them to claim one day or not as they saw fit. I offer this book's names in something of that spirit, an extra name that could be opted into or plausibly denied by each of these individuals as lives change over time. It also remains a way of asking readers to engage with the larger health and social issues being described, but to respect the privacy of individuals unless they have reached out first.[16]

The slow time-lapse stories unfolding in Mr. P's album were also shaped by a gradually changing landscape. Erosion touched human bodies as well as their environs, atmospheres, and infrastructures. They all wore down in ways that were materially connected. In fact, Mr. P and I first started up our conversation while standing in the doorway of a stranger's barn, watching the broken-down yellow school bus we'd been traveling on get pulled up a hill backward by another school bus. That road strained many engines, and bad weather chronically worsened already rough terrain. That particular afternoon, the hours sitting around the farm where our bus broke down felt like the opposite of a crisis. But that same trip for someone urgently needing medical care would have been a very different matter. One woman recalled how her surgeon planned to cut below the knee, but the vehicle carrying two necessary bags of blood sent by a loved one got stuck in flooded roads after a storm. The infection moved faster than the ambulance. By the time the blood delivery arrived, the surgeon had to cut above.

TRAVELING WITH SUGAR

One of the first expressions I heard for diabetes when I arrived in Dangriga was "traveling with sugar." *Sugar* is a very common phrase for diabetes—though "traveling with sugar" is not a set label, just one possible translation. In Belize's English Kriol, to "travel with" has long been a term for living with chronic disease.[17] This striking turn of phrase stayed with me as I saw how trips in search of care were a significant part of how many people with diabetes spent time, often traveling by slow public transportation to far-flung clinics, hospitals, temples, or other destinations in search of materials "to maintain" themselves and support their family members. "Traveling with sugar" also echoed common reflections that living with diabetes could feel like being on a strange trip or a very long road, chronic routes that people had to navigate for themselves without knowing where it all might end up.

In Garifuna idiom, one could also "travel" in a spiritual sense, through forms of inner reflective work or metaphysical communication with visiting ancestors. That is why expressions like "to take a trip" or "to get a passport" can double as Garifuna euphemisms for death.[18] I remember stopping by Ára's house on the night before she died, its familiar rooms suddenly filled with children who had made the trip from Chicago when they heard the news. They told the nurse I was accompanying not to worry about checking Ára's sugar unless she woke up again. "She is traveling now."

If some of the people I met were traveling with sugar, I was trying to travel part of the way with them: to be worthy company in moments when people invited me somewhere, to write down what they offered up, to ground my questions, and to learn what I could from faraway libraries or locations abroad that might fill in some blanks about the deep divides between us and the uneven conundrums people faced. Foods, technologies, and medicines were also traveling. Like the movement of people, objects' mobility could be capacitated or curtailed by larger infrastructures. Some of the most profound "travels with sugar" were the first journey across a room on a new prosthetic leg or learning to travel on one's hands, people teaching each other to move again as bodies and worlds change.

An ambulatory anthropology of sugar draws attention to how differently we each circulated through the same infrastructures, and how my own comings and goings contrasted so starkly with the mobility of others. Sometimes, but not always, I could borrow a pickup truck and offer rides to the hospital for emergencies. I accompanied hitchhiking friends to doctors and glimpsed the terrible frustration along certain junctures as air-conditioned resort vehicles sped by, but I have also been a passenger in precisely such private vehicles that passed by good friends. There was no eschewing the tourist infrastructures I moved through and no avoiding their troubled histories and ongoing implications they carried. And, of course, traveling with sugar can mean all of this too, trailing charged colonial legacies: travel with money, pleasure, illicit gains.

Tourists were hardly the only ones coming and going. "Garifuna people, *we travel*," Antonia told me emphatically. "We traveled from Africa." For many proud members of the Garifuna diaspora, traveling is an important idea far beyond health alone. It signals a deep history of fierce persistence against ongoing dispossessions and today includes a diasporic community of more than three hundred thousand strong around the world. "*Travelling* the ocean under British control" is the first theme that Joseph Palacio highlighted in his oral history work, when he italicized the word to signal its meaning as both a specific historical practice and a more abstract ideal of active navigation through a matrix of oppression.[19] "I Have Traveled" (Áfayahádina) is a well-known Garifuna song that describes the composer's good fortune: "While she has traveled and seen the world, she chooses to remain in her home village."[20]

Others wished for such luck. Reliance on medical technologies like dialysis often thwarted people's plans to eventually return home. Some in U.S. cities even considered themselves in medical "exile," stranded abroad with diabetes and its complications. Still others in Belize who were more tenuously connected to kin networks abroad nonetheless lived with full details of the medical specialists they could not reach.

Even a modest job in a U.S. paper cup factory could open a world of retirement resources to be leveraged back home later, such as when one woman in Dangriga had her specialty diabetes prescription pills (unavailable in Belize for any price) delivered monthly via FedEx from a CVS Pharmacy in Chicago.

Traveling organizations like the Belize Diabetes Associations of New York and Miami coordinate with wider networks from across the Caribbean and Central America to bring care teams to Belize each year. Many individuals who contributed to this said they considered these kindred transnational communities as the publics—along with caregivers and families living with diabetes elsewhere in the world—that they hoped this project might reach. Accordingly, I have placed certain reflections meant for academics alone in footnotes and online, trying to find language that might also travel.[21]

Of course, the word *sugar* already contains many journeys and histories. One version of how sugar's pivotal episodes altered the course of Garifuna history might go like this: Columbus planted sugarcane on what became the Dominican Republic in 1492.[22] By 1505, the first slave ships arrived.[23] The Caribbean archipelago at that time was one of the most heavily populated geographies on earth. By the late eighteenth century, some 90 percent of the Kalinago population and other Indigenous peoples of the Antilles had been exterminated by military campaigns and European epidemics, as island after island was converted into sugar plantations.

By the late eighteenth century, the last Indigenous-controlled sovereign territory in the Caribbean was Saint Vincent, an island strategically chosen as a fallback point because its mountainous geography allowed for fierce defense. It also became home to a growing community of mixed Indigenous and African ancestry (including men and women who escaped boat by boat from the sugar economies of surrounding islands), which colonial authorities soon labeled "Black Caribs." This group that came to call themselves Garifuna[24] defended their land against European invasions for nearly two hundred years, winning a long series of wars against the British. In 1796, the British military finally managed to exile the majority of the Garifuna families from their land, which they had called not Saint Vincent but Yurumein, "Homeland." This violent dispossession occurred because the English wanted their land for a sugar plantation.[25]

There are at least *two* plants relevant to the topic of global diabetes that were growing on Saint Vincent on the day of Garifuna exile, both

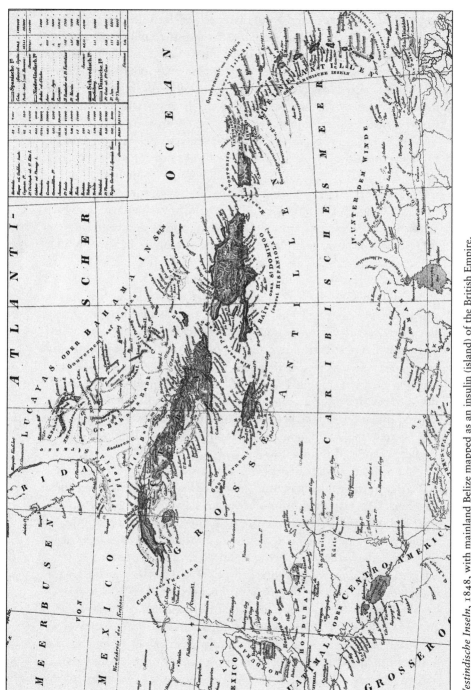

Westindische Inseln, 1848, with mainland Belize mapped as an insulin (island) of the British Empire.

of which British companies would later sell back to the descendants of those Garifuna people who were packed into the hold of the warship called *Experiment* and its fleet. The primary one was sugarcane. But another was a weedier specimen with tiny pale flowers that the British had bioprospected from Turkey long ago—*Galega officinalis*, the botanical source for metformin, which is today the most widely prescribed diabetes pharmaceutical in the world.[26]

An estimated three-quarters of the Garifuna population died during this forced removal from Saint Vincent to Central America, especially while being held captive on the isle of Balliceaux. Many of their ancestral crops were also lost during this time, although survivors managed to keep cassava plants alive in the ship's hold, watering them with their sweat.[27] But the majority of their medicines, foods, and vegetables fell into possession of British planters, who sent samples back to London for agricultural exhibits and testing by pharmaceutical companies. The British called this the Garifuna people's "transition."

In public health, the term *epidemiological transition* is often applied to explain the rise of chronic conditions (such as diabetes) in the late twentieth century.[28] In contrast, this book aims to craft a troubled, interrupted, and slowed-down version of this transition story: one that approaches the uneven distributions of diabetic sugar in relation to the ongoing effects of colonial legacies and modes of knowledge making. To do so, it builds on the arguments of numerous scholars who have considered the interrelations between colonial violence and rising diabetes elsewhere in the world, and considers ethnographic realities in relation to these shape-shifting histories.[29]

No one factor alone can explain the way the odds have gradually been stacked against healthy agriculture in places like Belize. But if you take a step back and play the history over again slowly, there is a before and after to how food systems have changed. For Garinagu, some of the relevant episodes upon arrival in Belize could include many small incidents: The colonial creation and subsequent neglect of Garifuna land reserves. The year the farming demonstrators got defunded. The year the government stopped selling the variety of rice that people knew how to grow.

Many tracts of land have been sold to foreigners to cover diabetes medical bills. The changing kinds of foods sold in local grocery stores also each had a history. More recent shifts only compound much longer histories of dispossession: Back in the 1790s, British authorities had dispatched natural scientists to define racial markers in hopes of disproving the Garifuna's dual ancestry as both Black and Indigenous in an effort to deny them legal rights to their ancestral territory. Even today, Garifuna people still struggle to be legally recognized as Indigenous by the state—part of a new era of land sovereignty struggles and agricultural transformations that this account explores, in relation to nutritional changes and gradually rising diabetes rates.[30]

For all that has changed since the days of Saint Vincent, there are certain disturbing continuities over the centuries: sugar remains a primary sign of violence and uneven injuries, and industrial profit continues to accumulate around preventable deaths and patterned land dispossessions. In this sense, the struggles with diabetes described in this book could be read as only the latest chapter in five hundred years of traveling with sugar.

In *Sweetness and Power: The Place of Sugar in Modern History,*[31] Sidney Mintz famously argued that the rise of a British "sweet tooth," related to changing factory labor that drove global demands for sugar, could only be fully understood as part of a global system that relied on the exploitation of land and labor on sugar plantations in the Americas. Yet Mintz actually began his investigations on this matter with a much more granular mode of anthropological storytelling about Caribbean sugar: the individual life history, which narrated the experiences of one person's trajectory working in cane. This approach revealed social dynamics without assuming any individual was modal or "representative" of a given population.[32] Mintz's later account of sugar as global commodity in *Sweetness and Power* was an attempt, he said, "to trace backwards" the norms he encountered in the course of individual life history work.

The realities of diabetes examined here might be considered living sequelae of the transformations that Mintz described, sugar *out of place* in modern history. In what follows, I try to bring these two ways of approaching the anthropology of sugar—individual life histories, and global histories of racial capitalism[33]—together in the same book. Talking with people and thinking with their own insights into their conditions, as my teachers João Biehl and Adriana Petryna show, "compels us to think of people not as problems or victims, but also as agents of health"[34]—and co-envisioned ethnography as an "open system" for public exchanges that may continue long after books end.[35]

In juxtaposing life histories with global stories of commodities in systems, the aim is an ethnographic version of world systems theory that stitches together glimpses of global processes and infrastructures with their living consequences for people. There is, inevitably, some trade-off in depth when trying to assemble bits and pieces from this broad scope, at times only gesturing toward enormous literatures with deep relevance—anthropologies of environmental change and food studies, ethnographies of medicine and global health, social studies of science and technology, settler colonial and postcolonial histories, debility and disability studies, work on maintenance and infrastructure, and Belizean and Garifuna cultural histories, among others. While a more narrow framing might make academic analysis easier, it would not do justice to the stories of individuals who are dealing with elements from all these intersecting arenas in trying to live with the erratic sugar in their bodies.

I approach such fraught storytelling guided by Mintz's insight that none of us exists outside the global legacies of sugar—to the contrary, he argued, we are each related in ways that we might not understand. In this view, the uneasy position of my own whiteness is not something to be disclaimed. It is a constitutive part of the global legacies of sugar in question, and a role I occasionally perform as narrative foil.

Whatever else the diabetes journeys recounted in this book suggest, they are also haunted by thwarted and incapacitated travels: life-giving mobility that got occluded or made unthinkable for others, even while often available to me. It is painful to recognize that after all these years of trying to share connective experiences and find commonality with the people who appear on these pages, the places where our paths diverged may be more illuminating than any of the junctures where they joined up for a short while. The unjust gap between my "travels with sugar" and those of others also sheds light on chronic infrastructures much bigger than any of us—ones that you are somehow positioned by too.

In an aging world system, there are "remainders of violence"[36] at play with power of their own, exceeding anyone's conscious intent. But exactly what that meant (or might come to mean) for this story was not easy to name. The more that people taught me about their actual ways of living with sugar, the more these suggestive parallels with bloody histories seemed to both provoke and defy easy conjugation.

Sweetness and . . .

What?

ERRATA: METHODS AND MISTAKES

I have always been unsettled by errata: strange little scraps of text appearing at the edge of feature news stories and journal articles, like misplaced footnotes that set straight some error from a past edition gone by. The irony of errata is a fundamental one: by definition, corrigenda are uncorrectable corrections. The flawed template has already gone to press; revisions are no longer possible. All that is left to do is append, painstakingly detailing these mistakes and noting how they might be written otherwise for future versions. Errata are always details out of time and out of place, residues of errors coming to public awareness at least one issue too late. Yet it matters, not just technically but somehow ethically, to note for the record any mistakes observed too late to actually be fixed.

These thoughts about acknowledging unresolvable past errors stayed close in mind as I learned more about painful colonial histories and their material legacies across the Caribbean and Central America. But as I set out to do ethnographic work in Belize, a more immediate scale of concerns also began to take over my daily routines and attention. In addition to meeting people around town and visiting the local hospital, I also began going on home visits with caregivers from a local clinic. Those home visits often felt like observing not only a healthcare system, but also its gaps—diabetic sugar was part of people's domestic worlds in ways that far outpaced its "medicalization." I was very careful to repeat again and again that I was not a physician or a nurse (although people still called me both constantly). On these routes, I worked to act within the parameters of what a volunteer would be permitted to do in a U.S. caregiving situation; by way of a guideline, I would only participate in errands and practices that an amateur would be allowed to perform in U.S. homecare, terms that I knew from working in home care during college. But I sometimes found it unsettling how much expertise and medical power people were at times willing to allot to me. I was asked to do things like remove stitches and give insulin injections—which, of course, I did not do—but I had to draw firm lines about the medical forms I was *not* willing to wield. The mere fact of being asked to assist with these technical tasks when stopping by people's homes was a discomforting window into what they were facing: many of those diagnosed with diabetes also worried that they lacked sufficient expertise to safely inject themselves or their family members with insulin at home. Yet that was what therapeutic "adherence" often required.

During this time, I tried to mark myself as an anthropologist by avoiding certain symbols of the medical profession—for example, I decided not to wear scrubs as an everyday uniform when accompanying nurses or doctors on home visits, even though I was asked to do so once by a clinic director, worrying this would deepen people's confusion about my role. Meanwhile, other things I had used in the past to mark myself as an anthropologist—such as a notebook, clipboard, or paperwork—are all signifiers that anthropology shares with medicine. These items seemed to confuse people more about my connection to the healthcare system, rather than clarify my purpose. So my digital tape recorder became important to me during this time, as a marker of "not-doctor." The tape recorder often made conversations more awkward but felt like an important tool to try to make sure that people were telling me things as a storyteller.

It became apparent that there was also a local notion of research ethics circulating. This was explained to me by my language teacher on my first day in one Maya village where I worked. She told me the last anthropologist who had worked in their village had not "given back," and as a result he had met a bad fate. (And it happened that this professor was suddenly killed at a young age.) This was how some people in the community read his death, and she kindly said that she wanted to warn me from the beginning, so I could go forward only if I felt comfortable with the risk. Her tone was nothing like a threat—more like a disclosure of the risks this research could entail for me. Was this also a version of informed consent? If something happened, it would not be her acting, she explained—it was not like the metaphysics of *obeah* or human-directed witchcraft. The language and cultural knowledge itself had a force that could take lives as collateral for upholding the ethics and reciprocity of our relationship.

But less righteous lethal forces were also at work. The stakes of negotiating different ethical fields felt much greater once people I knew started dying. Once in a while, I would go to visit someone for an interview and find out they had died. In addition to wider circles of less intensive interaction (people I interviewed once or twice), there were fifteen people I began visiting once or twice a week, every week, for a year—the kind of gradually built relationship in which you really get to know a person. Thirteen of the fifteen have died since then. I had not at all expected this intensity in advance, and because these events became personally overwhelming, they also changed the kind of impressions I gathered. Sometimes writing my daily fieldnotes felt like attempting to cast death masks of people in their final moments, trying to capture something dignified about their lives before they were gone. At one point I tried to think of these as tributes or memorials; but they are also something more uncomfortable than that.

At this time, I also began paying more careful attention to the Garifuna death rituals that were happening around me. Messages received from the dead were part of how people situated their diagnoses from the hospital. Many Garifuna rituals centered around a notion of feeding the dead by cooking enormous feasts for ancestors that are thrown into the sea or buried in the sand. Since I was studying diabetes, this use of food seemed important because it often involved the very dishes that people living with diabetes were commonly advised not to eat—white rice, rich soups with coconut milk bases, desserts, and rum. The same foods being used to keep memories of the dead alive had become dangerous for the living.

I felt a deepening sense of undirected anger and ineptitude as numerous people with diabetes I had known died preventable deaths in the fatal fictions of "noncompliance." Through experiences such as sitting with a mother who asked me to take a turn holding her son's dead body, I came to understand something more about the ways a lost sense of security might become a chronic imprint or bodily change in someone. Shortly before I left, someone tried to break into the room next to where I was sleeping one night. I later learned that the thief had most likely been a child; nearby that night, someone else reported a break-in where the footprints in the sand looked too small to belong to an adult. Only ham and a loaf of bread were stolen; a laptop was left untouched. Afterward, I thought often of the little ham thief. What does it mean for a child's hunger to coexist in plain sight of tourists' luxury resorts? What happens when such profound inequalities take root over time? It was a context in which being any kind of white person left one with an unshakable sense of complicity, crucial not to disregard and impossible to escape.

I did not know how to process that sense of underlying danger and inequality. Here I was trying to understand medicine in the context of Garifuna notions of death while also becoming paranoid about my own. I lost twelve pounds in four days to an acute illness in April, then got pneumonia. And shortly after someone had tried to break into the nearby window, I found out that I was—by sheer coincidence—working in a clinic built on the exact place where an earlier white anthropologist who worked in the village had lived. I did not find out until late in my research that he was murdered in Belize. The figure of the killed anthropologist was therefore a disciplinary legacy in both places where I worked, which I came to feel unwittingly but inescapably connected to somehow. Just by choosing to stay in the midst of bad omens, I found myself also touched by a kind of Thanatos, which felt entwined with the offerings to the ancestors and other dead unfolding around me.

At some point, this unsettling context of my fieldwork became more than the methodological realities of my research, but also a central heuristic through which I was coming to understand the things I saw in Belize: medicine in the communities where I lived; the way people I knew there sometimes thought of their illnesses as inevitable and the imminence of death as intractable; the way this intimacy often became part of how they communicated with their ancestors through rituals, food, and songs; and the way people bore their losses, by redefining love and communication as something that only grew more powerful in the face of death. Maybe this was participant observation in a way too: I came not just to observe but also to partially participate in an intermittent reckoning with death.

For me, these methods came to feel like a postscript of obsessively studied mistakes—some of which I observed in global institutions' policy documents, occasionally witnessed and at times felt complicit in, or myself felt mistaken for engaging with in the first place. Of course, to some extent errors are part of human relationships themselves and therefore inherent to anthropological research, perhaps even part of the conditions for ethnographic possibility and its "troubled knowledge."[37] Carl Jung believed that "mistakes are, after all, the foundations of truth," while Salvador Dalí wrote of mistakes, "Understand them thoroughly. After that, it will be possible for you to sublimate them."[38] Yet that does not change the fact that I still considered or experienced certain events *as* mistakes, whether witnessed or my own. Many of their consequences are unfixable. But I like to think that maybe they can be appended in a limited way through what I write about them now.

If the following chapters started out with methods from the classic anthropological genre of life histories, many slowly turned into death histories—a painfully apt term I owe to Jim Boon.[39] Some of these stories are just fragments someone wanted to share. But others, more sustained collaborations with those I at times came to think of as friends, are perhaps more like elegies.[40] Garinagu have always written beautiful elegies, sung on disquieting scales across porches and in living rooms as well as ancestral temples. As Roy and Phyllis Cayetano describe, in such Garifuna lyrics, "people and events can be recorded in songs like little pictures which become public property and remain, long after the former becomes a matter of history."[41]

There is a certain sense in which my writing now feels like a partial mirror held to such gestures of memory. Just looking at my field notes when I work at night, hearing the voices of dead friends from Belize in interview tapes, and looking at pictures from this project became an experience of constantly encountering ghosts and trying to find ways to engage the dead and their memory. The attempt feels heavily borne because of my sense of helplessness and complicity in being unable to prevent their deaths.[42] Yet at this point, finding a way to tell these stories feels like part of my own ethical response to what I saw—maybe the only one still available. Trying to write feels not only like a postscript to the ethical dilemmas I encountered during fieldwork, but also like a gesture toward appending the lives of these untimely dead. These chapters are offered as corrigenda in the (hugely insufficient) sense of a place where they might still be alive.

But I cannot write about normalized death from the outside; there is no outside. I could only study the unequal systems I was caught in together with others and note our vastly different positions within them. Many understood the imminence of their own deaths much better than I did at the time, testing me as a channel to an imagined public record or wider stage with agendas of their own. Gestures of transformation pressed against the jagged edges of things that none of us could change, the playful and painful bound together. I never managed to shed the contradictory roles that have been part of playing the role of ethnographer since colonial times, though I tried to perform them more collaboratively: aspiring mediator, tolerable resource boon, academic authority, implicated naïf.

In some especially tense moments, I sometimes found my face freezing into an overwrought smile in an effort to appear at least well intentioned in my foolishness. Garinagu men wear masks with smiles like these when they dance the *Jankunu* dance around Christmas, with seashells stitched to their knees. They make the white masks out of cassava strainers painted pale pink and decorated with forced frozen smiles, satirizing the colonial absurdity of slave-owning white people and uniformed soldiers.[43] Above their whiteface the dancers wear hats decorated with garish paper flowers and bits of mirrors. But maybe these *Wanaragua* masks also capture more than they mean to, or at least something they do not purport to be rendering. There is a certain helpless white smile of someone who wants to be good but does not know how to face the violence of the past they are tied to, which resembles both the mocking *Jankunu* mask and my strained smiles in those moments. (Upon meeting a stranger, many old Garinagu women will stare down your cursory smile and not return it until they know you well enough for you to deserve it. I admired the wounding honesty of this habit.)

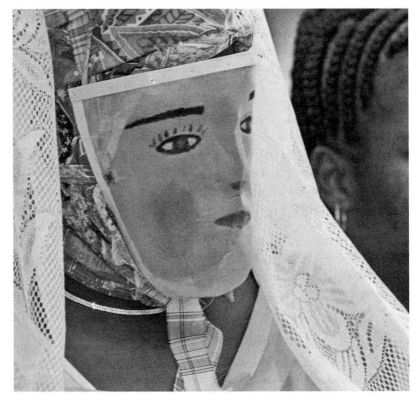

Masked character in *Jankunu* (*Wanaragua*) performance.

I have learned a great deal from the writings of anthropologists who work to unmask systems of structural violence. But for my own project, I gradually felt a more disquieting truth when acknowledging that I did not even know how to unmask myself.

SLOW CARE

Many of the individuals I met in Belize came to number among the millions of worldwide deaths now attributed to diabetes each year.[44] Somehow, the slow-moving quality of chronic conditions like diabetes—what U.N. Secretary General Ban Ki-moon once called a "public health emergency in slow motion"—seems to make it only more daunting to imagine reversing its spread in the future.[45] A range of disturbing statistics suggests that today's policy approaches have not slowed the rise of global diabetes rates or mortality; to the contrary, these figures appear to have accelerated worldwide each year they have been tracked. According to the latest projections of the International Diabetes Federation, the condition "affects over 425 million people, with this number expected to rise to over 600 million within a generation."[46] No health institution that I am aware of predicts that current interventions might be able to curb the problem on a population level. In this light, there is global resonance to what was probably the single thing I heard repeated most often by the Belizean and Garifuna individuals with diabetes who contributed to this project: "It is my children I'm worried about."

Every story in the rest of this book is really the same story that Mr. P taught me to see—chronic strains that slowly cause bodies to fall apart and the people trying to keep each other together. In fact, each chapter retells that same story again, from a different angle. When it comes to diabetes, this repetition is no narrative accident. Fatigue and relentless repetition are the defining features of what makes diabetic sugar harrowing—people trying to stave off bodily loss and failing organs day in and day out, year in and year out, over and over again, utterly foreseeable, likely coming anyway.

It was only people's work of maintenance, caring for each other in the face of all this, that never stopped surprising me. When one new mother told me that her dream with diabetes was to try to maintain for her kids, I paused expectantly, waiting for her to finish. She shook her head. "And so I must work hard to keep myself," she said. I waited with my pen poised for her to complete the sentence—to keep herself healthy, to keep herself going? But as we sat in silence, I realized that she meant the expression simply as it was—to keep herself, all of herself: the feeling in her nerves, her fingers and feet, eyesight, life. I closed my notebook.

A slow epidemic both is and is not like other forms of violence.[47] It plays with time. It breaks down stories, as Rob Nixon memorably wrote in his description of "slow violence"[48]—and unevenly wears on different bodies, Lauren Berlant emphasizes of "slow death."[49] But writing can play with time too—allow for taking a step back and making visible processes and their errata over a "long arc," as people and places intimately shape each other. If the slow violence of sugar continues to saturate many of these stories, its harms demanded the kinds of practices I often saw in Belize, which I came to think of as *slow care*—ongoing and implicating joint work in the face of chronic debilitation.[50] That is not a caveat. It is the guiding frame for the rest of this book.

Looking back at these families' survivance[51] with diabetes unfolds the small moments that make up this epidemic—allowing a chance to

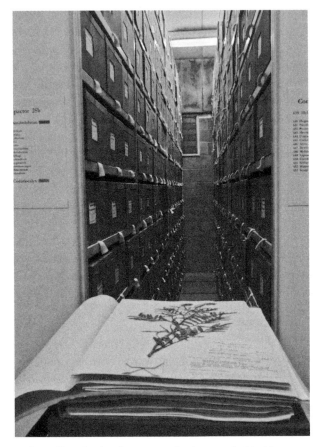

Galega officinalis, the plant source that became the blockbuster diabetes drug metformin, at the Kew in London.

pause and reflect on how these realities came to be, and to try learning from the moments of remaking and recovery already underway. Their struggles bring to life Mintz's argument that the point of drawing out social histories of sugar is to remind each other that "there is nothing natural or inevitable about these processes."[52] In contrast to how bleak many global projections can make the situation feel, the Belizeans profiled in this book taught me to approach the rise of epidemic diabetes *not* as a settled past or an inevitable global future—but instead (as an anthropologist once wrote of co-envisioned struggles elsewhere) more like "a story we are all writing together, however we appear before one another—ready, set, go."[53]

Past Is Prologue

Sugar Machine

Told me to keep my eyes open for the white man named
Diabetes who is out there somewhere carrying her legs
in red biohazard bags tucked under his arms.
—Natalie Diaz, "A Woman with No Legs"

Sugarcane sprouted bright green along the dirt road where I was look-ing for Sarah's house. Some patches were cultivated by people; but other stalks grew wild in ditches of their own accord, hybrids strayed from forgotten stocks. When colonial botanists collected cane specimens, they often noted which stands had "escaped" from nearby plantations. Sugar only needs to be planted once; then it can keep reproducing, unless interrupted.

Media headlines about diabetes always seem to show bodies getting bigger, but the stories I heard in this stretch of Caribbean Central America more often focused on fears of getting smaller. If you sat and talked with people, missing body parts were often central to how they told stories and measured time. Some felt phantom pains or dreamt at night about running. Others, like Mr. P, watched with dread as it happened in their families or heard about beloved elders lost piece by piece. Nurses said that feet bitten by venomous snakes were easier to heal than those poisoned by sugar.

In Belize, this common name for diabetes traveled across languages: *súgara* in Garifuna, *shuga* in Belizean Kriol, *azúcar* in Spanish, *kiha kiik* in Kekchi Maya, or *ch'uhuk k'iik* (sweet blood) in Mopan and Yucatec Maya.[1] Some people described the dismemberments as a quietly surreal spectacle their families were already living with amid a lack of public acknowledgment: "They cut my grandmother down to a lone torso." Others spoke of dying in small pieces, like "my arm died that time" or "her eyes died first." A Garifuna spiritualist with diabetes told me of the new addition to her ancestral prayers—protection for "Feet, legs, toes, hands, fingers, arms, eyes. Amen." When a Maya seamstress walked into a mobile clinic without realizing there was an embroidery needle sticking out of her numb foot, the visiting physician knew that she likely had diabetes before the two ever exchanged a word.

SWEETNESS

Sweet foot—a limb macerated due to diabetic injuries—is common enough that you can find the term alongside other diabetes vocabulary in the Belize Kriol dictionary:

> sweet fut *n.* abscessed foot due to diabetes. **Sayk a weh Misa Jan ga shuga, ih gi ahn sweet fut.** Because Mr. John has diabetes, it gave him an abscessed foot.
>
> sweet blod *phr.* 1) sweet personality. **Raja eezi fi laik kaa ih ga sweet blod.** Roger is easy to like because he has a sweet personality. 2) diabetes. **Dakta seh Ah hafu kot dong pahn shuga kaa Ah ga sweet blod.** The doctor says I have to cut down on sugar because I have diabetes. *See:* **shuga.**
>
> shuga *n.* 1) sugar. **Bileez sen lat a shuga owtsaid.** Belize sells a lot of sugar overseas. *See:* kayn. 2) diabetes. **Dakta tes mi ma blod an ih seh ih mi ga shuga.** The doctor tested my mom's blood and said that she had diabetes. *See:* sweet blod.[2]

Sweet feet I heard said when it happened on both sides, which had become Sarah's predicament some seven years before we met. In the Stann Creek District of Belize where she lived, an estimated one in four people (and one in three women) lived with type 2 diabetes,[3] and some five out of six amputations were due to sugar's complications.[4] Certain images sounded straight out of a war story, like when the hospital's incinerator broke down once and everything had to be buried. But at the same time, it almost felt like nothing had happened.

The home that Sarah invited me to visit again felt comforting and bright. Its paint flaked into pretty layers, like sycamore bark. The rooms smelled of coconut rice and fresh laundry. I never saw her play the tambourine, but its open crescent hung on a nail next to a mosquito net she had improvised from a bedsheet to prevent insect bites. (She developed this strategy after once hosting a botfly in her knee, which took almost a year to heal because of high blood sugar's complications). "My treasure chest," Sarah joked of the container she showed me. Amid the cozy jumble of a lived-in room, her glass box of diabetes technologies looked like a tiny museum case. Among bottles of pills and other archived medical treatments, it held a broken blue and gray blood glucose meter.

"I just don't know what caused it," Sarah said of her sugar, which was what she called the condition she had been living with since 1978. She had always been slender in build, like many people I met who defied any easy conflation of diabetes with obesity. When her first foot started going bad, she said, it had started with a corn on one toe. It had just gotten "miscarried away." Miscarriages also figured centrally in women's stories about the effects of untreated sugar, and mortality during pregnancy for both mother and child is another diabetes phenomenon that is likely widespread globally (though reliable statistics are hard to locate).[5] Sarah's sister living with uncontrolled diabetes had been somewhere among these uncounted women, dying along with her baby during childbirth.

Sarah fondly recalled the Kriol midwife, Mrs. D, who used to go door to door to visit those she knew were sick. "Every house. She would walk." She used to bathe and bandage Sarah's ulcers to prevent infection. After Mrs. D died of cancer, the centralized health system was never able to replace her day-to-day care work in the village—part of a bigger story about homecare visits growing less frequent across Belize as old midwives themselves died of chronic conditions. Sarah summarized decades of care in hospitals by evoking a cast of doctors with good medicine that came and went, and the boiled herbs she used in the meantime; raw Clorox she applied for pain when a protruding bone's edge pushed into the skin. As she narrated the accumulated cuts and recoveries, it seemed like her illness faded into the background, unlike the FM radio she kept that blared theme music from *Ghostbusters* or a reggae version of the Bryan Adams song *Heaven*.

"I would like to know how high it is," Sarah said of her blood sugar level. "Indeed." The last time she had been rushed to the closest town's hospital, it was "five change," over 500 mg/dL. "I have needles, but no strips," she said of her unusable Accu-Chek meter, which was quite expensive (seventy U.S. dollars) and designed to require special brand-matched parts (around fifty U.S. dollars for one month's supply). Sarah used to travel to the Guatemalan border town of Melchor—about five hours away by bus—to purchase discounted blood sugar test strips, but had not been able to lately. Her meter rested next to foil-wrapped pills, which she took tentatively because she had no way to gauge her starting point. Diabetes medications at times can make people feel more sick, if the day's blood sugar is unusually low or high. I was unsettled to realize that the very objects that could have helped prevent her worsening injuries were both *there* and *not there* in the room with us, sitting as if suspended in the glass box.

"Sugar machine" was Sarah's name for the broken glucometer. Even in her lilting voice, this hung in the air with an ominous edge. It was one of the ways we were speaking *in* history, if not about it; getting to Sarah's village meant passing the remnants of another structure called a sugar machine. We both knew that just down the road rested a steam locomotive from the 1800s, mounted on eroded bricks like a train running nowhere, which had once boiled sugarcane into molasses. It still stands next to the plantation's evaporating furnace, a hot-air exchanger, a Tredegar engine that pumped water from the river, and the crusher with its flywheel. Their rusted-out pipes and oil tanks were etched with places and names that I could barely make out under the moss: LONDON and RICHMOND, VA covered in lichen.

That particular sugar machine and its adjacent fields of bourbon cane were established in the 1860s, long before Sarah was born, by a man from Pennsylvania named Samuel McCutchon. He was friends with U.S. president Andrew Jackson, who used to travel on his ship *Pocahontas* to visit the McCutchon family's Louisiana sugar plantation. Lists of the enslaved people whom Colonel McCutchon owned in Louisiana fill seven archival folders. He was among the Confederate sugar planters who fled to then British Honduras after losing the U.S. Civil War. By some accounts, more Confederates fled to Belize in the post–Civil War years than any other receiving country.[6] In Belize, the workers in McCutchon's cane fields were mostly Garifuna, Kriol, Maya, and Chinese. He founded three sugar estates in southern Belize,[7] transforming the landscape. Ruins built by Confederate planters after the Civil War, some as far north in Belize as Indian Church, are among many remnants of sugar machines still found across the Caribbean and the Americas. It was said that Belize's rainfall was so conducive to quick growth that the cane bent over by its own weight and then grew upward again into a field of S-shaped stalks, as if the sugar had started to spell itself out.

SUGAR ROADS

One morning in 2010, Sarah told me that she hadn't been able to sleep the night before. "I just don't know what it wants," she sighed. I prodded with a vague follow-up, and she explained she had tried Clorox. The moment passed before I could figure out a delicate way to phrase my real question: But what was *it,* that had wants?

I used to think that "sugar" was a popular synonym that meant dia-betes. But over time, I came to think that these labels often slipped into each other but were not exactly the same. The effects of sugar routinely exceeded common understandings of diabetes problems. Sugar was alive in the landscape. It named something that escaped from the many containers—biomedical, historical, scientific—of expert accounting. I began to think that any stable account of sugar's contradictory mean-ings and excesses would miss the very thing that people like Sarah named as the conditions they were trying to live with.

Belize is among the less cane-saturated places in the Caribbean. Nei-ther Sarah nor her children worked in the sugar fields. Many people in this book never talked about field labor or would trace their diabetes to sugarcane. Yet they lived in a region not only dotted with its ruins, but also fundamentally shaped by its far-reaching material legacies: where people lived and how their ancestors arrived; the way land was parti-tioned and used today and what kinds of things could grow there; the system through which they bought foods and what foods those were. Other associations were less literal but more pervasive. When a woman drowned together with her four children after she dove into a shallow pool trying to save them, people made sense of the tragedy by attribut-ing her terrified actions to diabetic sugar: "The sugar made her panic." A man whose loved one had "gone mad" explained her breakdown in this way: "The sugar went to her brain." Sometimes sugar was not ame-nable to intervention, but simply a way of speaking about terrible things one could not change.

The way people talked *in* sugar, though rarely *about* it, brought to mind Michel-Rolph Trouillot's notion of *implicit memories*: "Tying a shoe involves memory, but few of us engage in an explicit recall of images every time we routinely tie our shoes," he wrote. "Remembering is not always a process of summoning representations of what happened."[8]

People spoke *in* sugar so often that I began to hear it as a kind of implicit memory. Trying to understand what hung in its silences, I called someone who worked in curating more explicit memories of sugar: Mr. B, one of Belize's resident experts in sugarcane history, who suggested a drive north. We met in a pickup truck with seats full of books. As we shook hands hello, Mr. B said that shaking hands with a cane worker can leave your hands itchy all day with the feeling of little fibers under your skin, and I tried not to feel unsettled though that sensation is a common symptom of diabetes. We talked on the road north to Libertad, past Corozal's British brick pillbox structures with gun windows.

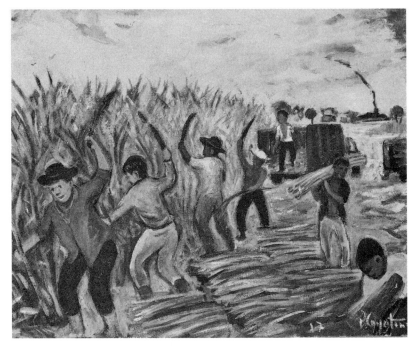

Cane Cutters, by Pen Cayetano.

Since sugar has no season, the fields outside the window were not uniform, each property in its own stage: burnt fields, high ratoon, the overgrown dense green known for snakes and bugs. Harvest leaves a field of stumps that have to be scorched to prevent stubble from sprouting from the stalk's joint-like nodes. Planting new sugar fields entails burying old cane billets in the ground, which sprout regrowth called stands.

When we got out of the car at Libertad, I thought how that field was the same one that many workers from Stann Creek District had once traveled to reach. Pen Cayetano, a famous impressionist artist in Dangriga, was among the Garifuna men who left home in southern Belize to work in the northern sugar fields of Libertad when he was a teenager. In his studio—fragrant with oil paint and smoked fish and bustling with family at work on art projects of their own—we sat on an overturned canoe, and he recalled how the sugar fields barely felt like vegetation at all: bright but not lush, sticky, known for the blind heat of the two o'clock sun. When I asked if he might want to paint an image of his memories of sugar work in Libertad for this book, he looked startled by my mental image of sugar fields as plantlike bright green. "You think I'd paint the sugar green?" He shook his head. "It felt *red.*"

By the time Mr. B and I walked through Libertad on a hot day in 2017, the sprawling cane fields and laboratory buildings were long overgrown. As we passed broken-down conveyor belts towering above stacks of rusting vats, it was not difficult to see why historians like Eric Williams viewed the sugar industry as a pivotal "synthesis of field and factory."[9] A single watchman kept an eye on the abandoned estate. He led us past a pumpkin patch he was cultivating near the old office, still hung with the rusted sign FACTORY MANAGER. Inside the derelict office headquarters, the wood desk had rotted and most of the inside walls had collapsed. But a metal filing cabinet in the middle of the room was fully intact, sinking into the dirt.

"Time and space have no meaning in a canefield," Jean Toomer wrote in *Cane.*[10] If efforts to enclose sugar in time and space often seemed to unleash further misrecognitions, I thought from Libertad, then I wanted to try following its wild entwinings instead. Somehow that sugar factory's feral filing cabinet became a helpful mental image for me as I gathered together the notes for this chapter, a container to temporarily order these bits of sugar's far-flung histories.

More intense stories of "sweetness and death"[11] elsewhere in time and place shaped how people ended up living where I met them. On Saint Vincent, sugarcane had become especially symbolic of Garifuna people's struggle to preserve their ancestral homelands at the end of the eighteenth century. As Paul Johnson notes: "Though never laboring as slaves, the Black Caribs lived under the continual *threat* of enslavement, and very much within the expanding sugar plantation system."[12] Legendary freedom fighters of what historian Julius Scott illuminates as the "masterless Caribbean,"[13] Garifuna fighters set fire to sugar fields to combat encroaching British settlers. Sugar's potent symbolism reached such a point that during one war, Garifuna leaders found it fitting for plantation overseers to meet their end "crushed between the cylinders of a sugar mill, the symbol of British greed for Carib land."[14]

Nearly two thousand miles away, in the mainland territory that later became Belize, commercial plantations were legally prohibited by the Spanish during the colony's early history.[15] Kriol people like Sarah descended from the enslaved families in Belize who once worked in logging, but were still caught and sold within a broader regional system founded on sugar markets. Most who ended up in Belize were traded through markets of the sugar islands, primarily Jamaica and Bermuda;

some labored on sugar plantations elsewhere in the Caribbean before arriving in Belize City.[16] Creating dependence on economies of imported food became integral to control within the logging camps of Belize, especially rationing sugar.

Farther north along the border between Belize and the Mexican Yucatán, sugarcane became a key crop that Maya laborers were forced to grow on *encomienda* plantations[17] and also an instrument of control and even torture. Thomas Gann gives the example of a "well-known merchant" in Bacalar known to punish Maya servants, "for no very serious offense," by shaving their heads and burying them up to their necks in the island's hot sand; "their heads were then smeared with molasses and the victims were left to the ants" to be eaten alive.[18]

When Christopher Columbus arrived in the Caribbean, colonial strategies initially favored capturing Indigenous peoples from the Americas and bringing them east to provide labor on sugar plantations in the Canary Islands. Sugar was used to ply local inhabitants and sow discord, as one chronicler on the third voyage of Columbus recalled when greeting the first Taíno boats: "I gave hawks' bells and beads and sugar. . . . after they knew the good treatment, all wished to come to the ships."[19]

While colonial strategies for both labor extraction and cane plantations' locations shifted dramatically in the face of subsequent epidemics, sugar continued to impact Indigenous populations of the Americas in a more subtle way than the better-known plantation histories of the Caribbean. Though sugar was often less of a key export (outside Brazil), mainland sugar plantations across Latin America provided a central source of funding for Jesuits and other missionaries focused on capturing Indian souls. They financed large-scale conversion enterprises largely by growing and selling sugarcane within what became the countries of Mexico, Peru, and Paraguay, among others.[20] Colonial and military projects of all kinds were indispensably funded and amplified by such sugarcane profits, giving rise to the axiom *"Without sugar, no colonies."*[21]

Sugarcane distillation laboratories also became sites for refining racial classifications of the era.[22] On conquistador Hernán Cortés's cane plantation in Mexico, which helped fund his later military expeditions across Central America, efforts to make sugar "emerge perfectly purged and whitened" were key to its market value. Some 90 percent of the sugar emerged in shades of brown, deemed low-value *prieta*—the same name people with dark skin still get called in that part of Mexico today. After boiled sugar was transferred with a "shoe-like scoop" for settling into sugarloaf molds, darker molasses leaking from the open bottom of the sugar cone was declared "poorly purged sugar [and] removed with a knife." Once severed, sugar's "foot form was separated from the rest to be returned to the purging house," the name of the building where sugar was whitened.[23] The foot of the sugar cone often accumulated heavy metals and other toxicants from the distilling machinery and collected any debris from the vats, at times including (as Edwidge Danticat notes) blood and bodily matter from laborers' injuries.[24] It was fed to enslaved people and horses.[25]

The English word "amputate" came from the Latin root *amputare*, meaning to trim plants or cut off the limbs of trees. Somewhere in the late 1500s or early 1600s, the word began to also mean cutting off human limbs.

"Sugar was a murderous commodity," Vincent Brown observes of the patterns of its violence during that era. Plantations functioned through "symbolics of mutilation," powered by people "who were themselves consumed" by sugar production.[26] Many enslaved families were forced to live in houses with roofs of thatched cane tassels.[27] "When we work at the sugar-canes, and the mill snatches hold of a finger, they cut off the hand; and when we attempt to run away, they cut off the leg," an enslaved character from Suriname famously describes in Voltaire's *Candide*.[28] In *Black Jacobins*, C.L.R James describes how some enslaved individuals were forced to wear a "tin-plate mask designed to prevent the slave [from] eating the sugarcane" in the fields.[29]

Historian Sir Hilary Beckles notes that the disembodiments related to diabetes therefore have especially discomforting resonance in Caribbean and Latin American regions today, as places long known for these trademark injuries of sugar are again called "the amputation capital of the world. It is here that the stress profile of slavery and racial apartheid; dietary disaster and psychological trauma; and addiction to the consumption of sugar and salt, have reached their highest peak. The country is now host to the world's most virulent diabetes and hypertension epidemic. [The British] parliament owes the people of Barbados an education and health initiative."[30]

Beckles, whose enslaved great-grandparents were owned by the ancestors of actor Benedict Cumberbatch, opens his book with homage to those Garifuna and other Kalinago and Maroon peoples who managed to elude plantation captivity and share sanctuary with others, honoring their "principal contribution to the freedom traditions of the Caribbean."[31] But he also wrestles with the legacy of those like his own

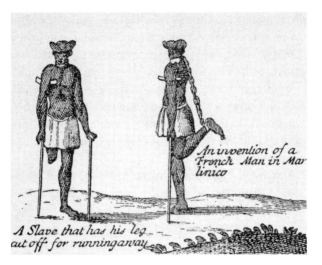

Left: Enslaved man who had his leg cut off for running away.
Right: Debilitation device meant to prevent slaves from escaping,
c. 1697.

ancestors in Barbados, who either could not escape to nearby Saint Vincent or tried and were apprehended in their journey.

Besides violently cutting off mobility, amputated legs were intended to be a grisly and shame-inducing public spectacle. Colonial-era sugar planters in the Caribbean even invented devices of psychic terror that mimicked amputation—forcing enslaved people to physically experience and imagine something of what it *would* be like if they were to have a limb cut off in the future.

"What's past is prologue," the old truism from *The Tempest* goes.

But what does that mean when it comes to sugar in the Americas?

"The machinery of the sugar mill, once installed and set in motion, soon becomes almost indestructible, since even when it is partially dismantled, its transformative impact will survive it for many years," Antonio Benítez-Rojo once wrote. "Its track will be inscribed within Nature itself, in the climate, in the demographic, political, social, economic, and cultural structures of the society to which it once was joined."[32]

The old pipe jutting over the river at Libertad looked like an oil pipeline, but it was built for molasses. For a brief time after 1989, a Jamaican company called PetroJam leased the old sugar estate and used its molasses to refine into ethanol for U.S. markets. But by the time I visited, only sugarcane was being loaded into the tugboats I watched preparing for export. Staring into the water that some call "the river of strange faces," I thought of Kara Walker's art installation in the old Dominos Sugar Factory in Brooklyn, where pools of dissolved sugar water reflected each visitor back at themselves. Now that sweet crude oil has been drilled in Belize, there are jokes that even the land has gotten sweet blood.[33]

WELCOME TO LIBERTAD read a sign at the edge of town. Welcome to Liberty. If you follow that road going north, a crumbled sugar distillery from the 1700s sprouts vines, a reminder of when Bacardi owned those fields and the ensnared cane workers were mostly Yucatec Maya men. Or go south, where remnants around the British brick sugar mill at Indian Church tell a story of robust Indigenous agriculture until the time of colonial contact, when Maya land use and diets became violently constricted and malnutrition skyrocketed.[34]

In another direction lies the sugar village of Calcutta. It was founded by East Indians branded "Sepoy mutineers" by the British and deported to Belize for participating in India's First War of Independence in 1858,[35] "sent to sugar estates in the north."[36] Or cut closer along the border, where the cane fields are transected by what people call "the sugar road." A signboard from Hershey marks the sugarcane's eventual destination for processing in Pennsylvania. Animal blood is no longer used to clarify industrial sugar, but charred cow bones are still a medium in the process many companies use to whiten sugarcane.[37] Before long, some of this refined sugar will return again to Caribbean and Latin American markets as sweet packaged food products, part of the global circuits of production and consumption that Frantz Fanon long ago foresaw as the next stage of exploitation: "The colonies have become a market. The colonial population is a customer who is ready to buy goods," which Fanon viewed as part and parcel of "that violence which is just under the skin."[38]

Colonial sugar economies were driven by "unequal ecological exchange," Jason Moore noted, not only human labor extraction.[39] Sometimes I tried to picture what the old forest in Stann Creek District looked like before it was logged and later burned to clear fields for plantations. Inhabiting a hobbled landscape, some interviewees told me they wanted to grow vegetables, but the soil along highway was too poor to grow anything but oranges and bananas. Was it always? This legacy was not only about land in law, but also about its biology. Once cane grows in certain ground, it depletes nutrients from the soil. This paves the way for further industrial monocropping, since it often leaves behind exhausted land that requires heavy doses of petrochemical pesticides and fertilizers in order to grow.

I didn't used to know the names of the chemicals they put on sugar in Belize, but I tasted them once. Biting to peel a cane stalk straight from the fields with my teeth, the white powder flaked dry on my tongue and dissolved without flavor. Later, a friend and I stood staring at the names of the agricultural chemicals advertised on a sign in town: Actara, Amistar, Cruiser, Curyam, Flex, Gesaprim, Gramoxone, Karate, Ridomil Gold, Syngenta. Somehow, the advertised list felt taboo to discuss: the shopkeeper did not want to talk about which ones he sold for sugar and which ones for other monocrops, like oranges and bananas. The term *pesticide drift* that I read about sounded like a sinister enigma. But lab tests in Belize measure it: glyphosate, better known by the brand name Roundup, was found in six out of six test sites in Stann Creek.[40]

"In 2002–2007, the sugar industry alone produced 5,074,261 to 5,950,123 gallons of liquid waste per year," the Belize Ministry of Health noted. Recent orange and banana blights had further driven the use of pesticides, the report added: "Wash waters and irrigation run-offs contaminate the watershed in the two southernmost districts—Stann Creek and Toledo . . . where runoff and chemical pollution affect adjacent water bodies."[41] Pesticides found in a Stann Creek water sample included cadusafos, ethoprop, acetochlor, fenamiphos, oxamyl, carbofuran, chlorpyrifos, dimethyl tetrachloroterephthalate, chlorothalonil, trifluralin, malathion, lead, and mercury levels that peaked where the Stann Creek river meets the sea.[42]

"They don't talk about it, but I think our diabetes is also caused by all the chemicals," Sarah's sister-in-law told me. Publications supporting her suspicion indeed existed in the literature—many chemicals are endocrine disruptors, which population-level studies report lead to a heightened risk of diabetes and weight gain.[43] But proof was not possible to demonstrate causality for *her* case of diabetes in particular, which is of course the point about not being able to tell where sugar begins or ends. An abundance of population studies elsewhere suggests that the growth in both type 1 and type 2 diabetes is exacerbated by exposure to pesticide runoff from agricultural and other synthetic chemicals and pollution in food, air, and waterways. The haze of what Vanessa Agard-Jones calls "accreted violence"[44] from agricultural pesticides remains a legacy throughout the Caribbean and Latin America. In this context of limited foods and abundant chemicals, Sarah's name for her glucose meter, "sugar machine," struck me as an apt frame for the way this region—if not much of the agro-industrial world system—is fast becoming a "diabetes machine."

CHRONIC LANDSCAPES

"I dug that driveway," Theo told me as we drove down a road that cut through plantations. We were headed in the direction of Sarah's village from some fifty miles north. Theo hit the brakes to slow down at the rusty bridge, craning to check for anything coming from the other direction. He said the bridge was so narrow because it was not actually designed for people or cars. It had been built as a railroad trestle for United Fruit's old banana train. That was why the two-lane highway contracted there and only one car could squeeze through at a time. The traces were hard to detect; United Fruit and their rail lines were long gone by then. There are new companies on the old plantations today, but the most radical change imaginable for this land now is a switch from bananas to other fruit.

I loved driving between Belmopan and Dangriga through the Maya Mountains with Theo because he knew things like that. I gathered between the lines of his stories that Theo, charismatic even as an old man, had been a heartbreaker in his younger years. He knew every village. Itinerant driving was his favorite line of work now, he said, but over the years he had also worked picking oranges, walked survey through Belize's forests, sung country ballads, traveled abroad, done odd jobs of all kinds, and traded fish when there still used to be a lot of fish in the sea. He described the days when there didn't used to be any bars but each house distilled its own liquor from rice or pineapples that was crystal clear. He showed me the neem tree with leaves that he boiled sometimes to help manage his blood sugar.

"I see children nine, ten years old dying of diabetes," Theo said as he shook his head, eyes on the road. He had diabetes, too, as did most of his friends. They were learning from each other's misfortunes. Theo told me how one of his toughest friends had been found mysteriously dead in a hallway at home. The death looked so odd, with the house suggesting signs of struggle, that the police ran tests to see if he had been murdered. But they could find no signs of foul play. Theo thought that probably his friend had woken up realizing he had low blood sugar (more immediately dangerous than high blood sugar) and had fought to crawl his way to the kitchen. He almost made it. Since then, Theo always kept a few pieces of hard candy in his pocket and in the car, to eat along the road and make sure he didn't pass out while driving.

Theo stopped at a curve in the mountains and bought two chicken tamales, handing me one. We stopped at a gas station to unfold the banana leaves coated in ash. Most people in Belize speak English, but it is filled with phrases you do not hear anywhere else. In Theo's words for the highway, the low traffic reflectors edging the forest were "cat eyes" and the speed bumps were "sleeping police." He showed me the field where he had faced a fer-de-lance in an orange tree and the place where he had emerged from months of working in the forest and learned his father had died. It always felt like whatever scene Theo was describing from decades ago was just out of sight of the window. Theo pointed out where the banana workers that United Fruit brought from Jamaica used to live along the highway and recalled how, as a Garifuna man working nearby, he was often mistaken for one of them.

By the time I had accompanied mobile care teams through those orange and banana plantations of Stann Creek, most of the workers were from Honduras, Guatemala, or El Salvador, with a handful born in Belize. This made it strange to be part of a group that arrived with an English-language diabetes education video depicting white North Americans in sweaters, who did not look like anyone (except me) on the plantations where we showed it. "Your pancreas is the size and shape of an average banana," one memorable line went, an anatomical cartoon of organs secreting keys and dots that flashed on the screen. A visiting Garifuna nurse prepared her glucometer for testing while the educational video—if anyone was able to understand it—was instructing the banana workers to avoid eating the exact types of food that were sold from the attached company store.

Only a few of the workers had high sugar that day (and were told to follow up at the hospital). I was put in charge of carrying the red plastic sharps box containing several hundred dollars' worth of used blood glucose testing supplies. The mobile team was attentive and kind, and their gestures seemed appreciated by the workers. But the machines already had theories built in, which made it feel like we were at once too early and too late: years too late to prevent exposures to pesticides or to the carbohydrate-heavy diets that seemed visible all around, but years too early to measure their effects. We all got sent home with bunches of green bananas. I handled mine carefully after seeing the metal claws used to dunk them in caustic chemicals, thousands of bananas floating in shallow baths under signs reading No Food.

Belize's beautiful landscape, spotted with mango trees and covered in flowering vines, often gives visitors the impression of a paradisiacal garden. This lush appearance makes it particularly paradoxical that much of the country would easily qualify as a food desert today, according to U.S. definitions (which are based on factors like miles of distance and transportation difficulties to purchase healthy food; limited, high-priced selection of vegetables at those locations; and overall poverty levels). Potentially arable land that could (but does not) support vegetable agriculture in Belize only accentuates the manmade ironies underpinning food deserts most anywhere.

The territory now bounded as Belize once produced food for an Indigenous population of two million. Yet today, this same land is unable to grow enough vegetables for Belize's current population of 380,000. Pesticides are often hailed as necessary for scale, but Maya techniques of soil engineering allowed for larger-scale agricultural productivity than the monocropping on that same land now.[45] Even a few decades ago, when individual Kriol families in southern Belize used to grow more kitchen gardens along the coast, some would travel to nearby ancient Maya ruins to obtain the rich soil from the areas where pre-Conquest inhabitants buried waste using methods to optimize the soil's later chemistry (including burning in particular sequences, and strategically distributing materials like nitrogen-rich seashells).

Today, the majority of vegetables sold in Belize are imported and pricey in contrast to surrounding countries. "You know," a man from the Yucatán told me, "in Mexico, poor people go into town to *sell* vegetables. Belize is the only country I know where most villagers go into town markets empty-handed to *buy* them." As the history book *British Honduras: Colonial Dead End* reprised of Belize: "Its land laws [are] far behind the Republics of Spanish America [that] have laws for the encouragement of agriculture, which in spite of revolution and misrule, have attracted immigrants when this Colony has repelled them."[46] Reflecting on this archival source, the authoring historian acknowledged that "the 'progressive' land tenure system in Spanish Honduras was almost a replica of the *ejido* system or Indian village commons."[47]

Anthropologist Richard Wilk's work helps to further unfold the complex history of foodways in Belize.[48] He calls the colonial food economy in then British Honduras "the first global diet, a kind of nineteenth century equivalent of McDonalds hamburgers," since agriculture was forbidden in the colony's early history because of fierce land disputes between Spain and England, and British settlers were made to rely on barrels of white flour and salted meats shipped from London. The economies supporting Belize's "rogue colonialism"[49]—run by men who called themselves not pirates, but privateers—actually have much in common with the privatization of late liberal economics.[50] A global industrial food economy—in ways similar to the forced imported food-ways and trade constraints that existed in Belize for centuries—is becoming increasingly common in many countries and getting further amplified by harmful trade policies, as Alyshia Gálvez observes of Mex-ico in *Eating NAFTA*.[51]

Even though I read those things in books, seeing them through the eyes of someone like Theo who had observed change over time brought a more human scale to what I could gather about changing foods and farms. From his car window, the "sclerotic landscapes"[52] and constricted food systems that scholars write about made more sense. Sclerotic arter-ies kept showing up in diabetes clinics, but from the road I could also see *sclerosis* even in the lush land that nonetheless choked free movement through it—like the United Fruit bridges and the roads that followed, still constricting the motion of food and people long after the corporation and its train tracks were gone. Some historians of science used to search for what they called the "machine in the garden," moments when industrial technologies entered nature.[53] But I realized that the banana train, miss-ing now, wasn't the machine in this garden any more than the crumbling mills and their rusting wheels. When it came to wild sugar and its land-scapes, what looked like the garden *was* the machine—altered infrastruc-tures and biologies, living sugar "absorbed" into bodies and absorbing them in turn, overgrown excesses of fixed and moving parts.[54]

But whenever I thought I had found some connecting plotline to think with across scales, the events I wanted to wrap a story around seemed to shape-shift again. Some months after our last trip, I was shocked to learn that Theo had been murdered in the same car we had driven in the past summer. Memories of those trips and the stories suddenly changed grav-ity. The last time I saw him, he was listening to country music and said his sugar felt low. He was going to buy a piece of fruit.

No matter how many times I read headlines in Belize like "Sugar and Bullets," I can't really grasp the scale of the numbers.[55] Yet according to national statistics, what happened to Theo is not strange at all in the sense of numerical probability. Murder was the most likely way for a man to die in Belize, followed by diabetes (for women, diabetes was still number one). What makes this reality especially hard for both Belizeans and scholars to understand is that the country's homicide rate was very close to zero only a few decades ago.

The rise of militarized forms of policing within the United States has deeply affected Central America, as has the growing demand for opioids headed for U.S. markets. Current homicide rates are well over the so-called civil war benchmark countrywide. At last count by the U.N., Belize City's homicide rates ranked third highest on the planet.[56] Some 90 percent of Belizean children have seen a dead body, compared to 20 percent in Mexico.[57] Yet unlike many nearby countries where violence is also a major issue, there is no legacy of civil war in Belize. Once I asked a prominent journalist who regularly publishes on what he calls the "violent triangle" of Guatemala, Honduras, and El Salvador why he leaves Belize out of Central America, even though its violence rates are comparable to or higher than those in the surrounding countries he focuses on. "Nobody understands Belize," he said.

Since many of my memories of Belize's landscape were learned through the windows of Theo's car, now the whole landscape felt learned anew through the memory of what happened to him there. Being afraid to move around at certain times or places was part of sclerotic landscapes too, and one of fear's many unpredictable effects. You couldn't easily see it on the surface, but on glucometer screens you could watch the way an untimely death made an entire family's blood sugar erratically rise and fall. Fear of safely moving through a place could make a daily exercise routine feel like weighing immediate security against future health. I began to learn how easily a country's relaxed atmosphere can be mistaken for an absence of social problems, rather than a hard-won effect of the way people absorbed hardship and undertook the labor of transmuting it for those around them. These realities are now also part of "what it means to be human in a place advertised as paradise."[58]

Theo used to say that he was jealous of friends who had HIV/AIDS instead of diabetes. He said the two chronic diseases shared similar daily demands—except that with AIDS, "if you take your medications in time, you can eat just about anything." And the difference that most preoccupied Theo: "With AIDS, they don't cut you up." He started laughing at this harsh contrast, the way blood with high sugar doesn't make others afraid, unlike AIDS. "They don't *want* to cut you!"

They cut him more than a dozen times, face and neck. When I listen back to recordings from his car now, Theo's storytelling as we criss-crossed Belize feels impossible to separate in my memory from what happened to him later in his vehicle. Slow violence bleeds into violence of other tempos. The stories he told me about food and landscapes as I looked out the window already held the quality of blurring past, present, and future, and now make me imagine looking back at him in the driver's seat with a similar sense of "simultaneous time."[59]

I recalled his carefully stowed hard candy in quick reach in the console and thought back to Theo's story about his tough old friend, who the police initially thought had been murdered but seemed to have died fighting his way toward the kitchen with low sugar. Everyone in Belize called diabetes the "silent killer," but I never grasped it as clearly as in that story of what police had mistaken for a crime scene. Staying on guard against other violent killers could share a gut-level feeling with diabetic sugar: There were measures you could take, but there were things far out of your hands, and life with it meant just knowing that.

Theo fought back hard, his gashed arteries undoing the delicate investments behind decades of care. The story that he had told me most often was about the time a few years ago he'd tried putting a teaspoon of sugar in his morning coffee, after hearing it was good for diabetes. But it had caused Theo's toe to "crack open like a statue." His son had brought him an aloe plant to massage onto the injury each day for months until the threat passed.

DIABETES MULTIPLE

One woman in Dangriga asked whether she had type 3 diabetes. In medical journals, "type 3" would reference theories of Alzheimer's as an additional or comorbid form of diabetes, linked to insulin disturbances in the brain that interfere with insulin's role in memory.[60] But for her, this meant something else. She clarified: type 3, the kind of diabetes that means your arms or legs get cut off.

Nobody needed a visiting ethnographer to tell them about "diabetes multiple," an interpretation I had once felt clever for proposing. In *Body Multiple*, Annemarie Mol examined different hospital treatments of sclerotic arteries—the hardening blood vessels linked to ischemic leg ulcers, often associated with diabetes—to reflect on how different bodies come into being, depending on the treatment approach chosen.[61] This insight also has crucial implications for observing care inequalities (though Mol doesn't choose to go there). Yet juxtaposing her book with this one offers a case in point: its front cover depicts an image of two legs being readied for precisely the surgery that helps to prevent diabetic amputations.

In one sense, this provides an uneasy demonstration of Mol's insights: physically different bodies get *produced* through differences in medical practices and technologies. By putting into play (or not) different possible treatments, diseases can become physically distinct entities. This can create multiple versions of a condition like diabetes—as when clinics in Belize amended the preprinted posters that listed the disease's warning signs, writing in by hand severe manifesting symptoms like "blindness" next to milder warning signs like "blurred vision."

Yet comparing how multiple *versions* of diabetes are produced by unequally available treatments and practices also begs another question: how connected material histories shape what care options come to seem "ordinary." After all, these different norms of treatments are not unrelated, thinking of *Body Multiple* from the Stann Creek District of Belize—"Stann" being the Dutch word for "Safe Haven," the name by which early Dutch settlers claimed this Maya ancestral territory. While there are several accounts of how ancestors of Garifuna people first arrived in the Caribbean, some historians believe they descend from African men and women who escaped from the Dutch slaver ship *Palmyra*.[62]

In some opaque way, the "ordinary" sclerotic surgeries in a Dutch hospital have a historical relationship to the absence of those restorative technologies in most of the Caribbean. They are obliquely connected by colonial histories of plundered bodies and lands that still today shape institutional resource flows—systems impacting how different forms of medical expertise and technologies developed. To extend Mol's logic to Belize, these "versions are both different and interdependent: multiple."[63] "The capital amassed in the eighteenth and nineteenth centuries through various forms of slavery economy is still in circulation," W. G. Sebald wrote, reflecting on what he called the "money laundering" of Dutch art funded by Caribbean sugar, "still bearing interest, increasing many times over and continually burgeoning anew."[64]

There is also another aspect of "diabetes multiple" that is not easy to trace with hospital observations about disciplinary differences alone. Technologies do not get used equally, even in affluent hospitals, for reasons that occur without the intent or knowledge of anyone involved. In textbooks about sclerotic arteries, for example, the choice of which procedure gets used should not relate unjustly to an individual patient's skin color. But looking at U.S. population data, it becomes clear that racial assumptions have been systematically enacted on patients' bodies.

Drawing from ten years of New York hospital data, one study analyzed 215,000 cases of people with diabetes arriving at the hospital with symptoms of peripheral artery disease.[65] It found that Black patients were 46 percent more likely than other patients to have received an amputation instead of a "salvage" procedure to restore blood flow to their legs. Black patients and women were also more likely to be amputated above the knee rather than at the shin. Above-the-knee amputations notoriously make recovery much more difficult.[66]

Perhaps most disconcertingly, these disparities were actually highest in the hospital units with mostly white patients, so they cannot be easily attributed to preexisting resource or equipment inequalities of segregated cities. Another study mapped the geography of diabetes-related lower limb amputations in Los Angeles, which is actually the largest Belizean city in the world by population. This mapping revealed that people were ten times more likely to experience diabetic amputations in the poorest areas of the city, which were also the most segregated. It shows a disturbingly patterned geography of "diabetes multiple"— inequalities that can make diabetes a physically different condition for people of color and for patients with fewer resources, those more likely to have limbs removed even when experiencing identical symptoms.

Certain scientists still argue that diabetes risk is "inherent" in the DNA of nonwhite people. This text instead follows Anthony Ryan Hatch's illuminating work in *Blood Sugar*—including his observation that "race is not biological, but racism has biological effects."[67]

In hospital labels, the technical name for diabetes is *diabetes mellitus*. It derives from the Latin word *mel* for honey, a reference to an old European medical trick of tasting a patient's urine for honey-like sweetness as part of the diagnosis. Physicians today commonly shorten *diabetes mellitus* to "DM." In contrast, the word *sugar* was adopted into Latin from the Arabic word *sukkar* around the time sugarcane was adopted into imperial Rome from its plundered colonies. And in the clinics and homes of Belize, people were constantly reworking this label of "honey diabetes." No, many insisted: they had *sugar* diabetes.

Not everyone I spoke with in Belize described their condition as "sugar." Relatively well-heeled patients, more able to manage, were more likely to say they had "diabetes." The terms slipped into each other constantly. But I noticed some patterns.

For many with diabetes, an event like dying young or losing a limb would register as a surprise, even an outrage—either would be shocking, for instance (by way of contrast) among those with diabetes in my white, middle-class extended family in the United States.

Sugar, on the other hand, I often heard in relation to societally *normalized* injuries and untimely deaths. Living in foretold death and injury meant that something terrible *not* happening was also newsworthy. Sometimes I found those comments more haunting than the bad stories. One man told me of his mother, "She died with all her arms and legs on."

The long fights to which a foot is lost to diabetes often remain illegible as "battle scars," Kiese Laymon writes in *Heavy*—and "unacknowledged scars accumulated in battles won often hurt more than battles lost."[68] Unacknowledged scars of sugar could be read as one of many distillations in the "climate that produces premature Black death as normative," in the words of Christina Sharpe[69]—or for others, as part of "the labor of living in the face of an expectant and a *foretold* cultural and political death," as described by Audra Simpson. "With settler colonialism came . . . a radical shift in Indigenous diets and their bodies. As a result their blood is excessively 'sweet' and has a high prevalence of diabetes—a bodily indicator of these spatial and dietary transitions."[70] Seeing disembodiments happen to others only deepens existing traumas, as Mojave poet Natalie Diaz captures of diabetes and surviving such losses: "Asks me to rub her legs which aren't there so I pretend by pressing my hands into the empty sheets/ Feels she's lost part of her memory the part the legs knew best like earth/ Her missing knees are bright bones caught in my throat."[71]

The racial logics of normalized injuries and death that distinctly characterize both settler colonialism and white supremacy[72] came together in sugar for some like my friend C, who was proudly Garifuna—both Black and Indigenous. She was among those who told stories of her doctor's shock when she returned to the hospital for a long-held appointment after the diabetic crisis he had assumed would cause her death at age thirty-four.

"He said, '*How are you still alive?*'" she really laughed, mimicking his wide-eyed incredulity. It was the hardest that I ever saw her laugh, so I laughed too, but looking back on it I only saw a surface fraction of the joke back then. I appreciated her comic critique of biomedical limits. But I missed the eerier echo of implicit memory: her ancestors had been facing expert iterations of that very same question—*How are you still alive?*—ever since the first European surgeons arrived on the warships sent to eliminate them from Saint Vincent.

Normalized death, extraordinary survival, transformations that became necessary to live on—whatever expectations *sugar* indexed, this was the closest thing to a refrain that I encountered across individuals' stories. People regularly showed up in clinics with blood sugar levels that textbooks said would be fatal. Doctors, caring, confused, faced with sugar escaping the biomedical rubrics of diabetes mellitus, would ask: "*How are you still alive?*"

STILL. THERE

When I loaded the microfiche about Confederate plantations built in Stann Creek, the first slide said in huge letters: "END." The reel must have been spooled backward on its last rewind, but it felt fitting—the traces of sugar that it held were the opening frames for the afterlives I was trying to learn about. My vision blurred while scrolling through Samuel McCutchon's papers: letters, maps, almanacs, sketches, clippings of machines he hoped to buy. His favorite was called "The Concretor," a device that turned sugarcane simultaneously into molasses and its byproducts into concrete building blocks.[73]

It was strange to see McCutchon's bookkeeping straddle countries and decades. In pre-emancipation United States, the enslaved people he legally owned were listed by name alongside his estimation of their dollar value. In southern Belize, he used the same notebook brands and page formats, but this time the price column marked a minuscule hourly wage. The lists contained many last names of Kriol and Garifuna families I had known in Belize. Chinese indentured laborers were listed in McCutchon's books only by numbers.[74]

But even in its enigmas, the microfiche was an archival loop that I could place back into its cardboard container. The Belizean landscape upon which those diagrams had been enacted, in contrast, presented a more unruly material record of sugar histories' afterlives.

In addition to *Saccharum officinarum*, "official sugar" (grown on most plantations), there is a species named *Saccharum spontaneum*, "spontaneous sugar." Once "introduced by sugarcane breeding programs . . . *S. spontaneum* has the potential to become a serious invader of cultivated land . . . host to a large number of pests and diseases."[75] With both rhizomes and seeds, it propagates freely. Such cane "looks like wild corn has mated with bamboo," bearing "fluffy, hair-like flowers."[76] Though becoming scraggly and less useful to humans, even "official sugar" breeds of cane can survive in the wild and move across landscapes.

In sugarhouse sketches, there are often circles marked "Still" centering the structure, its vats used for distillation. Seeing that term orient so many diagrams of sugar, the word's other meanings made me think of a core of time as well as space. Still: ongoing; unmoving; but.

The Confederate families flying flags of Dixie are gone from southern Belize. The sugar industry came and went in the southern region, leaving only rubble on the edges of a global system where Belize was a fringe node at best.[77] But sugar remains iconic of the larger shifts such colonial forms have unleashed on a global scale: motors of industrial agriculture and ecological extractions; chemicals used to grow crops on spent soils; plantations that led to corporations;[78] machines rusted in place in fields yet in ongoing motion across landscapes and inside cells of human bodies, even when left behind by all accounts. Long gone; still.

When someone's glucose is high, it is present not only in the blood but also in sweat, breath, saliva, urine, respiratory fluid, and tears. Once I was invited to a funeral for a friend's father after his death from diabetes and realized how many people in her family must be crying sugar.

In today's diabetes markets, even the sugar in tears holds potential capital. Some researchers have argued that such tears could be collected, dried, and cut into pieces for lab tests or public health metrics. "Persons without diabetic symptoms would be less reluctant to give samples of tears than of blood," one policy proposal read: "Thus a fairly accurate estimate of the prevalence of diabetics could be made with less resistance from the public."[79]

One could argue that in today's global markets, the sugar inadvertently cultivated in people's blood and bodies is more valuable than any sugar growing in the ground. These global sugar markets feed each other in ways that recall Lochlann Jain's insights about how "key aspects of the economy involve both causing and treating" many chronic conditions.[80] Importantly, Jain reminds us that such profit engines do not imply any malicious intent or human ill will. But when protecting local foods and environs has no global "market value"—while dietary and therapeutic products that both cause and treat diabetes are highly profitable—those incentives fuel systems that reproduce with a life force of their own.

A number of older people with diabetes I met in Belize diagnosed or monitored their glucose by smelling and tasting sweetness in their urine. Others first realized they had diabetes by noting insects gathering in the places they urinated, drawn to consume the sugar. For them, "sugar" was not an abstract unit mediated by technologies or paperwork—bodily sugar had a sensibility and flavor, a literal taste. And, of course, blood sugar reflects much more than the sweets someone has eaten. Since all carbohydrates turn into glucose in the body, foods like flour tortillas and white rice can cause high sugar levels in bodily fluids too. The ants can't tell whether a glucose molecule was broken down from cane or white flour, once sucrose or fructose. By then it is just sugar, and they are there to eat it next.

Sugar not only reveals scales but also *produces* them, like the genes described by Ian Whitmarsh elsewhere in the Caribbean.[81] When a diabetic ulcer refuses to heal, some hospitals actually apply a topical poultice of sugar, which for unknown reasons at times has more medical efficacy than many antibiotics.[82] Certain foods may be disproportionately eaten due to a history of exploitation, but people have also learned ways to make "dietary disaster" delicious, and often there is "clearly life surging around the sugary rite."[83] Sugar holds contradictory meanings: eating and getting eaten; histories of hardship and labor, but also of love, pleasure, and luxury; both wealth and poverty; security and danger; terror and intimacy; violence and comfort; age-old, growing new; hunger and indulgence; invigorated and devastated agriculture; ancient human staple and disobedient Frankenfood.

The symptoms and injuries of sugar likewise hold contradictory meanings and intimacies. When "a source of value is extracted from the population being injured,"[84] Jasbir Puar argues, wounding might be better analyzed as *maiming*, to mark the uneven ways that racial capitalism and settler colonialism play a role in "rendering populations available for statistically likely injury."[85] More than disability, she calls this *debility*—someone profits.

"Hurtful" was the particular word that Sarah used to speak about it. Her language is also helpful to think with—creating her own terms for recognizing pain, but distinct from the terms of "damages." Sarah's relational concept of the "hurtful" offers a different mode to recognize injuries and debilities that people were dealing with and actively seeking ways to share about more publically.[86] Something hurtful points *back out*, asking us to examine the external forces and infrastructures inflicting hurt. It's also already being dealt with—requiring recognition of the dignity with which injuries have long been borne, and implying that storytelling is also implicated in processes of cause and effect.

Listening again now, Sarah's words sound as much gentle rebuke as kind invitation—not just to the searching student who kept coming to talk without always being able to understand, but also for whomever she imagined my voice recorder was a proxy for reaching. I like to think that this included anyone ready to author diabetes policy without consulting the people actually living with it.[87]

Of course, playing back her words in air-conditioned rooms is not without its own double edge. It could be easy, from there, to think we were outside the sugar machine. But on the contrary: sugar plantations across the Caribbean and throughout the Americas played a major role in endowing U.S. and European universities like the one that sent a student like me to study and report back on distant nutritional deprivations.

Who profits when bodies break down from sugar? And which bodies? Is it even possible to examine such unequally distributed problems without profiting too? I used to think this project could find an outside to these contradictions. Now, I just believe in more honest wrestling with the ways we each get interpolated by sugar's legacies and ongoing effects.

"I'll tell you, I have a great time, girl." Sarah said she wanted to get a small Belizean flag to wave for Independence Day in September. "Are you going to the parade?"

In the face of irreparable histories, I wish I knew a better gesture than trying to co-create platforms for thinking with teachers like Sarah and the unauthorized expertise they shared. People are already speaking back—time and again, implicitly and directly—to common public health rubrics by which they are otherwise objectified, managed, and related to. They have ideas about the work of justice. But their insights often do not have a channel back to those who make science, design, and policy decisions that impact their lives. Which kinds of public efforts might help support and expand the vital grassroots care projects already underway? And which policy misrecognitions feed more limbs to the sugar machine?

In this view, any sugar machines that are possible to photograph— like the glucose meter with unaffordable parts that broke down in Sarah's treasure chest or the colonial equipment rusting among the trees near her house—are only synecdoches, little pieces of a five-hundred-year-old engine. But the larger apparatuses they support are the mechanisms and infrastructures by which the death and dismemberment of nonwhite people had come to seem ordinary—forecast as acceptable or just inevitable, weighed against profits engines and global markets. This again disturbingly echoes earlier logics of sugar, as Saidiya Hartman writes of such afterlives: "Death wasn't a goal of its own but just a by-product of commerce, which has had the lasting effect of making negligible all the millions of lives lost."[88]

Many of the "fixes" addressed to normalize sugar seemed not only to fail to contain its loose forms but also to generate additional harms: from pesticides that poison bodies even as they protect crops, to foreseeably insufficient and unevenly accessible care technologies, to the excesses of violence and insecurity that trail long histories of lost lands, foods, and families. With these legacies unleashing material forces,

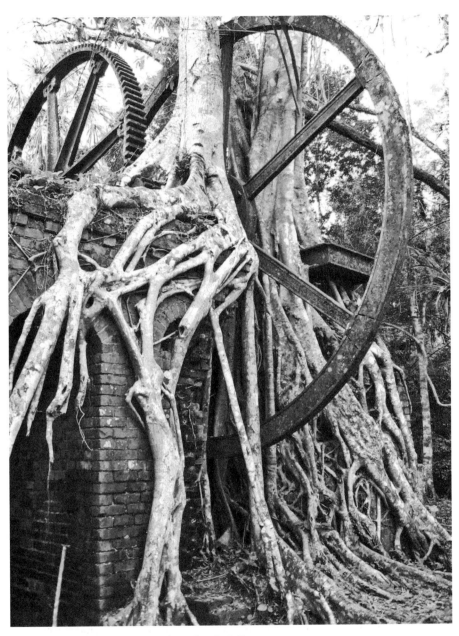

A Confederate sugar machine at Indian Church, Belize.

diabetic sugar's normalized losses emerge from a machine five centuries in the making—overgrown and breaking down yet proliferating and exceeding many remedies meant to triumph over it.

Over time, I observed experts try to put sugar in many different enclosures. In one archive, I saw pressed sugarcane plants get filed in niches labeled as "pigeonholes," each numbered. The Kew collection in London included many indigenous plants and vegetables from Central and South America and the Caribbean that are now extinct in the wild, making me realize I did not know of any extinct species of sugar. "Unfortunately, our sugar collection is mostly just tassels," one caring botanist told me regretfully as she handed me folders of wheat-colored bristles from the Americas, mostly from Mintz-era Puerto Rico. The botanist kindly added that she wished they had more cane stalks on file so that she could show me sugar's unusual joints. "Try to think of them like knees," she said. Much later, driving past a patch of cane sprouting along the road in Belize after a day spent talking about lost limbs, I thought of the London analogy's misfit; only sugar keeps growing back.[89]

Yet if sugar was still there, so was Sarah's family. And given the heaviness of history that preceded our encounters, I felt surprised by Sarah's generous parting words in 2010: "It's a great time to be together. You know, love one another, talk with one another. Feel happy to know that you know someone strange. Make the best of it, love."

What Is Communicable?

Caregivers in an Illegible Epidemic

The body isn't wrong, isn't "disabled."

The environment itself—gravity, air, solidity or the lack of it, etc—is what is somehow wrong: ill-matched to the body's abilities . . . verticality, stability, or mobility.

She . . . whose limbs struggle to accomplish their given tasks on earth is, in this sense, like an astronaut: far away from home, coping.

—Teju Cole, *Blind Spot*

By the time we met in southern Belize, Dr. W had already named it in his mind: the "Caribbean diabetic limb crisis." He said he hoped someone does a study about the trauma caused by diabetes amputations, and not just for patients. He said someone should also do a study about trauma for surgeons who are being put in the position of repeatedly removing pieces of their patients.

It took me a moment to put together the fact that Dr. W was one of those surgeons.

"You can't imagine how much I never want to see another person lose their foot," Dr. W would tell me later. "But I know that each day I do this, that's what's coming."

Sarah's younger brother, an animated man named Tobias, was among those I saw greet Dr. W with a warm handshake. He and his wife had traveled to Dangriga just to say hello to him. I began to grasp why, when Tobias recounted an odd story to me: A few years ago, he was walking and a bone fell out of his foot. He barely even felt it glide out from the lesion that a diabetic ulcer had eroded in his tissue. Tobias

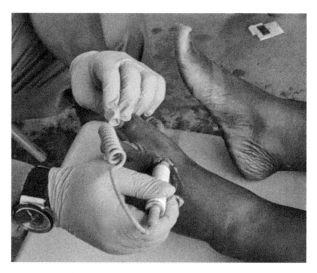

Dr. W at work, Dangriga.

picked his bone up off the floor—a joint below his toe—and took a picture of it. Then he placed the bone in a clean plastic bag.

Later, Dr. W described the photo and message he had received from Tobias: "He called one day from Belize and said, 'Hey Doc, this bone fell out of my foot this morning. It didn't hurt at all.' And I thought to myself, you know, this really isn't okay. It's almost . . . Frankenstein-ish. But it doesn't raise any real alarm. That tells me a lot about where things are, when people are kind of . . . used to it."

Archaeologists say the world's oldest known prosthetic appendages are mostly toes, fashioned nearly three thousand years ago in ancient Egypt out of wood, leather, linen-like plant fibers, and glue.[1] By 2010, I never met anyone who bothered for "just a toe." But if you looked at the sandals of the people gathering in line, you could see that a number were missing toes. Those waiting to see the doctors appeared to be from all walks of life: stylish fashions and threadbare clothing, many formidable in stature but others looking markedly thin, a mix of skeptical-looking teenagers and grandmothers in weathered hats. The arriving members of the Belize Diabetes Association's New York branch and their colleagues from Dangriga and the Belize Ministry of Health unpacked supplies for the day, arranging stations around an open pavilion. The team's mood was relaxed and convivial. Only their gear, plastic boxes packed with foot care instruments, hinted at the day's high stakes.

Dr. W's team brought a stack of photocopied papers, titled "Limb Salvage Form." These sheets displayed sketched outlines of feet: a right and left foot shown from both bottom and top view, with circles outlining the twenty-two quarter-sized places on a foot where podiatrists test for sensation to detect any signs of lost feeling. ("Can the patient see the bottom of their feet?" the paper asked, just above a question about the safety of shoes.)

The Belize Diabetes Association collaborates with Dr. W's Diabetic Foot Care team, which since 2004 has been traveling between their New York City base and a range of Caribbean countries. Their group focuses on foot maintenance checkups, only one station among an array of services being offered around the pavilion. When requested, they provide training to build expertise among local caregivers and the Belize Nursing Council. On occasion, Dr. W also performs follow-up salvage surgeries to restore a diabetic limb that may have already been scheduled for amputation. The medical word *salvage* has a particular echo in the history of social observers: some early anthropologists imagined forms of "salvage ethnography" to document people and practices they prematurely labeled as dying off.

The team's practices of salvage here, in contrast, signaled the very opposite of resignation to harm. In medicine, the term *salvage* means that all possible measures are being taken to ensure an ailing limb stays alive and attached. Limb salvage procedures often include vascular surgery measures to restore blood flow, such as unblocking blood vessels or placing stents. They most broadly demand the careful monitoring of feet to catch tiny wounds before anything reaches a crisis point.

This labor has its own lexicon. I made lists of unfamiliar terms in my notebook.

Claudication comes from the Latin verb *to limp*, the name for stabbing leg pains caused by restricted blood flow. This is often linked to peripheral artery disease, which most doctors just call PAD. Debriding means removing dead tissue to try to give the living parts around it a chance to grow back. The paperwork's "Deformities" box holds checklists of things you did not know could go wrong with parts of your feet you did not know existed: Dorsiflexed first ray means that the foot segment containing the first cuneiform and first metatarsal bones rides high; there are two other checkboxes nearby on the page to indicate a concerning equinus (flattening arch) or troubled calcaneus (heel bone).

(The feet's cuneiform bones are wedge-shaped, which is how they ended up with the same name as the ancient Mesopotamian pictographic script once etched on clay tablets with wedge-shaped writing tools.)

Hallux limitus is an arthritic condition of the big toe, with rearfoot and forefoot varus varieties. A bony prominence of the great toe joint causes severe pain and rigidity. There are varieties of toe deformities—hammer toes, claw, and mallet—and three types of corns that classically afflict them. The physicians paid close attention to each detail, trying to tune out the long lines of people waiting around them. Any concerning characteristic on a diabetic foot could morph into catastrophic injury if it went unnoticed and untended for a few weeks: maceration, tinea between the toes, ankle plantar flexion, an obstructed dorsalis pedis or posterior tibial pulse, bunion, drop foot, Charcot fracture.

And a very serious acronym: LOPS, or loss of protective sensation. Dr. W's team had set up a station to teach people strategies like using their hands to feel inside their shoes before putting them on, since feet numbed by diabetes can be felled even by tiny injuries. The need for amputation can often be traced back to a sharp pebble in someone's shoe or a bug bite in the wrong place. One U.S. study about the causes of diabetic limb amputation found at least twenty-three unique causal pathways at play (including 46 percent lost to ischemia, 59 percent to infection, 61 percent to neuropathy, 81 percent to faulty wound healing, 55 percent to gangrene, and 81 percent to initial minor trauma). Those numbers add up to 383 percent instead of 100 percent because most amputations are caused by several mechanisms simultaneously—which is also why remediating any one pathway will not necessarily save a limb. The biggest pattern this study found was that up to 80 percent of amputations were preceded by a "pivotal event," usually a minor cutaneous injury.[2] In Dee's case, the pivotal event that led to losing her left leg was stepping on a seashell. It was as small as a tooth, just one sharp edge.

It turned out that several of the team's visiting doctors were originally from other parts of the Caribbean as well—part of a larger Caribbean Diabetes Initiative—and had connected in New York with the Belizean group. People from Dangriga kept telling the team that the letters on their T-shirts, BDANY (Belize Diabetes Association of New York), resembled a Garifuna word meaning "your time"—and, by way of this little joke, let the BDANY members know they were grateful for their time.

"You have salt or sugar?" old friends called out to each other across the pavilion.

("Both" was the most common answer—diabetes along with hypertension.)

"I never thought you were sweet!"

No matter how many times we heard some version of the joke, everybody laughed.[3]

FOOT SOLDIERS

"She's one of our best foot soldiers," Dr. W smiled as he and Nurse
Norma hugged hello. Years ago, he had arranged for her to complete
diabetes foot care training. It was tough work: of the twenty-five nurses
who began the two-part training, Norma was the only one who returned
for the second year to complete it. In the months or years between visits
from the Belize Diabetes Association's New York team, Norma stood as
the front line of defense for those needing diabetes limb care in town.

Norma's brother says she has nine lives, like a cat. As a steadfast
nurse and head of the local branch of the Belize Diabetes Association,
she had managed to maintain herself with type 1 diabetes through many
decades and to help keep many others intact. In the southern district of
Belize at that time there were no known endocrinologists, podiatrists,
or other caregivers who had specialty training in diabetes foot care
except for Norma. Her particular expertise included tending to diabetic
toenails, a crucial skill: one clip at the wrong angle could lead to a
jagged ingrown nail and later necrosis. Toenails also archive: some
researchers measure their glycation to detect diabetes and its sequelae of
organ damage.[3] Trimming required complete attention, at once rough
and delicate. Afterward, Norma usually said something deadpan to her
patient that I could not follow in Garifuna, and they would both laugh.

The blue plastic tub labeled FOOT CARE quickly piled high with sterile
medical wrappers and used gloves. Carefully emptied, it soon filled
again. When a tall woman slid off her sandals and revealed four self-
bandaged ulcers across both feet, Dr. W stood nearby as a collaborating
physician tended to her. I knew the woman, Grace; she was part of a
group that had showed up previously when I advertised on local TV
and radio an upcoming presentation sharing early findings of this project on diabetes in Dangriga. I watched as the visiting doctor brushed
sand off Grace's toes, then used a Duplex Doppler device to listen to
Grace's feet for calcium blocks or other subtle acoustic clues, pressing
with a wand that amplified the sound of blood flowing through the
arteries.

Grace was already missing one of her big toes. Crumbled scar tissue and a protruding bone suggested that the digit had broken off with dry gangrene rather than a surgical cut. Making jokes about pedicures, the doctor took the foot firmly in hand and asked Grace to close her eyes. The physician used an array of soft-point brushes and metal hammers to detect where and how Grace's nerves had numbed or deadened. Then she rubbed Grace's feet vigorously with soap until enough dead skin sloughed away that the ulcers began to bleed at the edges, which might make regeneration possible. The newest ulcers were perfectly round circles, bright raw pink and eerily symmetrical. But the doctors were more concerned about how her feet sounded: they could barely hear a pulse near her missing toe, signaling diminished blood flow in the tissue that would make it much harder to heal.

Dr. W wished aloud to the team that there was some way they could give Grace two days in their New York hospital's hyperbaric chamber, the enclosed apparatus that can help otherwise impossible wounds begin to heal. "Is there any way you can get to New York, dear?" His invitation hovered in the air for a moment. But that afternoon, nobody knew a way to access a hyperbaric chamber. After Grace's remaining nine toes were wrapped in fresh bandages, her flip-flops would not fit over the dressed wounds. The doctors could only laugh in admiration at her raw tenacity when they saw her afterward climbing onto a bicycle. They knew the big toe is particularly crucial for balance, yet Grace moved with steady poise. Someone snapped a photo of her posing with gauze-wrapped feet pressed to the pedals, but their smiles looked privately worried. There was nothing left to do for the moment. We all watched as she rode away.

With an intensely focused look, Norma pulled another hurt foot onto her lap.

NON-TRAUMATIC MEASURES

The surgical unit where so many amputations took place had a sign near the doors reading OPERATING THEATRE. Everyone's use of "the theater" to refer to surgery rooms gave the events of amputation a surreal quality; I always found this label for medicine or war disquieting, like some script born elsewhere being played out time and again. *Surusia*, the Garifuna word for any biomedical doctor, comes from an ancient French word for *surgeon*.[4] The term should be a relic from the age of colonial warships when surgeons were literally at the front lines, but it has uncomfortable resonance in the age of epidemic diabetes.

Dr. W worried that even many caregivers do not understand what their patients with diabetes go through in rooms like this, which hold kinds of expertise that nobody wants to hear about: types of gangrene (wet, dry, gaseous), varieties of instruments (pneumatic bone saws, Gigli wires, Zimmer drills). "If you're not a surgeon, you've probably never seen an amputation," Dr. W noted. He recently jolted one audience of nurses and doctors at a Barbados hospital by starting his lecture with pictures of a procedure.

"And they were horrified. Horrified! Now, of course, they're medical people, and they've seen many things. They're not squeamish and upset about blood. But when you actually see an amputation, it leaves an impression on you that you will not soon forget. Then I took it from that point and said to them, 'so every patient who you know is going down this road will have this experience.'"

Dr. W explained that he was working on a new lecture. "During the [U.S.] Civil War, everyone was getting amputations because of major gunshot wounds. That is the only other time I've ever seen a picture where you have stacks of legs in a setting. What's the trauma here? It's almost like we have a civil war going on in these countries every year, [in that] we have the same number of amputations. In many cases, maybe more amputations. . . . So can you imagine us having civil war trauma, over and over and over again. Unrelenting, unrelenting. Unabashed. Uninterrupted."

Dr. W's civil war imagery made me recall how his medical specialty is more formally referred to as limb "reconstruction." In drawing analogies between diabetic injuries and war photos, Dr. W described a tension that many have grappled with: the twofold problem of looking or not looking at such visceral images, and how to weigh the choice to make them public or not when valences of shame haunt either option. "I could have looked . . . until my lamps went out and I still wouldn't have accepted the connection between a detached leg and the rest of the body," Michael Herr wrote of pictures like that during the Vietnam War.[5]

The problem is ugly at any point along its unsavory continuum: At one pole, there is the real danger that images of violence can be viewed and taken up in ways that verge on gratuitous spectacle or even repellent intrigue. Yet at the other end of the spectrum sits an equally chilling truth that gruesome things are already happening to some people, and many in broader publics would rather look away than face their part in the larger systems that depend on unequally patterned injuries—silence that often fosters complicity with even sharper injustices ahead.

All of us holding cameras were dealing with these dilemmas: What kinds of images were usefully sobering, which gratuitously sad? Who gets protected from the grisly side of diabetes? How do we represent this latest chapter in a familiar story of racialized bodies hurt by sugar—when we live in a global economy so deeply shaped by this legacy that even pictures of its echoes could become capital? Yet there was no denying a severe and growing problem that people were working hard to more accurately make public. How to convey that erased reality without dehumanizing anyone in the process of trying to make it visible?

Some patients began to display their injuries for cameras to try making the issue more legible—as you'll hear later, one dialysis advocate even began improvising "press releases" each time another part of his body was about to be amputated, calling up the major media outlets in Belize and asking people to make and reckon with images. As Laurence Ralph reflects elsewhere about "living *through* injury," sometimes "it becomes politically strategic to inhabit the role of a 'defective body' in order to make claims about a violent society." When individuals exhibit and even publicize their injuries to call attention to the broader social injustices shaping them, this can become part of a strategy that Ralph calls "what wounds enable."[6]

Belize Diabetes Association groups were facing related questions with immediate stakes: photos of imperiled feet help them to disrupt ideas of diabetes as a boring disease and thus to gather support for material care. For many members, this was not an abstract or theoretical debate about reproducing ideas of suffering. It surfaced instead as a dilemma that was unfolding in real time—as in the first week of 2018, when the Belize Diabetes Association Belmopan branch posted an arrangement of the new year's photos on their Facebook page.

The image was carefully composed to both shock and counter-anchor in dignity. It was prefaced by the pointed note "Permission granted by clients to share" and the hashtags #SaveAFoot #SaveALife, with pictures of four feet in limbo with mottled and missing toes, stitched to a larger photo of a T-shirt that said:

BEHIND EVERY PERSON WITH
DIABETES
THERE IS AN EVEN
STRONGER
FAMILY WHO STANDS BY THEM
SUPPORTS THEM AND
LOVES THEM
WITH ALL THEIR
HEART

"It seems as if the exotic things get the attention. . . . Having five people with Zika brings the media. It's very sexy, it's exotic, it's front-page news. People getting their limbs cut off, not really exciting," Dr. W reflected later on diabetes and the difficulties he's had for decades trying to bring public attention to it. In his words:

> I think the problem is that in this world of sound bites, diabetes is not that impressive or sexy. But the damage it does is absolutely horrific. . . . diabetes is expanding and growing at an alarming rate. It's chewing up your GDP. It's smothering countries. It's something that's really killing how your health system will work in every way.
>
> I think the problem is that it's not studied. People don't really know how many amputations are going on. First, there is an occult number: a number not well known. Number two, the long-term effects of it are not well studied in this population. Number three, the transgenerational issues that go along with that. The fear, the worry, the anxiety, the denial. . . . No one is measuring that. It's just like, yeah, diabetes. It's in this area.

A report from Belize's only prosthetic leg clinic noted that of the six amputations attributed to animal bites the previous year, only three had been snake bites. "The other three were attributed to rat bites becoming infected in diabetic patients. Bites from rats speak to the need for improved standards of living."[7] The report added: "Most diabetics from [our] Belize clinic ambulated in flip flops, sandals or ill fitting footwear due to poverty. In addition, they reported having their blood sugar tested once every three months! This very likely contributed to their becoming amputees in the first place."[8]

In the U.S. context, for which better data exists, about 80 percent of the country's total amputations are due to diabetes. But even the broadest literature review on diabetic amputation numbers I could locate did not contain data from a single low- or middle-income country. Despite this limited geography, even narrow studies suggest jarring numbers: About a third of people with diabetes experience an ulcer, and more than 50 percent of diabetic foot ulcers become infected.[9] A third of people who seek clinical care for ischemic diabetic ulcers (the most common type) will die before their injuries ever heal.[10] Diabetic foot ulcers "have morbidity and mortality rates equivalent to aggressive forms of cancer."[11] After having diabetes-related amputations, over 70 percent of patients die within five years—a death rate second only to lung cancer.[12] Following a major diabetic amputation, 50 percent of people will have another limb amputated within two years.[13] Despite these troubling fragments of statistics, though, there remains a dearth of global funding for diabetic foot care, due largely to lack of evidence documenting that there *is* a global issue.

"Internationally, accurate numbers of limb amputations performed are very difficult to estimate as there is no recognized database or organization collecting this information,"[14] one journal article about this global data gap recently summarized. The article also noted a brute-force fact that bears repeating: "Amputation of a limb is one of the most severe pains in the human experience."

Tellingly, some of the best statistics about the global severity of diabetic injuries have been collected by accident. Diabetic amputations have often turned out to be the number one cause of limb loss captured by databases meant to gather information about landmine blasts and other war-related injuries, as reported in studies with titles like "Diabetes or War?"[15] Researching the "yawning gap" between the need for diabetic foot care and sparse funding to support it, David Armstrong and colleagues recap: "There is a lack of federally and not for profit–funded research directed toward diabetic foot ulcers. This funding gap is disproportionately large in comparison with the public health impact of this sequela." The authors call this discrepancy "a clear and present medical and fiscal calamity. We must mind this gap as a locomotive of lower-extremity complications is approaching."[16]

The odd turn of phrase that ends their article underlines a strange fact: if the injuries and amputations that their team analyzed had been caused by actual locomotive trains, they would be robustly included in the global statistics that guide health policy funding. The World Health Organization's recent Global Burden of Disease report, for example, was designed especially to attend to the daily difficulties of living with chronic injuries. Its scale of "disability weights" emphasized the painful toll of amputations on daily life.

But the twenty-six possible *causes* of amputations and related injuries that the 2017 study painstakingly charted did not include diabetes. It did estimate global amputation burdens, though, for six kinds of traffic accidents (motor vehicle; motorcycle; cyclist; pedestrian; mass transportation, including bus and train; and other road incidents), as well as for venomous and nonvenomous animal bites, domestic violence, gunshot injuries, self-harm, war, and torture.[17] This led the report's authors to conclude that global injuries are declining and the world today is becoming a safer place. I wonder for how many countries in the world, besides Belize, that summation sounds plainly inaccurate.

The last time I visited Belize, I went to see a few friends one weekend and found that three of them had lost a leg since my last visit. The repetition was becoming so normalized that anxieties about "getting cut"[18] came up constantly in conversations. The pattern did not require an epidemiologist to notice that something was wrong. Of course, not everyone with diabetes dealt with limb injuries. But every person with diabetes did have to be constantly on guard, and those stakes felt high. I thought the struggles against shame that people described around amputations were related, at heart, to the non-counting of diabetes limb loss as a global phenomenon. Missing numbers do more than perpetuate missing material resources for care—they also change the feelings and ideas of responsibility that get associated with a given hardship. "In other words, the numbers inform how people tell their stories; the stories people tell shape the categories used to collect numerical data," Adia Benton observes.[19]

The standard legal definition of trauma is "a wound or a condition of the body caused by external force, including injuries inflicted by bullets, explosives, sharp instruments, blunt objects or other physical blows, chemicals, electricity, climatic conditions, infectious diseases, radiation, and bacteria, but excluding stress and strain."[20] Limbs injured or lost to sugar are thus not considered traumatic because they take shape slowly. When it comes to these non-traumatic diabetes wounds, in hospitals around the world, tough choices get made at the time of amputation. For instance, surgical teams must decide whether to use limited supplies of anesthesia to render a patient unconscious or to only numb them at the waist. In the conscious version you are awake and listening to everything. Bone has to be screwed to the table before they saw it. One woman in Dangriga told me she prayed so hard and felt her family's love so palpably that when the drill started up she felt the grace take over completely, and her ears filled with a loud ringing so beautiful that it became the only noise in the room.

"There are so many miracles," she told me. "Thank God."

DISPLACED SURVEILLANCE

Long after she officially retired, Nurse Norma kept going to the hospital to help provide diabetes foot care. She also made certain home visits, even though she no longer got paid for the work. She heard that specialized diabetes foot training will be coming soon and said she will start to relax her watch if she gets an apprentice. In a district where so many were losing limbs, how else could the only person certified in foot care training truly retire?

Humans alive today, in general—and nonwhite people, in particular[21]—are subject to constant surveillance. Algorithmic tracking and facial recognition tools are on the rise, alongside what Alondra Nelson calls "data spillover," cases when even materials like saliva submitted for ancestry testing or photos shared on social media can be harvested as data by interested parties ranging from pharmaceutical and life insurance companies to law enforcement databases.[22] We have never had more information collected about us by companies and states. This made it feel even stranger to come across the rare case where members of the concerned population actually expressly wanted institutional "surveillance" collected about key data—only to find that *this* data remained elusive.

"A lack of surveillance in Central America has stalled the development of amputation prevention services,"[23] one prosthetics maker in Belize noted. Here's the catch: it takes numbers to redirect global policy money, but it takes global policy money to assemble the numbers.

Belize has made more headway around these uncomfortable numbers than most Central American and Caribbean countries. A very small study incorporating data from Karl Heusner Memorial Hospital (Belize's only tertiary care hospital) was written up and published by concerned physician Uldine Wright, who recently returned to Belize from medical training in Cuba. She recounted a tally showing that among patients who came to the Belize City public hospital to treat a diabetic ulcer (often caused by an ingrown toenail or similar tiny wound), 89 percent of patients received an amputation.[24] Some 29 percent lost their leg below the knee, and 24 percent lost the limb above the knee. I heard informally that medical interns do many of these cuts. Eighteen percent of amputations were trans-metatarsal (toes or fingers with a piece of the foot or hand), while 18 percent lost only digits (mostly toes). Twelve percent of patients healed with debriding, and 0 percent healed with conservative treatment.[25] The second hospital that Wright also studied showed a less pronounced but still alarming figure: 24 percent of patients who arrived for diabetic ulcer care received amputations.

Even a tiny snapshot like this begins to suggest some sense of how normalized injuries impact care across the board—physicians upset with patients for not coming in earlier; patients terrified to seek care when they know the significant probability of returning with an amputation. There were tensions about which cuts were possibly avoidable or totally necessary, everyone struggling to bear their piece of the intensity.

From what I could observe, the caregivers most routinely dealing head-on with diabetic injuries were mostly Black and Indigenous women. They made up the majority of the community health workers and nursing and medical attendants with whom I spoke. Their expertise was formidable, but their labor offered little way out of the intense sensorium in which rural health workers practiced their craft. It took time to learn unwritten care strategies, a Garifuna rural health worker named June explained to me as she recounted the story of the first time she had cared for a diabetic foot: "I just told the patient, I'll be right back!" The older Garifuna nurse with whom June was apprenticing later praised how artfully she had concealed the pause when she went outside and vomited.

"If the patient sees that you are scared, they will be scared too." Nurses taught each other techniques to steel oneself to unwrap a diabetic foot, since "you never know what is going to be under there": for example, to be ready for larvae so that anything else is good news; or how to take the cap off the bleach bottle before you open anything else, and then just focus on the bleach smell. June described learning to swallow her dread while calming patients' reactions if they looked down at their foot by telling them stories about similar diabetic limbs that ended in some form of recovery. She said this was not the work she imagined. "Laugh, don't cry," she added.

I once fell into conversation with a team of care workers in Belize wearing matching bright green "EYES ON DIABETES" T-shirts. The printed design on their backs featured watchfully gazing eyes. I found myself thinking about how the assumed optics of functioning health surveillance had been displaced. In the gaps of accurate foot care epidemiology being conducted by global institutions, it seemed to me, not only were care workers "improvising medicine" to blunt the impact of diabetic injuries, with care practices full of the ad hoc force that Julie Livingston memorably describes around another chronic condition.[26] Members of these makeshift networks were additionally improvising select forms of surveillance, akin to the multiplied perspectives that some have called "para-sighted" optics—teaching each other new ways to see, keeping their own counts of emerging patterns, watching out for each other.[27]

People I met improvised daily surveillance of their own bodies: obsessively checking their skin for scrapes or soft spots, enlisting others to help check the bottoms of their feet, praying to spirits for help monitoring.

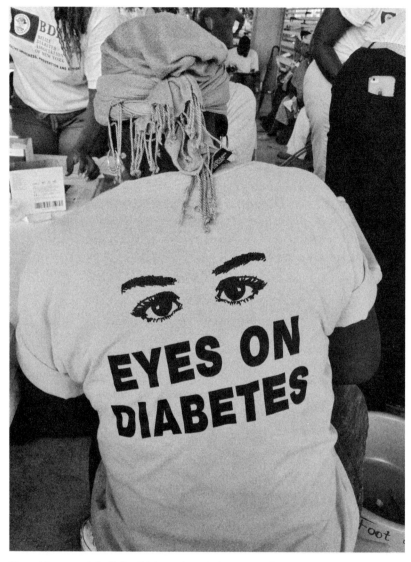

Nurse Norma and the Belize Diabetes Association on watch.

At one meeting I attended in the municipal building of Dangriga, the crowd of mostly women sitting in blue theater seats taught each other strategies for making a physician see their feet. "Untie your shoes ahead of time, while you're waiting. Then stick it right on their desk. Just tell them, 'Well Doc, I am about to put my foot right up on your desk!'" Everyone laughed, nodding. It was a good joke to remember: make the busy Cuban doctor laugh, buy an extra minute of their overstretched attention.

The Diabetic Foot Center Group that Dr. W founded and heads recently launched a new program in their travels across the Caribbean: visiting the proprietors of nail salons to teach them signs of diabetes ulcers. This network of beauty shop technicians is now helping to refer clients to hospital care when their hands or feet are in danger.

As Dr. W described initiatives like this, his words kept returning to two observations that are hard to square with each other: on one hand, the public has no idea what is happening; and yet, this is very well known by those who know it. What was happening in the space between these two truths? After we met, I planned to reach out to Dr. W back in New York, in hopes of interviewing him one day. But you know that you are studying a badly misunderstood topic when one of the field's top physicians takes time out of a packed schedule to email you first.

MIXED METAPHORS

"It's like an old friend, so I can talk about it," Dr. W said of diabetes. He considered it like getting to know certain people over time, where mystery grows along with knowledge. Indeed, when we first met in Dangriga, I never expected to find myself listening to multiple perform-ances of Dr. W's convincing Rod Serling impersonation as we talked in the Staten Island community hospital where he has long worked: *"There is a fifth dimension. . . . It is a dimension as vast as space and as timeless as infinity. It is the middle ground between light and shadow, between science and superstition, and it lies between the pit of man's fears and the summit of his knowledge."* We both laughed at his *Twilight Zone* reference, and then Dr. W switched back to his regular speaking voice. "But really, diabetes has its own dimensions. It's not an ordinary dis-ease. It's quite extraordinary."

This was a sharp contrast with how diabetes is often portrayed. Dia-betes is typically imagined as boring and mild. This banality is integral to the ways its disproportionate costs for certain populations get nor-malized as individuals' own fault. Simultaneously dull and virulent, the particular stereotypes surrounding diabetes are profoundly enmeshed in five-hundred-year-old racial imaginaries that nobody can call back. There will be no truce of representation.

In *Illness and Its Metaphors,* Susan Sontag famously described the disease metaphors that societies come to accept as common sense—

despite the ways such associations often blame and shame patients for their own illnesses, and frequently do harm to people's sense of self and their possibilities for recovery. "Patients who are instructed that they have, unwittingly, caused their disease are also made to feel that they have deserved it," Sontag worried.[28] At the same time, she added, "we cannot think without metaphors."[29]

This is why I admired Dr. W's skill at inventing counter-metaphors, which he mixed unabashedly. Consistency in literal images is not his objective—just consistency in bodies.

"What really bothers me is the look of loss on a patient's face when you tell them the reason they are going blind," he said. In the face of that, he was willing to try any metaphor on for size. "Diabetes is like fighting a bull. You need to grab it by the horns, or it can gore you." He explained that mixing metaphors was a talent he had honed over the years by talking with patients, learning what analogies seemed to stick in their mind and help them live with it better or mentally get a handle on some certain facet of it all.

"You can't outrun diabetes. You can only outsmart it," Dr. W said, smiling to himself. "That's a good one. It can be overcome, but not without a strategy." Different kinds of personification may be strategic for different things, he said. Many of his patients struggled with depression as their diabetes progressed. What framings might help really depended on the person. Alongside photocopies of medical instructions, Dr. W's team kept on hand a variety of prayers for grieving patients who were religious. Other times, it helped to cast diabetes as an external nemesis and the body as an epic terrain where great carefulness was required, without implying any personal shame: "When you enter the land of diabetes, Dracula is around."

As his Rod Serling voice suggests, Dr. W grew up with a love of science fiction. Dracula was one among a cast of diabetes monsters that Dr. W and his patients might evoke for each other. Sci-fi shaped how creatively he explained diabetes and listened to those dealing with its more extreme forms. It seemed to me as we spoke that perhaps science fiction had also prepared him for his encounters with sugar's stranger subtleties in his work traveling across the diabetes epidemic: the crucial plot clues in sci-fi tend to come from paying careful attention to the faint signs of something potentially sinister ahead.

Dr. W's other inspiration for his approach to dealing with patients was the seventies ABC show *Marcus Welby, M.D.*, about a humanistic doctor who went out of his way to connect with patients. While his three brothers wanted to be sports stars, Dr. W said, by age seven he dreamed of becoming a physician. His particular interest in lower limb reconstruction came a few years later, at age ten, when he was trying to dash home from his grandmother's house during a commercial break without missing any *Star Trek* and was struck by a car. He spent months recovering in a body cast (and never got to reschedule his plans with the prettiest girl in school, he sighed). That period of healing was one of the formative experiences that made him want to be a lower limb surgeon. The diabetes focus came to his work later, from observing patterns of injuries and sheer need in neighborhood community podiatry clinics. He has now been taking care of diabetic feet for over twenty-one years.

"I think we need to be more poetic about diabetes," Dr. W said. "Let me give you some images." He proceeded to reel off so many that I could barely keep up and had to distill them down later.[30] They kept slipping between metaphors and the uncanny clinical realities prompting them:

> When you hear diabetes, it isn't alarming. Even in this information age. Diabetes is the disease that nobody knows, because everyone thinks they already know. It's the known unknown. It's abstract in a way, but so tangible. Some people's arteries are so calcified, they show up on x-rays as bones. So we are seeing people turning to stone from the inside. It kills you slowly. Almost methodically. Almost systematically. Almost intentionally. It starts off not so bad. Some of my patients are afraid to see me because they live with the fear of losing a leg after seeing it happen to their parents.
>
> Diabetes can accelerate your age, large glucose molecules attaching to the outside of your cells. It can affect every cell of your body in a different way. There is always more mystery, the medical paradox. A patient will tell me sometimes, "Doctor, I feel like my feet are being lit on fire. Right now we're in this room, but my feet are in hell with the devil." The nerve damage keeps them up at night, and all I can do is give them GABA drugs, painkillers. Neuropathy: numbness, horrific pain, shooting, stabbing, burning. Ask people. You will hear a hundred different words for a hundred different kinds of pain.
>
> Phantom pains after an amputation: the trauma over and over of feeling a limb still there and seeing it is gone. It tricks your body. Diabetes is the great magician. It gives you illusions, hunger and thirst you can't satisfy. Diabetes is like a thief, or a trickster. It is a thief of limbs. It is a tragedy that keeps happening. Patients getting cut into pieces. It hits like an asteroid. It changes like a chameleon. As soon as you think you know what it looks like, it will change shape and hit you in another form: it's high blood pressure, it's kidney disease, it's blindness, it's a toe. It keeps morphing. It lives with you. It lives in you. It's almost like it's a virus, hiding.

Driving home from Brooklyn, I kept replaying Dr. W's eerie images in my mind. "Our bodies prime our metaphors," James Geary observes, "and our metaphors prime how we think and act."[31] I wondered how policies to guide public perceptions of diabetes care might look different if they were based on Dr. W's descriptions of learning to live with a volatile shape-shifter, offering no false claims that the work would be easy. His creative descriptions struck me as efforts toward what Charles Briggs and Clara Mantini-Briggs call "communicative justice"—working at the junctures of public storytelling about health conditions to try to change the ways they biologically manifest in bodies.[32] There was one image, in particular, Dr. W had voiced that I found myself returning to again: *almost like a virus, hiding*. Not quite like a virus. Slow, cumulative. But in certain ways . . . almost. In contrast to the rest of Dr. W's figures, that was an image of diabetes I had heard many times before.

PARA-COMMUNICABLE CONDITIONS

As rising diabetes became part of the social fabric in Belize, rumors began popping up that certain forms could be contagious. There were numerous stories about husbands and wives becoming afraid to sleep in the same room, with the specter of threatened limbs again appearing as the defining feature of these anxieties.

"Well, here it comes for me," Laura recalled thinking when she was diagnosed with diabetes in her twenties. "I knew it was coming for me, because my mom had it, my sister . . . we all have it." The personified pathogens that people kept using to allude to their diabetic injuries came from the language of infection: many said of diabetes sugar that they "caught it." Other phrases echoed histories of attempted escapes from sugar: "*It* caught *me.*"

I was surprised that rumors of contagion seemed to multiply, rather than subside, as time wore on and as people in Belize became more familiar with the illness and observed it more closely in their own communities. Public health authorities often emphasize education about the causes of diabetes as one of the most important tools to curb its spread. But in this case, it was not that people had never received diabetes education; it was that the one-size-fits-all biomedical education from abroad often did not fully square with the realities they saw with their own eyes. Diabetes moved like an epidemic. It killed like an epidemic. In the Stann Creek District, diabetes affected at least ten times more people than HIV/AIDS,[33] and everyone knew that AIDS was an epidemic. Diabetes was spreading quickly, and a "non-transmissible" disease is not supposed to spread.

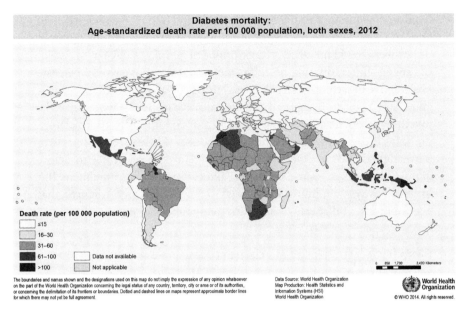

Map of global diabetes deaths, shown at community forum in Dangriga.

As historian Allan Brandt notes, "The problem of causation is critically important because it reflects directly on the fundamental moral issue of responsibility for disease."[34] This point hit home more concretely for me when I gave a public presentation on an early version of this project's findings to a small crowd in Dangriga. The audience came mostly from local branches of the Belize Diabetes Association and HelpAge, a local organization providing supportive care across generations. I began our conversation that day with a cursory slide showing the World Health Organization map of diabetes deaths. I had assumed that larger context was the part everyone would already know, but the global map seemed to be the only image I showed that surprised anybody. People raised eyebrows at each other. *Wait, versions of this are happening across the world?* Some people later reflected that they had gotten so used to stories attributing the Belizean rise in diabetes to their personal responsibility or local "cultural foods" that it shook up their perspectives just to take a step back and think of diabetes *as* an epidemic—a much bigger story, whatever that might mean.

There is a lot on the line in "explaining epidemics," as Charles Rosenberg once put it.[35] Global aid resources tend to move according to the moral rationales of humanitarian "crisis."[36] This kind of intervention "has come to define itself through exception," Peter Redfield aptly observes, though that framing quickly "loses its transcendent magic" when "diseases prove chronic."[37] One woman in Belize named Nel described how a team of U.S. medical students visiting her village had been fascinated by her ankle wound when they believed she had leishmaniasis (a tropical disease caused by sandfly-borne protozoa parasites), but stopped visiting when it turned out to be a diabetic ulcer. Senses of medical urgency (or nonurgency) also remain deeply contoured, as Priscilla Wald describes in *Contagious,* by "how both scientists and the lay public understand the nature and consequences of infection, how they imagine the threat, and why they react so fearfully to some disease outbreaks and not others at least as dangerous and pressing."[38]

The "entwined histories . . . of tropical medicine and racial thought" continue to shape how health issues get perceived, Warwick Anderson argues, together underpinned by colonial notions of contagion. [39] A cursory glance into the archives yields more than fifty years of ignored calls for a response to diabetes in the world. "Diabetes is no longer a rare syndrome in the tropics, and in many parts is being diagnosed with increasing frequency," Dr. Silas Dodu wrote in the *British Medical Journal* in 1967. Returning home to Ghana after medical school in London, Dodu linked the phenomenon he observed to the spread of "white man's food."[40] Several years later, the Pan American Health Organization (PAHO) sounded another alarm. "Right now the seriousness of the problem is reflected by the large number of diabetics who suffer, die, or become invalids," reads their 1975 diabetes report, "fatalities considered largely preventable because effective treatments for these diseases were known."[41] Their astute and progressive policy recommendations are disturbing today, because they detail precise knowledge and actionable suggestions for policies to prevent diabetes injuries from spreading further—published before HIV/AIDS ever became legible as an epidemic, and before most people described in this book were born.

Although wider diabetes policy responses largely stagnated after PAHO's 1975 call to action, other aspects of diabetes knowledge have grown more robust over the decades that followed. In addition to studying industrialized diets, more scientists now also track the ways that diabetes risks can be amplified by environmental exposures and chemicals. Some molecular pathologists call this "the new toxicology paradigm of endocrine and metabolic disruption" that reframes diabetes and related autoimmune conditions as a "hidden cost" to polluted landscapes.[42] This phenomenon first became clear through industrial accidents: for example, diabetes rates in a small town in Italy spiked in the twenty years after its chemical plant exploded.[43]

Altered atmospheres also get absorbed: a recent long-term study of 1.7 million U.S. veterans estimated that about 14 percent of diabetes cases may be associated with air pollution, regardless of what diets individuals ate.[44] Foods are impacted by air changes, too: crops such as wheat have less protein and more carbohydrates when grown in high-carbon atmospheres,[45] while rice can absorb heavy metals like mercury (which also contribute to diabetes risk) if the rice patties are fed by polluted water.[46] Chemicals used to protect crops also get inside humans: a study of 3,080 farmworkers in India reported that exposure to organophosphate chemicals significantly increased diabetes risk, apparently because insecticides meant to kill pests also interact with the microbes crucial to metabolic balance inside people's digestive tracts.[47] This is only one of several mechanisms by which endocrine-disrupting chemicals contribute to diabetes, which is a disease of the endocrine system.[48]

"We are porous selves within microbiomes and with microbes, sharing social lives even when we may not want to," notes Juno Salazar Parreñas.[49] Exposure to viruses can also trigger certain forms of diabetes and cancer.[50] In addition to the microbial life within us, there has also been more scientific attention being paid to the plasticity of human biology—including metabolic absorptions that connect human bodies and larger environs,[51] hunger- and stress-related epigenetic modulations,[52] and ideas of "infective heredity."[53] The notion of "situated biologies" proposed by Margaret Lock reflects these puzzles—Lock initially used the name "local biologies" to consider such contingent effects on each individual body, yet the worldwide patterns in rising chronic conditions presented her with a paradox: How are "local biologies" of individuals changing in such patterned ways across global scales?[54]

In this view, human eating is only one dimension within "nested metabolisms."[55] Bodies exchange matter through "metabolic landscapes,"[56] such as the paradoxical "choices" that Elizabeth Hoover examines in *The River Is In Us* when studies revealed that local fish and waters contain diabetes-causing toxics.[57] Chemicals also impact industrial farm animals and plants, as Hannah Landecker examines in "Food of our Food," which become part of human digestion as well when people eat them.[58]

Amid so many complex interactions, diseases are not binary either-or conditions. So how did our terms for addressing them come to be? It is worth taking a step back to ask how diseases came to be framed in such a dualistic paradigm to begin with.

The old paradigm of environmental *miasma* comes from an ancient Greek word meaning "pollution" (*muíaσµa*), which framed disease as coming from "morbid material" in contaminated local environs. In the nineteenth century, germ theory replaced miasma paradigms with a stricter dichotomy. Dominant models today still hold that there are two basic ways to think about diseases: they are either "communicable" or "non-communicable." In this binary schema, infectious diseases need to be addressed in terms of interrupting contagion between people, vectors, and environments via specific exposures to disease-specific germs or biological pathogens. Meanwhile, since non-communicable diseases are by definition not being transmitted between bodies, they are typically analyzed via the individual's own inborn genetic constitution or understood as resulting from personal choices and "lifestyle" behaviors.[59]

Public health classes often reference iconic histories of contagious disease surveillance, such as John Snow's team's identifying and disrupting patterns of water-borne cholera at the Broad Street Pump in 1854 London. Yet the shadow side of Snow's discovery remains instructive: it prefigured germ theory, which described *an* important way that bodies are exposed to disease. But some industrial actors tried to cast infection as the *only* way that exposures mattered, by seizing this new explanatory model to shield themselves from responsibility. In 1855, Snow was called in a legal case about deregulating industrial pollution in London. He testified that chemicals could "not cause disease; those poisons do not reproduce themselves in the constitution." When prodded further about reported symptoms of toxic exposure among workers, Snow responded: "Persons are often very much influenced by the imagination."[60]

To approach chronic disease patterns, we need ways to recognize and publicize potential exposures of processed diets and industrial toxicants, as well as biological germs—an epidemiology of what Adia Benton has called "connectors," rather than vectors alone.[61] That requires attention, Michael Fischer notes, to "the bioecologies at play" between porous boundaries and reactive membranes, commodity flows, and human and ecological health.[62]

In light of these gray zones, the either-or labeling of "contagious" versus "non-communicable" disease appears insufficient to describe the prevalence of human-made diseases now becoming visible around the world.[63] Diabetes is not an exception to, but very much *iconic* of growing chronic epidemics—such as cancer clusters[64] or the soaring prevalence of asthma and other autoimmune conditions.[65]

When I talked with public health practitioners and policy makers about such exposures, I found it helpful to have a working name for this in-between. I came to describe it as *para-communicable*—chronic conditions like diabetes that may be materially transmitted as bodies and ecologies intimately shape each other over time, with unequal and compounding effects for historically situated groups of people. Focusing on *para* causalities—the products and exposures changing *alongside (para)* people's bodies—draws attention to the imperative to acknowledge and rework those systemic harms. Exploring this approach also became a way to translate across different spaces of knowledge making—such as academic conferences where keywords to describe exposures were abundant, and the arenas of practice where they were often illegible or quietly fell out of frame.

This is not a return to miasmatic thinking, though. As historians have observed, cloudy causalities are indeed frequently part of what it feels like to live amid ongoing exposures—but confusion is difficult to regulate, and industries bank on this.[66] Nor can chemicals simply be reframed as contagious—they too do not follow a neat binary pattern. They have their own intervals of low-dose "latency."[67] Current regulatory paradigms that contribute to so many toxics on the loose are in part flawed for exactly this reason. Germ theory informed the ways in which chemicals were tested in the laboratory, but these simplified models of disease have often failed to recognize the complex ways a chemical can still cause harm.[68]

Sugar and food industries have also attempted to intentionally produce confusion, akin to techniques described in books like *Merchants of Doubt*.[69] Marion Nestle examined how Coca-Cola, for example, has paid doctors to back suspicious studies and run ad campaigns focused on how individuals with chronic health issues need to exercise more.[70] These corporate strategies raise special challenges for scholarship dealing with uncertainty. The key theorists of *syndemics*—a widespread model describing how multiple epidemics interact—recently expressed concern that the term can take on a miasma-like cloudy quality if it is taken up imprecisely or without follow-up steps to trace specific pathways and signatures of responsibility.[71] Anthropologists like Elizabeth Roberts[72] are seeking ways to build a counter-science, through sustained collaborations and a grassroots-guided "science of the in-between."[73]

Thinking back to "diabetes multiple," policy interventions (or their absence) may actually produce biologically different versions of diabetes, on the population level as well as for individual bodies. What an epidemic is *is* different—not just in scale, but potentially in its mechanisms and forms of transmission. The first two cases of drug-resistant bacteria documented in the United States both occurred in diabetic ulcers—apparently from separate instances of horizontal gene transfer, by which bacteria can nearly instantaneously swap genes with other living or dead bacteria.[74] One study of 150 diabetic ulcers in India found that "91% of the bacteria were resistant to three or more antibiotics," including feared bacteria like MRSA.[75] In cases where people live for months or years walking in sandals with open diabetic wounds on their feet, it is also possible that horizontal gene transfer occurred directly between the bacteria infecting lower limb ulcers and the bacteria living in local soils.

This tendency for unchecked diabetes injuries to foster drug-resistant bacteria may have implications for future antibiotic efficacy and diseases of all kinds. Yet if drug-resistant bacteria sound like an urgent global issue in a way that the foot ulcers fostering them do not, that is another example of why the diabetes epidemic will continue to grow.

GEOGRAPHIES OF BLAME

Media analysts report that a "full 73 percent of articles that mention the poor, African Americans, or Latinos blame obesity on bad food choices, compared to only 29 percent of articles that do not mention these groups."[76] As Paul Farmer has noted of the common figure of a blame-worthy patient, "All too often, the notion of patient noncompliance is used as a means of explaining away program failure." He related this to "immodest claims of causality"—how patient noncompliance is commonly assumed and made persuasive without evidence, but any alternative explanation requires a great deal of evidence for policy makers to find it convincing.[77] Looking at tuberculosis cases, Farmer asked how people with TB could be labeled "noncompliant" with treatment when 50 percent don't even know they have it. This is the same percentage of people with diabetes globally that the International Diabetes Federation today estimates have never been diagnosed.[78] These patterns resonate with the "geographies of blame" that anthropologists have documented around the politics of labeling "noncompliance" elsewhere: *Throughout the world, those least likely to comply are those least able to comply.*"[79]

"How am I going to make a diet? There is only one kind of food here," I often heard patients tell the visiting Cuban physician, who would laugh kindly but never really had an answer. In nearby Guatemala, Emily Yates-Doerr has described the ways nutritional experts carefully avoided talking about problems of macro-infrastructure that neither they nor their patients could change, since that advice could easily have registered as cold or uncaring.[80] The caregivers I met likewise avoided initiating conversations about "social determinants of health" directly with patients, in hopes of generating a healthy sense of optimistic possibility—focusing on the scale within their grasp. This mostly meant trying to equip patients to negotiate existing foodways. But who will rework larger food *systems*?

Some preliminary studies have proposed that diabetic foot ulcers could be better treated if patients were also provided with supplies of nutritious food.[81] Scholars such as Harvard economist Michael Porter have argued that such investment would be beneficial for health systems, which spend thousands of dollars each time they amputate a diabetic injury. That money could be better invested in nutrition programs to help prevent amputation.[82]

Yet even the food baskets that accompany HIV/AIDS treatment programs often contain cheap grains, such as white rice, which are precisely the kinds of high-carbohydrate foods that people with diabetes are discouraged from consuming. What would be in a diabetes food basket? (And should it be in the HIV/AIDS food baskets, too, considering how many patients with HIV/AIDS are also getting diabetes as a side effect of their drug treatments?[83]) Trying to imagine a food basket's hypothetical contents only highlights the bigger issue: to actually curb the rise in diabetes, healthy foods need to exist for sale at affordable prices in grocery stores, not just dispensed in baskets for those with already sick bodies or imperiled limbs.

This also casts different light on the limits of existing models. For instance, some global health programs piloted ways to attach medicines to cases of Coca-Cola in order for treatments to hitch a ride to rural regions beyond health systems' reach. But in the case of diabetes, this delivery proposal would be an unsettling image. Which is more disturbing: the idea of insulin and metformin pills traveling to remote areas they could not otherwise reach attached to cases of soda, or the present reality of the Coca-Cola arriving alone?

Every local diet that has been dismantled by industrial diets is unique—meaning that any guidelines about eating require local texture in order to be meaningful for people. One morning, I joined a group in Dangriga that gathered to share cooking ideas to modify Belizean and Garifuna dishes for those with diabetes. Inspired by Garifuna cooking projects like Isha Gutierrez-Sumner's *Weiga* (Let's Eat!)[84] and Belizean restaurants like Nutrilicious Corner,[85] some suggested that events around healthy eating with diabetes might get people talking.

It would be good, they said, to have a locally relevant alternative to the foreign pamphlets that gave the false impression that all diabetes-healthy foods were "white people food." Grace was there, mostly just listening. Recipe ideas that the group offered included blended greens with milk and nutmeg; boiled raisins with okra, bukut, and vanilla; oven-roasted carrots; beet salad with slivered watermelon; club soda with a squeeze of papaya; soursap leaf and orange leaf tea; and fish dipped in seawater (instead of table salt) for cooking, the way past generations did. Others had questions about local and ground foods, which of course came with no labels. Was toasted cassava safe for people with diabetes? They wondered if local labs could be equipped to investigate the nutritional content of certain dishes or to monitor their fish and water to guard against toxic chemicals.

I initially thought it would be fairly easy to apply for a grant to support the kind of local foods project they suggested. But it turns out that the U.S. National Institute of Health explicitly declines to fund research that generates locally relevant dietary and care translations; they reason that such outcomes would not be globally "generalizable." If only approaches imagined as "generalizable" receive policy funding, then most well-resourced interventions end up framing what is *inside* individuals as the problem to target, rather than putting resources toward remediating harms of people's lived environments.[86]

When I bumped into Grace later in line as she waited to see Dr. W, it seemed that her foot spoke not only of gaps in the surveillance around injuries due to diabetes, but of displaced watchfulness throughout larger global systems of food and medicine. Her injury seemed to evince the culmination of decades or centuries of policy and legal regulations that contributed to chemicalized water, air, and sustenance; and skewed food options, linked to unjust agricultural systems and long legacies of land dispossessions. Viewed in this way, every amputation is preceded by "a thousand tiny cuts," as Michael Montoya wrote of diabetes.[87] In fact, each end-of-the-line injury like Grace's (as well as its erasure in much global accounting) could be read as what Marcel Mauss called a "total social fact"—at once economic, political, legal, ecological, institutional, biological, alimental, spiritual, and familial.[88] A total social fact demands a total social response. Yet at present, only 2 percent of global health funding is spent on all chronic diseases combined.[89]

Some months after we last saw each other, I heard the heavy news that Grace had chosen to die with all of her limbs attached. After careful meditation, she made the choice to refuse the amputation of a gangrenous leg. "More people are doing that now," Norma said when she told me. Looking for a picture of Grace to send to her family, I found only a terrible archive of her feet. My mind kept returning to Dr. W's words from that day, when he wished out loud that there could be some way to get her to a hyperbaric chamber.

THREE ATMOSPHERES

At some point I started to think of decompression chambers as almost mythical places. Originally developed in the late 1800s in England for recreational and military scuba diving, hyperbaric chambers became widely used in hospitals for chronic wounds in general (and diabetic ulcers in particular) in Europe and North America throughout the 1960s and 1970s.[90] Their physics is akin to going deep underwater: the pressure inside hyperbaric chambers is measured on the machines' gauges in ATAs, Atmospheres Absolute of pressure. At sea level, you are at 1 ATA, experiencing one atmosphere of pressure. Inside of a hyperbaric chamber, each additional atmosphere corresponds to the pressure of being underneath an extra thirty-three feet of seawater.

This pressure helps to saturate blood plasma with healing oxygen. (Plasma is the hay-colored fluid in which the more familiar components of blood, such as platelets and red and white blood cells, travel through the body, helping vascular tissues heal.)[91] Even the most stubborn diabetic wounds might have a chance with this boost of intensive oxygen under pressure.

Bodies that stop healing are hard to imagine. Even a minor cut or scrape can't form a scab or shrink a little each day. A tiny abrasion might look like it had just happened for months, even years. Almost like the injury is frozen while time goes on around it, except that it can still become infected. Preventing infection is work that starts anew each day. But even very old diabetic wounds can often start to heal again if given a few sessions in a hyperbaric chamber. Some studies have even suggested that oxygen therapy is helpful not only for wounds, but actually for preventing the onset of diabetes in the first place.[92]

These devices activate the body's healing capacities through the saturation of oxygen-rich air, either directly inside the chamber or through a mask. Originally honed for safety by British naval experiments on herds of goats, today U.S. hyperbaric chambers are marketed even for pets, such as "equine athletes and pleasure horses."[93] At some centers, special breathing masks can accommodate the snouts of certain animal species. Humans, meanwhile, can wear a range of different models: some masks look like the clear bubble helmets intended for astronauts, while other images remind me more of scuba gear or nebulizer masks. Multi-person hyperbaric chambers can be sizeable, like a clinical waiting room with round submarine windows; others resemble an appliance like a huge microwave, with seating for five or more. Some report that the pressure inside feels very slight or even imperceptible but makes your ears pop, like descent in an airplane.

Researching the varieties of these decompression machines, I suddenly realized with some shock that there actually *had* been hyperbaric chambers in Belize all along. A chamber has been available for decades in a network sustained by Ambergris diving shops, in case any scuba divers experience the bends or other pressure-related sicknesses. As an additional safety measure, a second hyperbaric machine was also added to serve diving tourists on the island.

It turns out that the phenomenon of diabetic limb injuries across the Caribbean coincides with a geography particularly well equipped with hyperbaric chambers: Barbados, Belize, Cuba, Dominica, the Dominican Republic, Dutch Antilles, Jamaica, Martinique, Mexico's Cancun, Puerto Rico, Saba, Saint Lucia, and Trinidad and Tobago (among others), according to what I could find on websites like Caribbean Adventures and Dive Vacations. Most were located in places citizens would not think to turn to for diabetes care, such as marine parks, fisheries, nearby scuba shops, and inside army bases.[94] I watched a video of one, then asked Dr. W if he had time for a call, to make sure I wasn't misunderstanding.

"Are these the same machines that can prevent diabetic amputations?" I asked him.

The short version of his answer was "Pretty much . . . but it's really complicated."

The long answer would be something anthropologists might call a "socio-technical problem," since it's hard to separate technological limits from the way human societies position and use their devices.

In the United States, health insurance often covers hyperbaric treatment for diabetes ulcers, billing approximately $350 per dive as long as the specialist is accredited by the Undersea Medicine and Hyperbaric Society. But in parts of the world labeled as lower income, insurance reimbursement apparatuses are more complicated and oxygen more expensive per tank. And diabetic sugar's wounds, unlike diver's bends, are almost never a one-time fix. Additionally, most scuba divers with decompression sickness quickly recover. But the most serious diabetic ulcers might require session after session of dialing the machine up to three Atmospheres Absolute—the pressure of being under approximately sixty-six feet of seawater.[95] This means more compression and more oxygen—and thus more cost and possibly greater risk, since decompression therapy always carries the chance of a rare (but ever possible) side effect of seizures or a serious issue caused by the intense pressure. It is best to be near a full medical facility and nearby teams of physicians in case something goes wrong.

Dr. W was very hopeful that more portable devices featuring aerosolized oxygen in transportable bags may become accessible for diabetic wound treatment around the world in the near future. He sent me a link of a YouTube video showing the new technology, and we left it at that. From what I could read between the lines of "it's really complicated," Dr. W's decades of work across the Caribbean had taught him that a transportable device his team could carry with them would work well. But it had not proven easy to get citizens access to infrastructures of hyperbaric chambers that exist in their own countries.

For instance, when Sarah's brother, Tobias, had texted Dr. W that picture of the small bone that fell out of his foot, the only thing Dr. W could think to do was invite him to travel over three thousand miles from Belize to New York City. The treatment for Tobias's foot lasted over a year. When receiving optimal care in a hospital, diabetic ulcers still have surprisingly long median healing times, between 147 and 237 days.[96] In Tobias's case, treatment with Dr. W and his colleagues included not only dozens of sessions in a hyperbaric chamber but also a wound vacuum-assisted closure, antibiotic beads, and grafts to treat the bone infection. Dr. W helped him find a place to live near the hospital, and his network of colleagues found a way to cover the treatment costs. Tobias's neighbors and family all chipped in to help with his plane ticket.

Human solidarity is an elusive thing. One of the most famous early social thinkers to theorize it was sociologist Émile Durkheim. It is a lesser-known fact that Durkheim's influential ideas about social coherence were shaped by his obsession with the era's new sciences of bacteria behavior.[97] He suggested that community and communication shaped each other—since social groups impact how perceptions turn into concepts, "communicable to a plurality of minds."[98] In this view, communicability—the ways that biological conditions are transmitted between bodies—is impacted not only by our communication about them, but also in turn by the communities that take shape (or not) to respond.[99]

This, too, is integral to what I came to see as the para-communicability of diabetes: not just a different framing for explorations of causality but one that implies a more wide-ranging model of public response; "not to ignore difference, but to create alter-relations with one another," in the words of Kristen Simmons.[100] Hyperbaric availability for scuba divers is precisely designed to offer a safety net so that pleasure seekers can indulge in risk, yet have the option of rescue if they would die without it. This logic of care was not being extended to those dying from diabetic injuries. Between these two scenarios lurk many uneasy questions: What counts as an extraordinary measure, for whom? Whose lives are valued as worth rescuing and at what cost?

When I called the largest hyperbaric clinic in Belize, I learned their machine simulates dives of up to 165 feet. Staffed by a specially trained physician, the chamber is "multi-space," meaning it can hold more than one person and accommodate others coming or going midsession. When I asked if it could be used to treat diabetic injuries, the curator replied that scuba divers at times receive care for coral-related injuries, and indeed it could also be used on diabetes wounds. It cost three hundred U.S. dollars per session. She added that for patients with U.S. health insurance, the copay went down to one hundred U.S. dollars.

It has become customary to talk about globally unequal infrastructures in the language of "Global North" versus "Global South." But this geography kept taking on more complicated shapes, when trying to describe either outposts of U.S. insurance–accepting technologies available to those in the know in Belizean dive shops; or the checkered maps of cities like New York and Los Angeles, where diabetic amputation rates increased exponentially in correlation with poverty and segregated spaces.[101] These internal inequalities get smoothed over in maps based on countrywide averages. Hyperbaric chambers were another uneasy reminder that even in the same places, we live in segregated atmospheres—racialized climates that pattern out both inside the United States and within most any country, including Belize. And as James Baldwin once wrote of the psychic and bodily effects of racial segregation: "One is always in the position of having to decide between amputation and gangrene."[102]

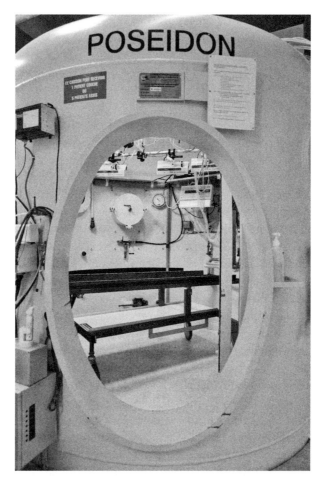

Stock photo of a hyperbaric chamber in a dive center.

My first impulse was to visit one of Belize's hyperbaric chambers, as if that would somehow resolve the contradiction. I had never been to San Pedro and wondered if Norma might go with me. But when I broached the subject as we chatted on the phone one morning, Norma said she had never heard of that machine and didn't think one existed in Belize. I looked down at my notes from the dive network's clinic, unable to put their price list together with the insights from someone who had spent so many years in diabetes wound care—all the patients Norma had worked with over time to pull back from the brink of loss, and all those like Grace she had seen die without hearing of any possible remediation measures that existed.

It didn't feel right to press harder about the idea of a trip together. But I found enough words to repeat to Norma how it was the kind of machine Dr. W had used to treat Tobias's foot in New York. The phone line got silent for a minute. We probably each had our own fantasies and doubts about the potentials of such an elusive apparatus. In the moment of quiet, I wondered if Norma was trying to imagine it, too: the pressure, the oxygen, the slow hours of boredom and excitement. The blood starting to move again through skin and tissue that had seemed dead. The feeling when sensation comes back.

I kept remembering how everyone laughed when Grace struck a jokester pose for someone's camera and then waved without looking back as she rode down a dirt path on her bicycle. There is no consensus about the larger worldwide pattern her trajectory is part of: the World Health Organization attributed 1.5 million deaths to diabetes at last count, but the International Diabetes Federation estimated this number to be 5 million deaths each year.[103] Recalling that last glimpse of Grace, in my memory she is riding straight into the place where it has come to seem normal to annually lose track of millions. People moving through these strange infrastructures bring us to another scale where, as Teju Cole writes, "The death toll is always one, plus one, plus one. The death toll is always one."[104]

This is it. This is the plague of our lifetimes.
It is by no means simple.

It's like a long hallway, or a maze.
In Belize, you know the Blue Hole where people deep dive?
When you go into the depths of it, you find that it's a whole other
    world.
I see diabetes as being like that.

I think people in the public need to be taken by the hand
If you could convey any of this in writing
Sometimes it reminds me of the Twilight Zone

Welcome to the strange world of diabetes
It is very different than what you have been taught
Come take a look from the inside
It's not what you think from out there.

—Dr. W, New York City[105]

PART TWO

Crónicas

Crónica One: Thresholds

Traveling an Altered Landscape
with Cresencia

To return once more to diabetes . . . it can strike man or
woman, threaten them with coma, often hit them with
impotence or sterility, for whom pregnancy, should it occur,
is a catastrophe, whose tears—O irony of secretions!—are
sweet.

It seems very artificial to break up disease into symptoms
or to consider its complications in the abstract. *What is a*
symptom without context or background? What is a
complication separated from what it complicates?

—Georges Canguilhem, *The Normal and the Pathological*

People living with diabetes and hypertension in Belize often lived with
"sugar and pressure" levels beyond the ranges programmed into devices
like glucometers and digital home blood pressure cuffs. But the Caribbean heat and sea air along the coast also regularly interrupted delicate
electronics from within, especially on very hot or humid afternoons.
The caregivers doing home visits often had difficulty discerning whether
a machine stopped working because of irregularities inside a patient's
body, or because of the mechanical weathering particular to a seaside
atmosphere, or both. On a few days, the most common blood sugar
reading was "Error."

The clinic's Accu-Chek glucometer had a different glitch; it couldn't
read blood sugars over 600. But Cresencia had a joke she told herself
whenever she saw the machine's message of "Hi" (short for high sugar).
She received it with intimate familiarity, rather than the designation of
clinical crisis its designers intended, and would respond in her mind: *Hello.*

One day in a southern Belize hospital, I heard my thirty-four-year-old friend ask the nurse if she could stick her own finger with the lancet so that drawing blood didn't hurt as much. The Accu-Chek said her blood sugar was 218, fairly high; the normal range was then considered to be between 80 and 120 milligrams per deciliter. "Too low," Cresencia said of her measurement, wondering aloud if that was the reason she had vomited after breakfast. "When it gets low, my body isn't used to it; 300 down gives me a lot of problems. I get sick and want to throw up. I can't stop shaking." Her ideal range was between 300 and 400, she said. The sick feeling Cresencia experienced whenever her blood sugar was within "healthy" range was the primary reason she had stopped taking medicines. "When I do the insulin, the insulin makes my body shake, shake, shake. Cold sweat," she said.

Cresencia's account echoed a persistent and disturbing trend: the great majority of the people with diabetes I interviewed in Belize seemed to have a story about how their doctors were shocked by their impossibly sky-high blood sugars. Caregivers repeatedly told them it was very lucky and wholly inexplicable they were not dead, let alone still walking around. "I've seen people with sugar of 800 busy doing laundry, telling me they feel good," one nurse told me. When a Cuban doctor was taking blood sugars at the diabetes clinic in Belize City one morning, we agreed I should write down the numbers as she read them out loud to sixteen otherwise anonymous patients. (The physician said that she considered it a pretty bad morning.) But even in a tiny and arbitrary sample, the set of numbers raised unsettling questions: 62, 93, 114, 180, 197, 201, 280, 396, 400, 530, 553, 665, 670, 682, 699, 718.

What does "normal" sugar even mean here? Only two of the sixteen people registered in the range defined as normal (80–120). Or maybe only one of sixteen, if applying the narrower range of normal (80–110) that was promoted for a short time—a reminder that changing how a threshold is *defined* also alters the biology that is perceived, treated, and materially produced in turn. (One reading, 62, was too low—actually more immediately dangerous than high sugar. Erratic swings in glucose levels over time propitiate both extremes.) The majority of the sixteen people whom the physician tested that morning registered blood sugars over 300 milligrams per deciliter—such high levels that, if chronically sustained, "severe complications are almost certain." But that was the low end of the range in which Cresencia spoke of feeling normal. When Cresencia was given insulin to bring her glucose back to "normal" and down from what the hospital considered dangerous, she began to vomit.

THE NORMAL AND THE EXTRAORDINARY

Diabetes was one of the key examples that physician-philosopher Georges Canguilhem wrote about in *The Normal and the Pathological*. He was fascinated by the many microevents that preceded the first time sugar could be found "pouring over a threshold" in the kidneys, the moment when detectable glucose (always present in human blood) suddenly leaked into urine and became legible as a disorder.[1] He argued that "the pathological cannot be linearly deduced from the normal,"[2] the way graphs tend to depict it. Instead, health was "a margin of tolerance," Canguilhem wrote, "for the inconsistencies of the environment."[3]

Today, "inconsistencies of the environment" are so pervasive that Canguilhem's ideas about the "ex post facto science of the normal" have become important for approaching ecological losses as well as human health, David Bond observes; in fact, he argues, disasters often produce what comes to be imagined as the lost baselines of "normal" environs.[4]

The Belizean reef underwent coral disease and bleaching events in 1995, 1998, 2005, 2010, 2015, and 2016. Surviving patches have already lived past what scientists once estimated as its "thresholds of temperature tolerance,"[5] survivability tested in ways that reminded me of "normal" blood sugar. Yet when "changes in degree become changes in kind," Donna Haraway observes, "all the stories are too big and too small."[6] There were "waxing and waning thresholds of life"[7] being demarcated all around: "epidemic thresholds," like the one the World Health Organization declared that diabetes had crossed; "pain thresholds," debated around when and how diabetic nerve damage should be medicated; "thresholds of exposure," which defined permissible levels of toxic chemicals. Adriana Petryna calls drawing such lines for tractable action "horizoning work": "perceiving critical thresholds, determining baselines, and carving out footholds" as part of a "fine-tuned awareness of jeopardy amid incomplete knowledge, and for labors of continuous recalibration amid physical worlds on edge."[8]

A little at a time, capacities might gradually change beyond what once seemed like hard limits. "Life tries to win against death in all senses of the verb. . . . Life gambles against growing entropy," Canguilhem wrote.[9] Exceeding experts' predictions, at times the intensities of death in life could create powerful modes of alter-survival.[10] When diabetic deaths and injuries were statistically "normal," stabilizing outliers exceeded the pathological—opening instead toward the possibility of

LIMB SALVAGE FORM

Note placement of:
- calluses,
- pre-ulceration areas,
- ulceration areas, or
- areas lacking sensitivity.

NAME:

BP

FS

*Circle or check findings as they apply.

			[] Right [] Left
Hx of amputation?			[] Right [] Left
Hx of ulceration?			
Right:	[] No	[] Yes	Date:
Left:	[] No	[] Yes	Date:
Pt able to see bottom of feet?			[] No [] Yes
Pt wearing properly fitting shoes?			[] No [] Yes

Vascular Findings: (+) Present (-) Absent

FOOT EXAM

[] Foot exam WNL	Dorsalis Pedis Pulse	
[] PAD exam WNL	Post Tibial Pulse	
	Foot Hair	
	Capillary Refill	

(If abnormal, indicate which foot.)

Foot ulcer?	[] No	[] Right	[] Left
Abnormal shape?	[] No	[] Right	[] Left
Charcot foot?	[] No	[] Right	[] Left
Toe deformity?	[] No	[] Right	[] Left
Thick or ingrown toenails?	[] No	[] Right	[] Left
Callus build-up?	[] No	[] Right	[] Left
Edema?	[] No	[] Right	[] Left
Elevated skin temp?	[] No	[] Right	[] Left
Decreased circulation?	[] No	[] Right	[] Left
Loss of sensation?	[] No	[] Right	[] Left
Muscle weakness?	[] No	[] Right	[] Lef

PERIPHERAL ARTERY DISEASE (PAD)

History of claudication?	[] No	[] Yes
Pedal pulses present?	[] No	[] Yes
Notes:		

Footwear

Checklist used by visiting Diabetes Foot Care Group, Dangriga.

transcendence. Some people in Belize explained to me how they lived with their symptoms as miracles.

When a woman named Tila, for example, noticed the two perfect pink circles that opened spontaneously on each foot, she recognized the symmetrical marks. She took fastidious care of the wounds in collaboration with her doctor. But Tila could discern nothing that she had done to "deserve" her diabetic injuries, as she explained, and their strong resemblance to Catholic stigmata helped her to bear the fact that they would not heal.

She said that she knew others in town with similar marks. "Many are chosen."

"I used to take insulin, but I tell them, no more," Cresencia had told me on the first day we met in the town hospital. It was February then, many months before she would first be called Miss Lazarus. "Now they just give insulin to me whenever I am dying." She laughed and adjusted her pink nightgown, sitting on a clinic bed that looked too low for her. A blurry Xerox taped to the wall behind her, labeled "The

Diabetic's Prayer," had caught my eye while I was visiting the hospital. That was when I had approached Cresencia for the first time, explaining my research and asking about the sign. She looked up at the wall with curiosity.

THE DIABETIC'S PRAYER
Our Father in heaven
Thank you for being
Our Teacher, Our Healer
Help us overcome DIABETES
By staying light through
Diet and exercise.
By living right
Through not smoking nor
Drinking
By thinking bright
Through positive thinking

And lead us not into
Temptation but deliver us
From stress
So we could live life to the
Fullest.
In Jesus name we pray,
Amen.

"That's not mine," Cresencia said of the prayer. It was labeled with the names of two collectives that shared materials, the Philippine Diabetes Association and a nongovernmental organization (NGO) in Tobago.

She shrugged. "But we could talk a little."

I joined Cresencia along some of her travels as she sought care in the following year, usually wherever she invited me. In addition to kitchens, temples, and clinics, Cresencia kept collapsing on the roads and on the beach. Some events were attributed to spirit possession and others to coma caused by either low blood sugar or by diabetic ketoacidosis (a state linked to high blood sugar and missing doses of insulin). The similarity of these semiconscious states confused the local Kriol nurse, who had to send for someone who spoke Garifuna to distinguish between trance and diabetes crisis each time Cresencia was carried again to her clinic.

How does expertise get constructed in different ways around death and survival? The crucial thresholds in this story all relate to that question. Caregivers presented these threshold definitions as "natural" facts, using them as tools to navigate uncertain biology. The specific ways they were defined often took on a meaningful life of their own, "healing despite sickness"[11] along the borders between religion and medicine.[12]

One of anthropologist Victor Turner's famous theories described the betwixt-and-between threshold states that he called "liminality," building on the work of Arnold van Gennep. He wrote: "The attributes of liminality or of liminal *personae* ('threshold people') are necessarily ambiguous, since this condition and these persons elude or slip through the network of classifications that normally locate states and positions in cultural space."[13]

Many anthropologists have since reflected on these ideas of *liminality* and *thresholds*—spaces of transformation, open on both ends. For Turner the way out of the liminal state was through ritual. But in situations of chronic conditions, it was not always possible to find a ritual that worked. Getting caught in its betwixt-and-between, neither-nor state can recall what it's like for patients to live with chronic diagnoses, Jean Jackson argues, classified by biomedicine as "ambiguous beings."[14] Yet a "liminal figure—one that haunts the very field of power that excludes her"—at times also sheds light on those fields' definitions in turn, Angela Garcia offers.[15] "Such a liminal position can animate a critically different reflection on medicine and society, a reflection that need not accept things as they are," Arthur Kleinman once reflected.[16] Ieva Jusionyte adds that certain thresholds of states may look like peripheries but in fact act as the core, consolidating political power along their borders.[17]

I once crossed one of Mexico's southern borders with Cresencia and her aunt, which elicited a different kind of threshold making: On her customs form when we crossed the border, Cresencia had written in her nationality not as Belizean (like her passport) but as "Garifuna."

Chetumal's sugarcane industry had come and gone long before our trip that summer. Passing back through the border town between Mexico and Belize once again in 2017, I stood a few blocks from the sea on the wooden porch of a makeshift museum and thought how the last time I was in that town, Cresencia had guided me. The memory seemed so improbable by then that I found myself pulling out my passport later, as if to verify that the black and blue stamps were still there from an overnight trip in August 2010.

From the porch I kept remembering our younger selves stepping off the bus, an old repurposed Kansas Bluebird arriving from Belize City: Cresencia wearing a new yellow T-shirt and carrying a pillow and her Aunt S with high braids—two Garifuna women leading with unhurried steps,

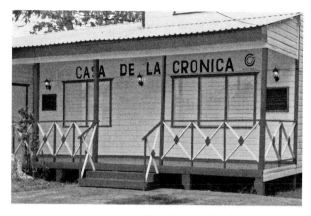

CASA DE LA CRONICA, north of the Mexico-Belize border.

and an eager graduate student smiling awkwardly next to them. I spent most of our lunch anxious about whether it would seem humane or patronizing to pay for our shared meal, then found out they had paid for my *panades* without my knowing. I told them at the time that I felt bad about their generous surprise, but actually I was elated. The gesture cast me as a somewhat welcome burden for the moment, and I was grateful to be included in their routine journey to seek medical care along the border.

Seven years later I looked up at the makeshift museum's hand-painted sign, CASA DE LA CRONICA. The institution began in 1847 as home to the town's *crónista vitalicio,* who was tasked with keeping public health "vital records" of local births and deaths. But what accumulated over time became something more: relics of town histories and family pictures, little artifacts that people wanted to share, trying to leave traces of themselves as humans in between the cracks of health statistics.

At some point I started to think of the accumulating chronicles in this project more in the vein of *crónicas,* slowly told tales of individuals' daily struggles to live with lasting conditions. A language of the threshold, the word came back across the border from Mexico to Belize with us (though most in Belize speak first languages other than Spanish). But the term *crónicas* helped me think about slow-moving storytelling grounded in and guided by the travails of people like Cresencia. In English, this gets separated into two distinct terms and ideas—*chronicle* (a slow-building written account) and *chronic* (a slow-progressing condition). But as retracing Cresencia's long-ago route to Chetumal reminded me, *crónica* already means both story and disease.

ANCESTRAL DISCONTENT

As Cresencia and I stood outside the house in her home village of Sagoun back in 2010, a cluster of women had laughed about how many units of insulin they would need to counterbalance the ritual foods they were each given to eat according to the ancestors' instructions. (No one actually had any insulin; that was what made the joke funny.) I could hear close female family members humming in Garifuna through an open door, their pinkies linked as they stepped in a shuffle. A curtain of articles of clothing separated them from the food, the wire stretching across the room bent low under the weight of domestic items belonging to the dead to whom the ancestral mass was dedicated: floral skirts and folded bedsheets, checkered blouses and dark trousers, a row of brassieres in yellow lace and white nylon.

On the other side of the partition, a table was lined with banana leaves, barely visible under all the dishes. As the women's songs floated across the curtain of clothing, I counted dozens of plates heaped with food: quartered watermelons, halved pineapples, split papaya with black seeds in tiny spheres like frog eggs, bowls of white porridge, *hudut* plantain dumplings steeped in coconut milk, plates of manioc and other pale roots, whole gray fish with open eyes, rice and beans, roasted chicken, huge triangles of brittle cassava bread balanced between plates, a mottled brown cake with crusted syrup glistening in the candlelight. Alongside plates on the floor were glass Coca-Cola and green Lighthouse beer bottles refilled with rum or holy water, all stopped with tufts of cotton.

Since her ancestors had just been summoned to save Cresencia from death the previous week, she was not forgotten in the meal. Cresencia was handed some roasted chicken and a piece of purple yam when the dead instructed that specific bits of food be passed around and eaten by designated people. I saw the leftovers put into a massive silver bucket placed in a wheelbarrow, to be buried in the sand or thrown into the sea. "It's a miracle," people who hadn't seen her yet kept saying as they approached the place where we sat in plastic chairs at the edge of the yard. Because they chose to speak in English instead of Garifuna, I could tell their words were for my benefit too. "People are calling her Miss Lazarus. These doctors sent her home in an ambulance from the hospital to die; now she is walking around with us again."

"ThankGod," Cresencia would smile, saying it like one word. She had lost more than half her body weight: a tattoo on her wrist was now shriveled, its few initials illegible inside the knife-pierced heart. When asked what the letters stood for, she laughed and called me a rude girl.

Her tall frame stooped, Cresencia weighed just eighty-eight pounds then. Against her blue daisy-printed Garifuna dress and kerchief, her tight features had a sharpened kind of beauty. Her hands were graceful, though one finger was missing due to a hitchhiking accident years ago. The infection that developed when she went to get stitches started with a soft spot under the skin but later required the amputation of a finger. Part of the hand below had also been removed, and it almost looked like nothing was missing. Each of her eyes had also been operated on earlier that year, by two separate university teams of visiting U.S. doctors who ran a vision project in Belize City. Both surgeries helped to slow the blurring vision caused by diabetic retinopathy but left pink veins and a thin raised line of scar tissue across the white of one eye, subtle markings of injury and repair.

By the time we left the ancestral mass, there were blue shadows on the sand. The two of us were walking over the beach, headed away from the sound of drumbeats, when Cresencia suddenly collapsed as if struck. "Aye!" she cried out and fell down next to me, the fruit and sesame candy she had been carrying scattered across the sand. Her spindly arms made sharp angles. She looked unconscious as I sank onto the beach next to her. I could feel the blue scarf that Cresencia's cousin had tied around my hair earlier coming undone. Before I could call out for help, women in dresses ran across the beach toward us. They supported Cresencia and walked her back toward the drums, removing her glasses as she swayed and shuffled with short staccato steps. The music did not stop. Some acquaintances circled around me, telling me not to be afraid and gently laughing at my anxious offer to get Nurse Suzanne to come with her glucometer. "There is a spirit in her," Terese explained to me.

In the center of the circle, Cresencia's slumped frame suddenly became animated in the arms of the two women who had supported her weight, and she gestured toward the darkening sky. Later, I would read that this shift in states has a name: a transition from stiff, glassy-eyed *adereha* possession to animated *agoburiha*, a full spiritual possession—in one linguist's rough literal translation, "to become re-ancient." Cresencia spoke with the high, thinning voice of the dead, her face transformed with an old man's puckered lips and squinting eyes. "It's her great-grandfather Artelio," a prominent community and spiritual leader named Igemeri told me. He had been officiating the day's offerings to the ancestors. "Artelio—he's the one who healed her."

That night, it had been four years since Cresencia was first diagnosed with diabetes and eleven days since the doctors in Belize City had given

her up for dead. Two weeks earlier she had arrived at the ER in a diabetic coma, after being transferred from the village clinic to the national
referral hospital in Belize City. There, the doctor told Cresencia's family
that aside from her usual high blood sugar, the tests were all normal.
Even after her blood glucose was stabilized, however, she had not
revived. Several days of crisis passed, hours of waiting parsed in insulin
injections. There was nothing left to be done, the doctor said—he could
offer no further treatment. He recommended releasing her to die at
home. She was still paralyzed on one side of her body, emaciated and
incontinent, drifting in and out of a coma.

"They give me up then. Hours to go," Cresencia would tell me later.
"My aunts were all crying, my whole family." Her relatives could not
accept the doctors' seeming resignation and decided to attempt a rescue
intervention. They chartered an ambulance to take her back home for an
urgent ritual. In retrospect, it's a striking image: the ambulance speeding
away from the nation's top public hospital and the country's leading
specialists, carrying an unconscious woman hours through winding
mountain roads and back to a modest home in a village on the sea.

After her father died with diabetes when Cresencia was nine, her
mother raised her along with six brothers and sisters in a wooden house
on the beach. It was in front of this same house that a group of village
women had gathered to meet her ambulance. Gaunt and too tall for the
stretcher, Cresencia arrived in Pampers. The women cared for her as a
child again, cleaning and changing her. Cresencia began murmuring in
Garifuna when they bathed her with clear rum of the highest proof
(which is often used to initiate commune with the spirits but can also
double as a powerful disinfectant and base ingredient for many topical
medicines made of herbs). This abruptly eased her symptoms when the
insulin and other drugs had not helped, signaling the possibility of a
spiritual cause.

Since Cresencia's parents were gone and most of her siblings lived
elsewhere, it fell mainly to her aunts, cousins, and caring neighbors to
manage the emergency care. The required rites, normally planned in
advance with elaborate protocols and collaborations, were in this case
a makeshift operation—a *chugú* held under a mango tree rather than in
an ancestral temple. It was not officiated by a *buyei;* since the death of
renowned Dangriga *buyei* Sarah Gonguez, there had been no Garifuna
shamans at that level living in Belize. For everyday spiritual matters, the
people of Stann Creek increasingly depended on *óunagülei*, or "mes-
sengers" (who have medium capacities but have not fully completed the

arduous steps of professionalization necessary, in conjunction with inborn abilities, to become a *buyei*). For major events, one could be summoned from Livingston in Guatemala. But in Cresencia's case, her family improvised, placing palm fronds and banana leaves on the sand, and with only two days' preparation, the most crucial elements were in place: a pig sacrificed, certain foods prepared for offering, rum obtained, drummers gathered to guide their dancing.

Unable to move, Cresencia remained in bed during the outdoor dancing of the *mali*. They "knocked drums" for many hours, she said. That was when Artelio, Cresencia's great-grandfather, possessed her for the first time. When he spoke through her in this state of trance, the news was reassuring: she would be fat again, restored to health. Artelio reported that the primary agent of sickness killing Cresencia had been a spell deceptively made to look like diabetes, something put on her. He worked to remove it. "That was one miracle!" Antonia reflected out loud to me later, flapping a green towel over her shoulder to create a small breeze. "Came here dying; now she is okay. She spoke, her grandfather spoke through her and said what the problem is. When it happens you cannot remember what you said, only someone who was there has to tell you later. Have you ever seen the movie with Whoopi?"

At first Cresencia sat up. "Can she walk?" asked an aunt; but the spirit chided, "Take your time! Do not rush. She will walk, but not yet." Later Cresencia stood up, but then sat down again. The next time she stood up and managed a few tentative steps before resting. Her strength returned in uneven waves. By the end of the night, Cresencia was dancing along with everyone else under the mango tree.

"It felt like a snake inside of me," Cresencia later described the bodily sensation of sorcery to me, touching her stomach lightly. She spoke quietly, the word *something* permeating her English for metaphysical terms that were not otherwise translatable. "They put something on me. There is good and there is bad. Sometimes you don't think about the bad part. But sometimes you have to think about that. . . . Sometimes you don't have nothing and still people want to do a lot of stuff, like they are God." She paused. "They are not." Artelio, assisted by two anonymous spirits, had successfully removed the spell that mimicked the symptoms of diabetes, she said. "He took it out," Cresencia explained, "slowly, slowly."

Yet this healing was conditional, and it came at a cost. Cresencia had been living for several years with another woman, Allison. To stay healthy, Artelio instructed, Cresencia would have to move back to the old family house where she had been raised. "The spirits don't want me to live back there anymore with my friend," she told me, her tone a mix of regret and resignation. (Friend was the word she suggested I use in writing, when we strategized about how to describe the spirits' heteronormative conditions for intercession.)

Now that Artelio's spirit had returned once again, I sat in the circle of people surrounding Cresencia on the beach and thought of Allison, alone in her house. Cresencia, wearing a housedress patterned in threadbare flowers, slumped in a plastic chair with a posture not her own. She gestured into the night sky with open palms. Two bare bulbs hung from a yellow extension cord above her head. Behind her, the thatched kitchen glowed, and in front of her, commanding women in formal button-up dresses packed a low wooden bench and laughed at the spirit's slapstick humor. Occasionally, someone would translate for me: "He said that my brother who died in a car accident is here," or "Phil is so jealous of the old lady" (said of a drunk spirit whose wife was on the bench among living men). Some people were summoned to the center of the circle by the spirit to be asked questions, teased, given messages. "This is why we are not afraid," Igemeri said to me. "We can be with our ancestors this way, talk to them."

Probably because I was able to understand only scattered words of the ancestors, as time passed I became restless and apprehensive that Cresencia might go into a coma again after drinking so much beer. Rail-thin and just back from the brink of death, she had suffered renal failure only days ago. "The spirit wants some Johnny Walker," Igemeri explained to me after Cresencia had already drunk several Belikin beers. A bottle of Black Label was obtained from someone's kitchen cabinet and poured into the calabash gourd in her hands. Igemeri reassured me that the ancestors would consume the spirit of the alcohol with no risk to Cresencia's body, but I remained tense until the tremors ending the three-hour spirit possession ceased. The spirit had trouble exiting after the long session; after being splashed with rum and encircled in smoke, Cresencia was taken to the back of the house. When I saw her again ten minutes later, she was serene and sober, stretched out in a hammock. Eating a fish in the darkness, she smiled and asked whether I would be afraid of her now.

While some people were "too strong" to be caught by spirits, Cresencia had been possessed many times even before Artelio first appeared ("sometimes my grandma, sometimes my dad"). Geographically, the house she had shared with Allison was on the farthest edge of the marshy road. Cresencia's recent miraculous healing had drawn her back in multiple senses from "being on a threshold," an ill-defined between, revived and reintegrated into the proverbial whole of *communitas* that an anthropologist would predict. But which community? Whose idea of a whole? Her grandfather's intercession—like biomedicine, and indeed any form of medicine—was extended with values and caveats of its own. If Cresencia's healing involved what Victor Turner once called "the human coefficient"[18] integral to the way ritual processes unfold, then Allison became its remainder.

Before Cresencia moved, I used to visit at the place they shared, which she referred to as "on the other side." The unpainted wooden steps leading up to the door were lined with potted aloe plants and sprigs of herbs sprouting from coffee cans. Allison wore her hair in loose braids pulled back in the heat. She worked steadily at a local resort, and with the house's full kitchen, Cresencia could eat well there, often making soups of meats and vegetables. They watched TV in a back room and played loud *paranda* on the stereo—ballads so upbeat that it took me a while to realize they are almost all about death. I was frankly intimidated by Allison's imposing figure and wry countenance, and except for pleasantries I can only remember really speaking to her once, when I got up the nerve to ask about the cloves of oyster-white garlic with sprouted roots that were tucked around the room and clustered on a ledge above the inside of the doorway (another threshold). But Allison just laughed, with a gentleness that surprised me. "To keep out the bad spirits," she said.

CORAL GARDENS AND THEIR METABOLISM

Conquistadors landing in the Caribbean used to note that the white sand beaches looked like sugar. But the sand they likened to sugar turned out to be dead coral, most grains having passed through the digestive system of a parrotfish. It was part of the fishes' metabolism.[19]

In *Coral Gardens and Their Magic*—Bronislaw Malinowski's colonial account of agricultural practices as related to gardening techniques, ancestral meals, land fertility, and uses of coral from the nearby reef—Malinowski had a strained reaction when he observed people in the Trobriand Islands feeding their ancestors by burying food in the earth. He wrote, with more than a hint of judgment, "The Trobriander's misapprehension of the fundamentals of human procreation is here matched by his misunderstanding of the processes of nutrition and metabolism."[20] Of course, this interpretation reveals most of all Malinowski's own assumptions about what the processes of nutrition and metabolism entail, informed by the sciences of his era: a single human body, processing intentionally eaten food.

Where does any one body's eating begin or end? I kept thinking about the sand and waves filled with bits of plastics, blended with the offerings buried to feed Cresencia's ancestors. It takes decades for food containers to photo-degrade into the tiny bright slivers found on the beach and in the waves. Little pieces of garbage get eaten by fish, moving up the food chain. The ancestral offerings represented a restorative force, a means of summoning spirits to rebuild; but the plastic remainders inside animals and in the land and water where the food was buried were a more enigmatic kind of "co-presence."[21] I wondered, was this also feeding the land and the dead? What about the living?

In this view, not only do human bodies metabolize their ecologies—but our environments in turn metabolize both humans and the long-lasting traces of people's activities. A focus on this kind of "absorption," Harris Solomon writes in *Metabolic Living*, "can open up key questions in the context of chronic diseases related to food: Who and what become the eater and the eaten? What is nutrition and what is poison? Who and what set the boundaries of inside and outside, delineating organism and environment?"[22]

By the time I knew Cresencia in 2010, more and more hunks of coral were washing up on the beaches of Belize undigested by parrotfish. About half the reef had died, and the coral skeletons that I saw took many forms: white spine-shaped columns, airy hunks of calcified sponge, and brittle broken fans. According to scientists, the Mesoamerican Reef—like most coral today—is also showing signs of metabolic disorders. It has trouble with its own food supply: the algae-like zooxanthellae that coral polyps harvest for carbohydrates, "much as farmers harvest corn,"[23] struggle to survive in warming oceans. High temperatures "cause the metabolism of the algae—which give coral reefs their brilliant colors and energy—to speed out of control, and they start creating toxins. The polyps recoil. . . . When heat stress continues, they starve to death."[24]

This loss of sustenance is the primary cause of coral bleaching, reef death, and the displacement of resident fish and other aquatic species. Other processes further compound the impacts of climate change on sea life: sea levels are rising, the oceans are becoming more acidic, and unchecked mining and foreign building projects are accelerating coastal erosion in parts of Belize. Some residents describe these shoreline erosions in terms of consumption, too: "The sea is eating the shore."

Certain old myths used to say the bubbled seaweed that people call Sargasso never died, but most locals recall it has always appeared along the coast in Belize at certain times of year. But after 2010, thick, pungent tides of dead Sargasso carried by the Gulf Stream began washing up along Belizean shorelines. While raking the decaying yellow and brown weeds, people I knew debated if the die-off possibly had something to do with the BP oil spill. Or maybe the carcinogenic plasticizers used to hide the oil. Or the underwater heat waves killing off life of all kinds. Over time, though, the toxic superblooms in Belize keep getting worse. By 2019, anthropologist Siobhan McCollum describes how miles of Sargasso was washing up on the beach in a matter of hours with an overpowering stench. Some in Belize attributed part of the issue to industrial fertilizer runoff from agricultural plantations as far away as Brazil.[25]

Phosphorus and nitrogen have been historically reaped from poor regions and brought to wealthy empires to replenish fallow agricultural fields and plantations with depleted soil. By the mid-1800s, England and the United States, in particular, were vying for control of guano islands in South America (especially Peru), across the Caribbean, and around the world. Influenced by the sciences of metabolism of his era, Karl Marx wrote that this movement of life-supporting soil nutrients from poor places to wealthy ones—what Marx called metabolic "rift"—interacted with human politics and the ecological displacements of capitalism, as it "disturbs the metabolic interaction between man and the earth."[26]

Although phosphorous and nitrogen are now industrially produced and chemically manipulated as well as mined raw, the afterlives of their nutrient cycles have cascading implications for metabolism across scales. The putrid-smelling algae blooms they fuel often kill off other sea life, including overstressed coral that in turn fossilizes some of the excess phosphorous in the calcifications of its polyps. Dead coral is thus sometimes also mined for industrial phosphorus, which in turn gets sold as fertilizer to add nutrients to keep plantation soil viable.

Belize is relatively unpolluted compared to most places on the earth today. The country has one of the smallest carbon footprints in the world.[27] To me, this beauty made observing its harmed ecologies all the more unsettling: even there, it was also happening. In a place that evoked what postcards try to capture, traces of mutation felt both invisible and hyperreal. Certain lagoons still held moon jellyfish and algae that glowed blue when disturbed, but the gnarled roots of many mangrove trees caged disturbing quantities of plastic debris. The distant sea looked a pristine azure blue on clear days, and manatees with brown

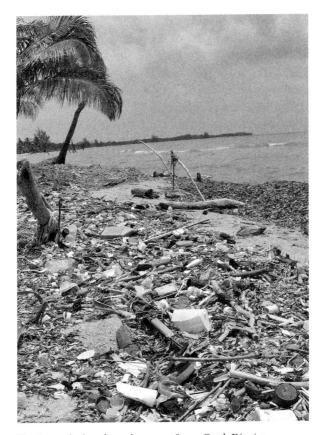

Plastics washed up from the ocean, Stann Creek District.

noses sometimes swam up to the docks. Other times what I mistook for a first sign of a sea animal on the horizon ended up being garbage. The most visually prominent of this tidal trash were plastic bags, floating in the waves like listless jellyfish, and Styrofoam, known in Belizean Kriol as *sea bread*—as if even the earth was being fed a sick diet.

According to the U.S. Environmental Protection Agency, each "floating city" of approximately three thousand cruise ship passengers discharges an average of 210,000 gallons of sewage and one million gallons of gray water into the oceans each week. This includes toxins and oil, discarded and expired chemicals, batteries, fluorescent lights, explosives, paint thinners, and solid waste such as plastic bottles and food containers.[28] Toxicologists note that plastic leaks bisphenol A and other endocrine-disrupting chemicals into the environment. What Sarah Vogel has called the "politics of plastics" is part of how people and chemical environs become literal parts of each other's biologies, disturbingly embroiled in human capacities for plasticity and change.[29]

Seeing dead fish floating in the water, I wondered: what counted as an environmental "sentinel," in the past or now? In 2010, a sea turtle washed up in southern Belize with crude petroleum in its mouth. One nurse told me that when she was growing up, some days they used to hear the sounds of dynamite in the distance, as foreign entrepreneurs hunted for oil underwater along the Belizean reef. In the aftermath of the explosions, a tide with dead tropical fish and paralyzed stingrays would be swept onto the sand. Belize has worked to curb the worst of these practices, but ambient exposures from other times and places linger.

An older man named Edwin once showed me his favorite trees in Sagoun. He talked about global warming a lot but mostly about the little ways he saw climate change making its way into daily life. It was ruining the best mangos, the rare blue kind that grew behind his sister's house. And the price of fish was rising steeply, almost doubled. It made him worry about the ocean. Edwin was born in a fishing village during the "times of abundance," back "in Lucy days" when a trawler named *Lucy* used to ply the Belizean coast buying up whatever fish were caught.

But now that fish and shellfish were starting to get scarce, he had more trouble buying what used to be an everyday food. This was changing the kinds of protein people could afford to eat, especially poorer people.[30] Some people thought the fish scarcity had to do with the rise of shrimp farms and their antibiotic-laden wastewater that was killing local sea life, while shrimp are primarily exported to enrich diets abroad. Edwin hoped the shortage could be attributed instead to climate change's contribution to new patterns of weather: he said his fishing friends noted an increase in winds from the southeast that drove the fish into deeper ocean or to coasts elsewhere. That was the most optimistic scenario. Competing theories held that they had simply died.

Even for an outsider like me, it was disturbing to observe grilled fish becoming more scarce on kitchen tables and in local shops because of rising prices. In some places it was easier to find the "fish" sold in spray bottles—FISH being the common generic name in Belize for chemicals that kill biting insects by design, but also kill aquatic life as a side effect.[31] Seeing them lined up on supermarket shelves made me picture a dystopian future zoo of aerosol animals, with a room of cans holding samples of whatever toxic mix helped to kill off the creature on its label.

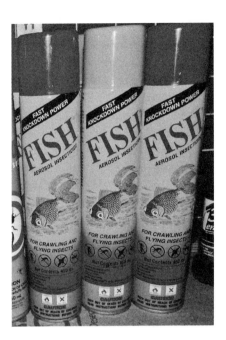

Last FISH at the grocery
store, 2010.

Whenever we went grocery shopping together, one friend and I made
jokes that took on hints of compulsive ritual, as if to remind each other
what was missing. We were probably just projecting much deeper anxieties onto those fairly trivial canisters, supercharged by the fact that most
of the chemicals on the loose around us were not labeled at all. But everyone was still breathing, drinking, and eating them. One local study about
the effects of DDT compared thinning eggshells and reproductive implications of the chemical for various groups of crocodiles in Belize. But the
research team could not find a "control group" of unexposed animals for
comparison; many of the contaminated crocodiles were sex shifting from
males into anatomical females, likely due to the organic pesticides in their
waterways.[32] The same hormonal pathways that trigger such changes in
aquatic animals have been linked to diabetes as well as breast and prostate
cancer in humans,[33] but the effects for people were not being measured in
this context. Many biologists and researchers from wealthy institutions
abroad came to study wildlife ecologies in Belize, but very few scrutinized
what the ambient chemicals harming crocodiles and jaguars might also
mean for the health of human residents.[34]

Issues like this are part of the reason why some observers today argue
that diabetes should be considered as an issue of not only "global health"

but also "planetary health."[35] This concept has grown in popularity so quickly that it now has its own journal of *The Lancet*. (For some, the language of "planetary" is uneasy too—the optics through which we know this scale were largely born of the visual technologies of nuclear war, Joseph Masco observes; and the rallying call toward shared causes and effects can gloss over how unevenly collective risks are distributed, many add).[36] Yet the debate did lead me to reflect on how *global* is also a paradoxical word. It is supposed to mean a thing in its entirety—yet by definition, a globe is modeled as hollow inside, a static shell. In contrast, *planet* models something *animate*, in the sense Kath Weston describes[37]—emphasizing the earth as a living character, not an inert stage for human politics.

These are key dimensions of health that certain earlier generations of social thinkers were often not forced to reckon with. "Well, if there has been so much change, it is not the climate that has changed," Michel Foucault once wrote, commenting on a description of weather in Virgil, "the political and economic interventions of government have altered the course of things."[38] In this framing, nature was assumed to be a receiving template for governance. But the realities that this overlooked even in Virgil's time (and certainly in Foucault's) are becoming more difficult to bracket. A living piece of earth is many things besides an inert territory; unruly oceans and atmospheres may not respond at all to the strategic designs of local sovereigns within the state in question or on a human timescale.

Yet what is a human timescale? In one of the most startling passages of *In the Wake,* Christina Sharpe evokes a rarely noted material dimension of transatlantic histories: "the atoms of the people who were thrown overboard are out there in the ocean even today. They were eaten, organisms processed them, and those organisms were in turn eaten and processed, and the cycle continues." Sharpe describes how such cycles are linked to *residence time*: "The amount of time it takes for a substance to enter the ocean and then leave the ocean is called residence time. Human blood is salty, and sodium . . . has a residence time of 260 million years."[39] Cresencia's ancestors' 1797 trip to Central America suddenly sounded closer on this timescale—only a quarter of their group (2,026 people) was still alive by the time they reached Honduras, the others buried either on Balliceaux or at sea. It made me recall watching the *chugú*'s food-filled canoes move through the waves, traveling toward deep ocean to feed the ancestors.

Yet maybe cross-reading metabolic connections with Cresencia's practices of caring for the dead was part of my own attempt to understand her survival. For her part, she did not need scientific measurements or theories of metabolism to think of her ancestors as present or to know that the past continued to exert a material force. Perhaps the very opposite: the spirits' most persuasive evidence, for her, began when they offered her means for continuing to live beyond the point when science ran out. Cresencia had learned how aspects of high sugar might be harnessed as transcendence. She continued having intimate encounters with the dead there, including many who had already died of diabetes. When family spirits were offered the rich foods they loved most, sometimes they revealed to her what to do next.

SUGAR GIRLS

Although she had grown up there, Cresencia did not settle easily back into her childhood home. She had no stove or way to prepare her own full meals, which made cooking anything a daunting prospect, let alone preparing any diabetes-healthy foods. She did have a fan and an electric plug-in kettle for heating water to make heavily sugared coffee and tea. Because the house had no electricity or plumbing, she ran a long, thin extension cord from her Aunt Dee's nearby house to power these small appliances. She spent most of her afternoons on the steps of Dee's porch, where she could catch a better breeze from the sea.

Whenever I approached Dee's house for a visit, chickens scattered between the abandoned ovens on the beach. You could almost tell how long a household in Belize had been supported by someone working in the States by counting the abandoned appliances surrounding it. Like the falloff point in carbon dating, the oldest artifacts proved the most accurate; a sixties-style oven was nearly guaranteed to have been sponsored from New York, but a Toshiba TV from the past five years yielded almost no reliable information, as these were now omnipresent in Belize, within the possible budget of someone with a resort job. The majority of the village's abandoned large appliances were four-burner ovens, which a few women used as well-insulated storage cabinets. Along the dirt road or in yards, one occasionally also saw sinks, refrigerators, and washing machines. I never knew whether people kept them out of nostalgia for the family members whose love they represented or simply because it would have been expensive to haul them away. Tourists often complained about these being eyesores, but at times I found their incongruous outdoor presence familial. The appliances cumulatively gave the ocean scenery a domesticated and cozily furnished air, as if the entire expanse of beach was the overgrown floor of an open-air kitchen.[40]

Cresencia and Dee took care of each other in the limited ways that a dying young woman and a spry old lady can, sharing not material help but small, loose gestures of grace. When Cresencia had been bedridden, Dee had made her coffee the way she liked it, thick with sweetened condensed milk; and when Dee spent two days vomiting in a pigtail bucket, Cresencia moved her pillow to the steps and quietly kept her company by the sea. Years ago, Cresencia had won several hundred dollars in the local lottery, and Dee recalled how her niece had a little of her windfall already waiting to share when they saw each other on the bus. "Cresie" (as Dee more often called her niece) made the generosity feel light by making a funny honking sound like *haauh* as she pressed the bills into Dee's hand, and they both dissolved into laughter. Back when Cresencia could work, she often bought little surprises for Dee, like a packet of clothespins. Despite their age difference, they shared many of the same hardships: each had diabetes; neither had any children or financial support from immediate kin; and both now found themselves unable to work, getting by on a trickle of income and the generosity of friends, extended family, and neighbors. They were both afraid of losing their legs and tended any wounds carefully to prevent infection.

Yet despite this painstaking work, Dee had been tending a gash on her leg for months that refused to heal. Some days the pain in her legs was almost unbearable, she said, and applied lime juice for the pain. Years ago Dee had been at her sister's side in the hospital on the day both her legs were amputated. This surgery, made necessary by diabetic necrosis, left a sobering impression on Dee. She recounted how relieved she had been when the doctor told her that she did not have diabetes then. But the next time her blood sugar was checked ten years later in Guatemala, it was sky-high, over 400; Dee was indignant. "This disease is for the animals. It is not for us Christians. So how did we get this?" Among the roaming chickens on her beach property was also a neighbor's one-footed rooster. It always left strange tracks around her house, one row of bird footprints and one row of little holes in the sand.

Although Cresencia was close with several of her cousins and aunts, including Dee, this was not the same as having the support of an immediate family member, especially a mother or one's own children. Being bereft of parents and immediate family has a specific name in Garifuna, *méteñu*. When such intimate family members die, it is considered a loss from one's own physical being and said that they die *from you*.[41]

Cresencia, already in *méteñu* by the age of twenty, had been pregnant twice when she was younger, but both times ended in miscarriage.
Particularly in a context where blood sugar tends to be hardest to control, it can be extremely difficult and at times even dangerous for a
woman with diabetes to have a baby. In Cresencia's case, it had not
proved possible. Cresencia had never found out for sure whether she
had type 1 or type 2 diabetes, as different diagnoses came from different
doctors, but pregnancy without comprehensive treatment is challenging
with either. The difficulty of giving birth with type 1 is so significant that
the disease was long considered a "contraindication" for pregnancy.
After insulin was discovered in 1921 and diabetes "was progressively
transmuted into a chronic condition . . . the once-dreaded combination
of pregnancy complicated by diabetes has become a clinical commonplace, requiring skill and tenacity but no longer an outright miracle to
end with a healthy mother and child."[42]

Historian-physician Chris Feudtner explores this figure in *Bittersweet*,
including both the new promise and the frustration for "insulin mothers," who in previous generations were usually either dead before adulthood or unable to get pregnant because of diabetes. One of the major
characters in his account of Boston's Joslin Diabetes Center was Priscilla
White, who worked closely with these mothers. She noted that even with
careful insulin adherence, there were many things that could go wrong:
"Stillbirths and macerated fetuses of the giant type are nearly as characteristic of diabetic pregnancies which are allowed to come to full term
today as they were in the pre-insulin era. Potentially child-bearing diabetic women . . . are concerned with the following problems: their chances
for (a) conception, (b) surviving pregnancy, (c) for reproducing living
children, and (d) for transmitting their tendency to develop diabetes."[43]

This sobering list had much in common with the reality that Cresencia faced. A recent study comparing pregnancy loss, maternal death,
and birth defects for both type 1 and type 2 concluded that despite
mothers' much lower blood sugars with type 2, "in terms of pregnancy
outcome, the seriousness of their condition is similar if not worse,"
although the "pathophysiology underlying the higher perinatal mortality in women with type 2" remains unknown.[44]

For many women in poverty, this represents a particularly devastating aspect of diabetic sugar: for some, a new generation literally cannot
be born. After the loss of her second pregnancy, Cresencia was left neither a mother nor a child of the living, roles that centrally define the
ways Garifuna women have secured community respect across many

chapters of their history.[45] One word for children literally means "those who will carry on."

I first mistook the little spray-painted numbers on the property Cresencia shared with Dee (and other numbers on older houses) to be informal addresses. But they turned out to be digits of disease control programs that had previously passed through, marking each of the houses that were sprayed with a rotating arsenal of insecticides such as DDT. Long after it was banned from the United States in 1972, DDT continued to be used in many Central American countries such as Belize, including for global health interventions related to malaria control.[46] Even many years after spraying, DDT's chemical residues continued to be found in nearly all sampled blood, breast milk, air, and 70–100 percent of soil samples in southern Belize—concentrated especially in sediment, raising concerns for those who eat shellfish.[47]

If not for the crossed-out numbers still visible on the planks that Dee had not yet saved up to repaint, I wouldn't have known an old campaign had passed through. The toxic powder that homes were once sprayed with has been statistically linked to elevated risk for many of the experiences and conditions that Cresencia went through—developing diabetes, lost pregnancies, and later reproductive cancer. What Michelle Murphy calls "distributed reproduction" across scales is linked to long periods of invisibility and latency, integral to how "chemical violence" can subtly linger in bodies over time. The DDT coating Cresencia's childhood house was only the most clearly marked. "Or it could be the effect of continuous, multiple, accumulated, multigenerational exposures crossing a threshold," Murphy writes. There was no way to know for sure whether Cresencia's losses were part of how the "chemical past thus manifests in the present through an absence: lives not born."[48]

No answers, just memory. Sometimes Dee and Cresencia would exchange gentle jokes about the two she had lost. Two boys, she said. When Cresencia would go out at night, her playful way of taking her exit sometimes included asking Dee to watch them while she was gone.

Tracing one of Cresencia's favorite routes, I usually walked along the sea to get a little breeze through the heat on the way to Antonia's house. Nurse Lee told me that many people in the village used to work for the citrus companies, loading boxes of tinned oranges onto giant cargo ships bound for Liverpool. Whenever the tins of citrus fruit later washed up on the beach in the village, people would gather the providential groceries from the tide's flotsam and jetsam.

Years ago, before she got diabetes and went blind, Antonia worked in the "section plant" of a factory where citrus fruits were dug out of their skins and canned. She was very tall, over six feet, with a boisterous laugh and a rowdy sense of humor. There was usually a towel folded in a neat rectangle on the top of her head or draped over her shoulder, to swat against the flies or heat. Antonia was generous with everything. "That is the way we live with each other, in love," she said. "The poor ones live on lone grace." She continuously fed me whenever I visited: gibnut meat, rice and beans, cassava bread, tortillas and creole buns, "milky ways" (my favorite, a kind of local popsicle made in a plastic bag). From her I learned a whole taxonomy of mangos—Lady Slipper, Hairy Mango, Number Eleven, Judge Wade (tiny green mangos that resemble overgrown lima beans)—circulating in an intimate economy of their own. I usually found Antonia in the same chair of her comfortable home, which had sparkling white tiled floors and caught the sea breeze through its open doors. But she also remembered when the houses were made of palmetto and cabbage bark. "There is a history there too. I was born on the ground."

Antonia shared her stock of diabetic pharmaceuticals when necessary with Dee and, occasionally, Cresencia. They looked after each other. Once, when they all converged at Antonia's to have their sugars taken, she burst out laughing. "The Sugar Girls," she said.

Antonia never had her own children, but she helped to raise six or seven. "It's a sin not to raise any children," she said. Most of them now lived in U.S. cities (although one had been in the U.S. Army, fighting in the Iraq War as part of her path to U.S. citizenship). Antonia was very proud of them, and most kept in close touch with her. The first failed surgery for her eyes had been in Guatemala, while the second operation took place in Chicago. When they make *hudut* in Chicago, Antonia said, Garinagu women there beat their plantains in a bucket with wooden baseball bats because it is impossible to buy a real *mata*. She enjoyed the United States, but it was a tough year. The man whom Antonia loved, "my gentleman," died suddenly soon after she returned home from Chicago, the same year she had lost her mother. "Now it is just memories that is left behind," she said. "Only that."

When I first met Antonia, I initially assumed that her blindness must be related to diabetic retinopathy (linked to microvascular wear on the eye's fragile capillaries that can cause blurred vision and blindness). But it wasn't until we were talking one day about her futile surgery in Guatemala that she went further back in time to explain the events leading up to the operation. "I used to have some pretty eyes, pretty brown eyes. See?" She pointed toward her unclouded eye. "But they condemn it."

Antonia explained that the second operation to try to save her eyes took place at the University of Chicago. "The doctor said the surgery is very good, because they find 90 percent vision. And where the 90 percent vision gone? Because it's evil . . . the vision just go back, like that." She had soon become blind in both eyes again. Antonia described having received a letter from Nigeria with evil things in it. When she opened the letter and read it, her eyes were condemned by the evilness inside, she repeated. She had learned about the source of her illness through vivid dreams in which her ancestors spoke to her, indicating the responsible parties. Antonia stared toward the open door. "I should have been looking for a bush doctor. But I didn't know . . . I was not supposed to go and operate my eyes, I supposed to go look for a bush doctor so that they can cure me." But Antonia had sought biomedical care first, instead of looking for metaphysical intervention; that was why the hospital's treatment had been futile, she explained.

Now, "it's too late," she continued. "But I believe in the good Lord so much. Move to move, I pray to he. I think if I could see, then all this I wouldn't *see*. You understand me? *I see all of this*. But I don't think about it that hard, though. . . . I just talk about it sometimes, not all the time," she said lightly. "Us humans, you know, we have to talk. *Because we know what's wrong with us*. But afterwards, I don't worry about it. Because I am not alone. I am not alone, Amy. Every day I see something different. Every day, every day, every day."

She described the images surrounding her as we spoke:[49] the room was crowded with children—so many that she could not see the door. "We call them the guardian angels," she said. Dressed in baby blue or pink, some of them were holding flowers. She spoke of other images she had seen: saints in heavy wool robes, "pretty shine rods." At times there were only colors, a calming sea of blue or "white white, like new snow." Some days she saw the children get into a beautiful bus and travel away into a river. Boats of food also floated down the river, never getting wet. Once, she had dropped a tissue in the bathroom, and she saw Saint Anthony illuminating it for her as she reached down in the dark. When she wanted me to publish her full name in my book (though I haven't for other reasons), it was not what she called her "damaged eyes" she had in mind but the powers they enabled. "The lady with the miracle."

Antonia's words reminded me of Jorge Luis Borges's account of going blind as an adult. He continued to see certain things and described being

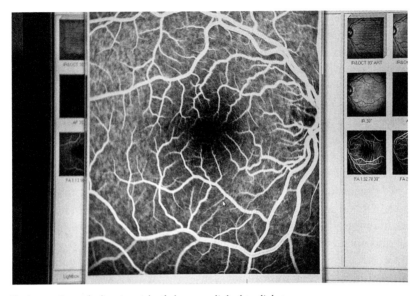

Retina angiograph showing risk of glaucoma linked to diabetes.

unable to sleep at night because of the intense colors surrounding him, in his case usually a bluish mist. "The world of the blind is not the night that people imagine," he reported; actually, Borges could no longer see the color black at all. He became fascinated by the work of other blind artists: Homer, Milton, and James Joyce (for whom he titled a poem on blindness, opening with the line: "Between dawn and dark lies the history of the world"). He ultimately came to call his condition "a style of living." "Blindness is a confinement, but also a liberation, a solitude propitious to invention, a key and an algebra," Borges wrote. "I have lost the visible world, but now I am going to recover another."[50]

LAND TENURE (IS THIS LEGAL?)

Anthropologists have studied many complex aspects of Garifuna land tenure: uxorilocal residence, patronymic nomenclature, matrifocality, consanguinity. But from what I could understand, diabetes was actually also playing a big role in land tenure. Many in villages who migrated to the United States made a living by doing homecare for elderly white Americans, then retired back to Belize without receiving that same luxury. "Who will care for us?" one woman joked—a painful joke because she had worked for decades as a hospice aid and could not afford one herself. "You know," one resident told me once of Sagoun, "a lot of people have to sell their house to pay the medical bills. Ninety percent of them with diabetes. Somebody gets his foot cut, can't do anything for himself, needs the money. People make that part of the deal [with the person who buys a property]: 'Just let me live here until I die.'"

Over the decades, the disturbing pattern accumulated. Many properties that Garifuna families would have much preferred to pass on to the next generation were being sold to pay for chronic medical expenses in general, and diabetes complications in particular. And most of the people buying these lots of land were not Garifuna.[51] Diagonally across one PROPERTIES FOR SALE board, someone wrote in graffiti that could not quite be erased:

!!IS THIS LEGAL?

These processes are part of what scholars have termed "the gentrification of Belize," reporting that approximately 80 percent of all the coastal land in the entire country has been purchased by foreigners for the development of resorts, condos, or vacation homes. "Rapid and uncontrollable development for residential and commercial purposes is an escalating threat to Belize's coastal zone," Belizean environmental scientist Colin Young has noted.[52] Over time, foreigners and entrepreneurs hoping for "beachfront property" removed many intertidal mangrove thickets and littoral forests at the edge of the Caribbean.[53] Although technically illegal, the practice was widely practiced over decades. The earth and soil that mangrove roots once buffered continues to wash into the sea during storms.[54] This afflicted landscape interacted with other bodily erosions. They shared chronic plots, as Veena Das writes, "both in the sense of a narrative plot and a plot (as in a plot of land) on which a story might grow."[55]

The road leading into Sagoun was surrounded by tracts of farmland in various stages of disuse. One could usually distinguish the active agricultural plots by certain signs: a machete resting under a tarp that someone had draped between trees to create shade or the refurbished scarecrow wearing a Cal Tech hoodie. The scattered farming still ongoing was performed mostly by older people, less a source of sustenance than a labor of love; no one I knew considered their own farms a commercial enterprise. Tending plots was squeezed in around financially viable pursuits. A once diverse array of crops had now narrowed to starches, especially cassava, crucial for making the wafer-thin *ereba* bread required for any ancestral ritual. Some suggest that patients with diabetes should eat certain preparations of cassava, as a lower-glucose and higher-vitamin alternative to white rice or bleached wheat products like bread. But the ancient staple had become something of a people's delicacy, taking a bit of extra work to acquire in a continuous supply and labor-intensive to make because cassava contains trace amounts of cyanide that must be removed during a lengthy process of grating, sifting, and draining through serpentine basketry before baking.

Whole swathes of the land along the road were now marked by uncultivated farms, the orange soil of waiting family plots tangled with dry weeds. Passing vehicles kicked up clouds of dust from the gravelly earth and damaged asphalt, powder crusting the low plants and palmetto trees with a coppery film that could sometimes completely obscure any traces of green. Until a heavy rain rinsed this away again, the dust-coated vegetation gave the vague impression of an elaborately wrought antique or an old sepia photograph of living farmland.

Given these tensions, and how much community land was being lost to outsiders, I thought that local residents were surprisingly kind—or at least adhering patiently "to the terms of an ancient truce between inhabitants of heavily touristed places and the people who pay to visit them,"[56] as Sharifa Rhodes-Pitts writes of gentrification elsewhere. Describing other ways things might have been, Rhodes-Pitts adds: "But this is the evidence of an unnatural history—it was not always this way, it came to be that way for a reason."[57] Trying to denaturalize how this diabetes-producing landscape came to be, and for what reasons, I read more about the history of land in the region as part of trying to grasp these changes.

While most of Belize has long been known for its dependence on imported foods, Garinagu had been prolific farmers on Saint Vincent and continued this lifeway upon their arrival in Belize.[58] In 1835, it was reported that the "Caribs" of southern Belize (as the colonial authorities of the time referred to Garifuna people) were "carrying on a constant traffic by sea with Belize [City], in plantains, maize, poultry, etc."[59] Observing coastal Garifuna communities across borders in the 1840s, Ephraim Squier reported that "all along the coast, generally near the mouths of various rivers, they have their establishments or towns . . . well supplied with provisions, especially vegetables, which are cultivated with great care."[60] In Belize, the Laws of Force Act in 1856 was put in place to economically integrate and control this threatening population, which remained "largely independent, self-sufficient, and unincorporated into the colonial structure." This act legally "provided unequivocal recognition of the validity of location titles, [and] the Caribs' provision grounds were not included."[61] White settlers from the United States and Europe were given "retroactive legitimacy" to the lands that the Garinagu in Belize had been farming for fifty years.

The Crown surveyor at the time reported hoping "that we will by this measure attract near Belize a valuable body of labourers." Historian Nigel Bolland reads this as a move "to convert the Caribs from a largely self-sufficient peasantry into a labor supply" for mahogany extraction and "to work on the developing sugar estates in the south of the colony."[62] When Confederate refugees from the United States arrived in waves throughout the 1860s and 1870s, an additional special discount on land was given for people "of Anglo Saxon origin" to try to create an incentive for white settlers to choose Belize over Honduras or Guatemala. In this era, the "nonwhite population—Maya, Caribs, and Africans—who had pioneered agriculture in the colony . . . were either denied titles to land altogether or had to pay twenty-five times as much for Crown land as the white immigrants."[63] Meanwhile, in southern parts of Belize, Wilk notes, "Garifuna (like the Mopan and Kekchi) were given 'reservations' of land. . . . Over time it also justified a 'hands off' policy. Hardly *benign* neglect, this meant that through the twentieth century these communities were denied basic services including medical care, roads, education, water, and sanitation."[64]

For a period of time when men began taking wage labor jobs and increasingly living away, Garifuna women of the area continued farming plantains, cassava, and rice.[65] By 1983, Joseph Palacio observed that, in addition to fish, bleached white flour and rice (part of a growing reliance on unhealthy white starches purchased by the pound) were the most important staples in the Garifuna village.[66] Anthropologist Nancie Gonzalez also noted the decline of herb and vegetable "kitchen gardens" that used to be "ubiquitous" during her work in the Garifuna town of Livingston, Guatemala, in 1965. She described how "biscuits, tortillas, and pancakes with baking powder or soda, as well as coconut bread made with refined white flour and yeast, are considered 'typical' Garifuna foods and figure prominently in everyday meals. Informants believe their own people have always made them."[67]

Now that many people in Sagoun have hourly jobs (in town or at one of the numerous local resorts), reliance on imported food continues to grow. Tourism has become an important new way of earning money for many families in villages. Yet as Louisiana native Natasha Trethewey remarks of another Caribbean coastline: "Opportunities followed growth, but so did environmental havoc."[68] In the words of the Belize National Garifuna Council:

> The people are frustrated by the great difficulty they experience in securing tenure for land. In addition there has been a lack of support for agricultural and economic development efforts. As a result the ties to the land are weakened as people are forced to migrate in search of alternatives. Far from accepting some responsibility for the situation, the powers that be see this as justification for depriving people of their land. . . . virtually all the lands immediately around [some] villages have been alienated and not necessarily by the people themselves.
>
> Absolutely no allowance has been made for village expansion let alone development by the villagers themselves. The lands are nearly all in the hands of outsiders who are attracted by the tourist potential of those areas with the result that our lands are being sold abroad on the internet. Because the foreign concept of land ownership differs from ours, our traditional access to these lands is blocked as "no entry" and other signs are posted for our attention. Apart from the fact that outsiders have an easier time in securing recognized ownership of our lands, not much regard is given to the environmental and social impact that their development schemes may have on the residents.[69]

Many local people valued employment in tourism, but the growing presence of foreign expats and retirees also generated ambivalence. Unsurprisingly, along the stretches of Caribbean beach where white foreigners built multimillion-dollar mansions within sight of local shacks, inequalities bred crime. Resort vans drove toward hotels advertised as "paradise," but on a nearby wall someone had graffitied the words GHETTO LIFE. At one village bar where the majority of the clientele tended to be North American and European expats, the hit folk song "Just Another Gringo in Belize" always aroused impromptu sing-alongs.

It was interesting to see how this Spanish word circulated in an English-speaking place, because in this particular region I never heard the word *gringo* used by anyone who *wasn't* an expat. In Mopan Maya the color white is *sak*, anciently associated with the cardinal direction of the global north. In Yucatec Maya, another word for white people is *satay*, which is related to a pre-Columbian Maya root word dating back to the ancient hieroglyphics that meant "loss or destruction." It can be used to describe not only foreigners, but any living thing that is expected to die out after a single generation.

In Belizean Kriol, white people can be called *bukra* or *bakra* from the Efik and Ibo root word *mbakara*, which linguists believe comes from Abon death cults, gradually evolving to mean "divide and conquer" in general and "white [plantation] master" or "slave hunter" specifically. Interestingly for studies of race and nation, a Garifuna term for "white person" actually *is* nation—*násiun*, from the Spanish *nación*.[70] When Belizeans compliment the lightness of very pale skin, they usually refer to its color not as white but "clear," which I found doubly unnerving, as if the person could see straight through you. But *gringo* ranked low on the list of disquieting words for white foreigners that existed across Belize's many languages. Expats who referred to themselves this way frequently seemed to treat the term with a wink, a joke they were in on—but (at least in the particular places I worked) it was used almost exclusively by white people in self-reference, an affectionate pet name for themselves.

At a few far edges of the new expat construction, you could see traces where old trees had once been rooted. Watching it happen, it was hard not to try imagining the landscape that used to be and other kinds of lives it had supported. "Stumps don't always die, but they no longer thrive; the offshoots do the work of the tree," André Aciman writes of such edges. "Cut short, this might-have-been life didn't necessary die or wither; it just lingered there, always unlived and beckoning."[71]

ON THE OTHER SIDE

When she moved from the house on the other side, Cresencia left her medical records behind with Allison. The file contained hundreds of papers charting the past five years of Cresencia's search for medical help, neatly stacked in an oversized yellow envelope of the type that hospitals often use to jacket x-ray films. It held bureaucratic forms and slips of paper in all colors and sizes, conflicting diagnoses and dappled MRI images, and pharmaceutical prescriptions in many handwritings and various fonts and languages from countless doctors across over half a dozen cities: Dangriga, Belize City, San Ignacio, Belmopan; Guatemala City and Melchor across one border; Chetumal, Mexico, across the other.

One muggy afternoon, Cresencia called Allison and asked her to bring the medical file over to her aunt's house so that I could examine its contents for this project. Sometimes I wondered whether Cresencia had chosen to leave these critical documents behind when moving just to break from the medical frustrations that their pages charted, at least for a while. In addition to the disappointments that the file condensed through its systematic documentation of so many hospital procedures, ineffectual drugs, and fruitless recommendations, she had also saved the receipts from all her mounting medical bills—records that together constituted an archive tallying precisely what years of bioscientific disappointments had cost her. Or perhaps leaving the file "on the other side" when she moved was instead a way of signaling an enduring tie, as if all the ghostly x-rays and MRI images and inscrutable photographs of her digestive organs represented some technical and intimate jigsaw puzzle of herself that remained in Allison's possession and might one day be reassembled.

Biopolitical analyses often position clinic bureaucracies or medical files as constitutive of a clinical gaze or related forms of control.[72] But these papers had been cut out of institutional archives and had an intimate value, part of the material culture of her illness; Cresencia was living her file. Looking through its pages was shocking. By the time we met, she took Tylenol only occasionally to ease the pain of walking and sometimes drank the tart resin-colored juice of wild noni fruit. She told me there was a time before when she used to take metformin pills and shoot herself with various insulins, alternating the injection sites between her arms, legs, and stomach. But somehow I had not really processed the years of drug regimens and treatment experiments involved in her care history until I saw their bureaucratic traces spread out all at once before me. She had traveled to virtually every clinic in the country, both private and public, and taken every antidiabetic drug on the national registry. There was also an extraordinary amount of duplication in the file, since Cresencia kept moving between doctors in search of one who could help her. New specialists often unknowingly acted on the same hunch as their predecessors—for example, she pointed out seven separate HIV tests in her file spread over two years, as doctor after doctor insisted on checking her status because she was so skinny. People who did not know Cresencia often called her *maaga*, a Belizean Kriol word that comes from the Scottish word *meager* and has historically meant something like "too thin to be healthy"—a characteristic that in Belize subtly implies some degree of social abandonment, since no one has fed you, and that today often refers to AIDS, the cause of many deaths in her village.

I was surprised to see that doctors had variously interpreted Cresencia's diabetes as type 1 or type 2; later I began to gather clues about the implications of this. One physician visiting Belize said that across many countries, their team was seeing an increasing number of adults with type 1 who were initially misdiagnosed with type 2. This was serious news because someone with type 1 diabetes should not take certain medications (such as glyburide pills) commonly prescribed for type 2. Doing so can lead to serious systemic complications. A simple amino assay lab test could distinguish the difference—but with most people getting diagnosed with glucose meters outside hospitals, type 2 is the working default assumption.

In addition to the specter of side effects, there were also suspicions of fake medicines. This reached nowhere near the scale of counterfeit pharmaceuticals that Kris Peterson has tracked elsewhere,[73] but I heard worries about uncertain quality in small moments in Belize. One doctor in Belize City explained that he often saw generic metformin and glyburide being sold in towns for prices that were "just too low. It's not possible." He worried that anything priced that cheaply might not have a full dose of the listed ingredients.

The Belizean government had no laboratory to systematically test suspect drugs, he said, though some of his colleagues were hoping to establish a channel to mail samples to Jamaica for full chemical analysis. Many such pills actually contain particles of Jamaica already: its bedrock is a widespread source of calcium carbonate, quarried from a particular geological strata that yields medical-grade limestone used as a common pharmaceutical filler.

The fact that supposedly "inactive" pill ingredients can subtly interact with active ones is another reason the same chemical compounds might be experienced differently between brands or individuals. I didn't hear patients speak about the range of drug quality directly as much as implicitly navigate whether certain formulations "worked" or were "good pills." Antonia, for example, kept three kinds of metformin: one sent from a niece in the United States, one acquired somehow from Mexico, and one from the local clinic in Sagoun. The latter was her everyday medicine, for when she felt fine. The one from Mexico was a higher dose, one thousand milligrams, which she kept in a large Kool-Aid jar. The variety from the United States was labeled as containing only eight hundred milligrams, but she felt the pills were stronger. Trusting their efficacy most, she saved them for days when her sugar was dangerously high, "when I need it to work."

Yet taking "drugs for life" is a complicated thing, especially when lab work was not always easy to access. Metformin can actually accelerate kidney failure if kidney function is not carefully monitored. Some dialysis patients later wondered if this had worsened their issues.

Insulin for type 2 was even more fraught. "Insulin is like a taboo to them," one internist in Belize City told me. "They say it makes your skin fall off. People have advanced complications by the time they start on it, and then they think the treatment is what makes them worse." Yet insulin is also one of the most risky drugs in existence. In the U.S., "studies have shown that the use of insulin has been associated with more medication errors than any other type or class of drug."[74] This is especially true in a context where people might sometimes go hungry and not have a consistent routine of eating to gauge their dose by—or glucometer access to carefully measure their blood sugar, numbers necessary to titrate insulin according to an algorithm. Prescriptions were written for people to take a certain number of units of insulin—in Cresencia's case, thirty-five units of NPH twice a day—but there were no additional instructions about how to modulate their doses for days when food was scarce and blood sugar might index an interval of hunger.

Insulin is powerful enough to kill a person in a single overdose; in fact, caregivers have expressed concern because it can be virtually impossible to tell accidental overdose from intentional suicide.[75] Nurse Suzanne flat out refused to prescribe insulin for most type 2 anymore and grew upset whenever reviving comatose patients, for whom insulin had been prescribed elsewhere without follow-through for its safe use. "I have seen a lot more comas from insulin than from diabetes in this village," she said. "Do you know what it's like to think you might lose a patient because of a drug you gave them?"[76]

The most frequent concern that I actually heard people express about insulin, though, was the fear of "getting addicted." Its accompanying syringes didn't help this rumor, but there was also more to the worry; mobile clinics could be ephemeral in their care, with foreign teams of nurses and doctors visiting for a few days during the year as part of "medical mission" groups and then leaving again after dispensing a supply of medication that would not last until they returned. Patients paying out of pocket might run out of money, and even regional hospitals could occasionally run out of certain supplies. "I don't want to get addicted to the medicine, because maybe sometimes you can't find it," one Maya man with diabetes told me firmly. "My brother used to take insulin though," he added. "He is right over there." The man gestured toward a nearby tree. When I turned, I was expecting another wisp-bearded mechanic to interview instead of a concrete tomb.

"We don't like to take insulin," Antonia said to me once, speaking in the collective voice she usually reserved for explaining new Garifuna vocabulary or some enigmatic bit of ritual. "It's like shooting your heart."

It was the following fall when Cresencia first came to believe that traveling to the United States was her only real hope of survival. "I tried to have a little thing, to raise some money last winter," she told me. Many Belizeans sought help for unaffordable medical expenses through small fundraisers: selling plates of food to friends or strangers, climbing from bus to bus holding collection jars plastered with pictures of intubated loved ones in hospital beds, or telling their medical stories on the radio or newspaper and concluding with bank routing numbers so that well-wishers could send support directly. Even the Belize Diabetes Association sometimes fundraised by selling the very fried foods their pamphlets instructed members not to eat: conch fritters, johnnycakes.

But in the case of Cresencia's makeshift fundraiser, a tragic and mundane coincidence had occurred. It so happened that she had purchased and prepared a huge quantity of food to sell on the very day a group of famous cooks in the village had made their specialty dishes right down the road. "A whole cooler full of barbeque chicken," Cresencia said, her voice cracking. She started to cry. "All my savings." It all spoiled, she said, again and again. "It all just spoiled."

DR. SALDO

One morning in August, I met Cresencia and her Aunt Lisa on a refurbished school bus, and together we headed for Mexico. My skin stuck to the pleather seat covers in the long hours of tropical heat, but Cresencia (who had made the trip many times before) was well prepared with a pillow from home. She slept soundly against a half-open window. I knew we were getting close to the border when the land flattened out into the limestone shelf topography I associated with the Yucatan: parched shrubs, abrupt hills, chalky soil. The bus sped north past the cement homes clustered around Orange Walk and continued through Corozal, slowing at speed bumps where vendors were selling bottled seaweed juice. The bus was decorated with a fluorescent reminder: MUY AMIGO SERÁS, PERO EL PASAJE LO PAGARÁS.[77]

Later, when the bus carried us into downtown Chetumal, the world seemed to suddenly shift to a macroscale: throngs of people, wide roads teaming with cars and SUVs, tall buildings (the highest structure in Belize is still an ancient Maya pyramid), and endless traffic lights (nationwide, at last count, Belize only had three). Many considered the sixteen-hour round-trip journey to the border town Mexican shopping centers worthwhile because there were no international franchises or even corporate food chains in Belize; the country's population was just too small to make such ventures profitable for global corporations. There had been two previous attempts to open fast-food places in Belize City, first a KFC and later a Subway sandwich shop, but both had gone out of business before the time of my research. This means that parts of Belize had some of the highest rates of diabetes in the world without having a single corporate fast-food chain. But can a country be "McDonaldized" without even having a McDonald's? I watched Cresencia and Lisa staring intently out the window as our bus passed dozens of Mexican megastores, interspersed with the massive parking lots of a Sam's Club and an Office Depot. "Welcome to the U.S.A.," Lisa said.

That night, the three of us shared a windowless room in a small downtown hotel named for a noncanonical saint. The cement blocks of the room's walls were painted yellow and decorated with the proprietor's oil painting of a nude woman who appeared to be a representation of Teri Hatcher. You had to flush the toilet with a bucket, but the room had a small TV. We took turns flipping through the five black-and-white stations. It was too hot to sleep, and in any case the alarm on Cresencia's cell phone was set for 4:00 A.M. Same-day appointments at the private clinic were on a first-come-first-served basis, so we piled into a taxi while it was still dark, arriving before dawn to hold her place.

When we arrived at Clinica Zaragota, a security guard waved us into an empty lobby bathed in a dim glow. We waited in a hallway with glistening tiled floors for the first receptionist to arrive. After Lisa found a coffee-vending machine on the way to the bathroom, we all drank cup after tiny paper cup of heavily sugared *café con leche*. It helped curb the hunger and exhaustion until we ran out of peso coins. After that we waited more or less in silence.

The three of us dozed intermittently in our chairs as the clinic slowly came to life. The pharmacist came in first and then a receptionist who tentatively scheduled Cresencia for an appointment at an unspecified hour. I collected several magazine-quality pamphlets on the services offered at the private clinic, and Cresencia quietly pointed out each of the diagnostic tests she had already had, which were listed by price inside a glossy folio. She had told me before that these tests were significantly cheaper in Chetumal than in Belize, offsetting the rather substantial cost of a hotel stay (twelve U.S. dollars) and fare (a total of fourteen U.S. dollars each direction) for the three school buses it took to reach Mexico.

As the clinic hallways began to fill with passing nurses, doctors, and clusters of other waiting patients, Cresencia looked increasingly anxious, fidgeting in her chair. Suddenly Lisa tapped her shoulder and gestured toward the door, relief visible on both their faces. I realized that the middle-aged man she nodded toward must be Cresencia's doctor and that they had traveled hundreds of miles without knowing for certain whether he would even be working that day. "There he is," Lisa said. "Dr. Saldo."

It was too early to laugh at her quick wit, although she and Cresencia exchanged a wry smile. But since then I have thought often about the nickname that Lisa invented for Cresencia's private Mexican doctor as we waited in the clinic that morning. *Saldo* was both a play on his first name and a joke that cut to the heart of a deeper irony. Most English speakers (like Cresencia and Lisa, and me for that matter) first encounter the Spanish word *saldo* on ATM receipts or when buying phone credits, so it has a certain popular association with money; one could loosely translate it as "balance," although if you look up *balance* in a Spanish dictionary, it will most likely say *balanza* or *equilibrio,* words that cannot be used to figure accounting. *Saldo* has no English equivalent that is quite right, the sum of accounts left over after an exchange—a residue, a trace, a remainder. I came to think of the great lengths Cresencia had gone to seeking private medical care in Mexico in terms of this biting joke—the thing that was left now after so many exchanges, the last residue of a withdrawn medicine. It seemed fitting to keep Lisa's dubbing of "Dr. Saldo" as the pseudonym for Cresencia's doctor here. Perhaps an English translation could be something like Dr. Money or Dr. Remainder.

We had been waiting in the hallway for almost five hours by the time a nurse called us into the doctor's office. I was struck by how personalized the desk looked, after so many months observing Cuban doctors in Belizean clinics, who were not around long or consistently enough to decorate. But Dr. Saldo had his own office and a cabinet filled with a vast collection of backward-facing elephants made from crystal, ceramic, and clay. He also had an array of pharmaceutical company paraphernalia that I suddenly realized was missing from Belizean public hospitals; like the McDonald's or Office Depot, apparently the tiny country's population was simply not big or wealthy enough to make it a prime target market for corporate saturation. Although we often think of drug companies' influence as potentially corrupting, I realized that the absence of exploitation by cutting-edge Big Pharma and its generic competitors could be a form of exclusion, too, and that access and rights to medical treatments are increasingly bound up with therapeutic market forces that were largely missing in Belize. But in Mexico, the doctor had an enormous assortment of branded pharmaceutical posters, anatomical trinkets, alarm clocks, and snow globes, each etched with the name of a blockbuster drug. Lipitor alone had furnished a sculpted photograph holder, a statue of a Mayan temple with the name of the pharmaceutical carved into the platform in faux ancient lettering, and a key hanger decorated with metal etchings of a sun eclipsing the moon.

"How are you, Cresencia?" Dr. Saldo asked when we sat down in the opulent cushioned chairs surrounding his desk. Later he examined her as they talked, speaking some English, she some Spanish. Unsurprisingly, her blood sugar was sky-high after a morning spent drinking sweetened coffee in place of food. Instead of chiding her, he listened closely as she spoke of her inability to keep down solid food over the past months and recorded everything in a thick file detailing their previous visits together. She had lost six pounds since her last visit. At one point Cresencia became too choked up to speak, and with the moment feeling too charged for me to ask her to explain her reaction, I searched her face and tried to understand why she broke down into tears as we left his office: Was it the sudden promise that these new prescriptions and tests might finally help her? Because she already suspected they wouldn't? Because he remembered her name? What would it mean risking to hope for a cure again?

Waiting for a school bus headed back to Belize, Lisa and I milled around a labyrinthine market, both a little on edge, while Cresencia vomited in a nearby bathroom. The market offered many things for sale, but Lisa chose to speak of the colorful produce as we waited: seemingly endless tables of cilantro and other leafy greens and various shades of peppers, carrots, and squashes. When Cresencia rejoined us, her eyes looking bloodshot and still holding the prescriptions tight in her hand, this was also her first comment. "Look at all the vegetables," she marveled in a slightly hoarse voice, and we climbed back onto a chicken bus headed for the border for a return trip that would take until around midnight.

Outside the bus windows, the road began to change. There was no time to stop for food after we crossed the border again. A lady with a basket selling drinks stepped down the aisle. Many passengers bought Cokes, hungry. I sipped mine and leaned against the metal of the school bus, watching our reflections in the rectangles of glass. We looked like a soda commercial.

GREAT WHITE HAZARDS

Seeing flourishing markets just across the border in Mexico helped me separate out certain things I had noted in Belize but had taken to be characteristic of relative scarcity, rather than of limits specific to the economy of a tiny nation. Yet like the pharmaceutical supplies and corporate franchises, vegetables seemed to be circulating robustly in Chetumal. Belize's population was too tiny to function autonomously in the same way as Mexico, a target market—and this appeared true for local growers as well as global corporations. In the words of one guidebook: "A walk through any Belizean market with its tiny piles of withered produce (mostly onions, tomatoes, and potatoes), is an accurate representation of the way in which such food is viewed here. . . . all too often what you get is a starchy mass."[78]

Richard Wilk has carefully examined this paradox in his ethnography of food in Belize. He noted that foreign development NGOs and consultants often try to "fix" the country's historical reliance on imported foods with technical interventions: training farmers, using soil enhancers, teaching local people to grow British-style gardens that quickly wash away in the tropical rains. These interventions repeatedly fail to examine the actual market structures of a tiny nation that make local food economies untenable. Wilk writes that such experts "are acting as if Belize really has a *national* economy, like the USA or Germany, so development is a matter of government making the right local decisions. They treat Belize as if it were a country, a continent, a place with its own economy. But Belize has always had an *international* economy, its borders open to movements of people and capital. . . . All the important decisions about Belize's position in the global economy—even today—are made *outside* the country."[79]

Wilk describes the endless interventions and the NGO "technical assistance" teams who have come to Belize trying to boost agriculture without realizing "that the problems were structural and political, and had nothing to do with the farmers, the climate, Belizean pasture grasses, screwworms or vampire bats—all of which had been blamed at one time or another."[80] "The problems that frustrated their efforts," he explains, "were simply *not under their control*. They cannot be solved in Belize because they are part of *global politics*. No amount of TA (technical assistance) for famers in Belize will change that."[81]

I thought of the bustling vegetable market in Mexico again the following week, when a nurse at the public clinic asked me to bring a stapled packet of educational photocopies to Cresencia the next time I visited her. A well-meaning retired U.S. nurse on vacation in Sagoun had dropped off the informational packet about diabetes for her there, after she and Cresencia had spoken in the village one day. I glanced quickly at the "Live Life! Scorecard" on the front page of the educational packet ("Healthy Living Made Fun and Easy!") and thought to myself what little equivalence it had to Cresencia's world before slipping it into my backpack. I didn't know the tourist who had left it for Cresencia or what their relationship might be, and assumed it might represent some gesture of care even if its contents were not applicable to actual realities.

When I pulled out the wilted photocopies later that week for Cresencia, I expected her just to set the educational photocopies aside on a corner of her bed and perhaps even make one of her wry jokes about the irrelevance of their contents. But instead she grew quiet and spent several minutes reading the pages closely. The cover page featured a long list of daily meal necessities for diabetes, recommendations like " 5 or more servings of veggies (about 3 cups total)—best are any dark leafy greens/lettuce, cabbage, broccoli, cauliflower, brussels sprouts, carrots, sweet potatoes, onions, garlic, leeks, tomatoes, asparagus, red/orange/ yellow bell peppers."

It is hard to convey how extravagant the list sounded in Stann Creek, where out of this list only tomatoes and onions would be sold at the average grocery store. About two-thirds of these items would have to be imported from Mexico and therefore would be a notable expense for someone struggling to make ends meet to eat *one* serving a day—let alone five. But watching Cresencia's face change, I realized that the pamphlet's breezy advice, given out of context, was something more than the ineffectual but harmless gesture of care I had mistaken it for. Making her fight for life sound so easy was not empowering; it was devastating. "No sweet beverages," the photocopies advised of her daily breakfast. "NO Great White Hazards—white flour products, white rice, white potatoes, or excess sugar." I realized that the prohibited categories were virtually a list of the staple foods available in the village. Looking up from the educational photocopies with a distant expression, Cresencia told me that sometimes the pain was so bad that she wanted to die.

That well-meaning nutritional advice was not just an isolated incident but part of a larger countrywide trend in scattered, ephemeral, and haphazard foreign education about diabetes. "Health development" spring trips had become wildly popular throughout Belize, as teams of university students, church groups, nurses, and other foreigners with good intentions (often untrained) visited for a few days and provided medical screening, education, or treatment to people in rural Belizean villages. In 2011, anthropologist Christian Vannier accompanied one such university team on its spring break trip to examine their visit's long-term impact and ethical implications. "In addition to our trip, there was a different university running the same medical tourism trip directly before and directly after us," Vannier reported. He described going to a remote village for chronic disease screening only to find they were the second team to offer diabetes education there that week.

"In fact, some NewHealth staff joked that during the spring and summer they worked ten to twelve hours per day with no days off due to the sheer amount of U.S.-based universities coming to Belize and setting up health screenings or clinics for diabetes and hypertension," explained Vannier.[82] One doctor coordinating such a trip worried that "dol[ing] out these medications with only a modicum of information or education represented a significant breach of medical ethics and an extremely unsustainable method of chronic disease control." Yet the same doctor also noted: "The trip is going to happen every year. . . . It's simply too popular and the medical school views it as a feather in their cap."[83]

In following the university team, Vannier discovered a troubling paradox: "Though many patients did not have a relationship with a local doctor or hospital, many demonstrated an extensive knowledge of the chronic disease with which they lived. Individuals knew the causes, symptoms, consequences, and treatments of diabetes and hypertension." Visiting groups often assumed that more knowledge would lead to "empowered" health decisions, but instead "patients demonstrated an extremely negative view regarding their overall physical health and mental well-being. The medical doctors were surprised. Strong knowledge [about] the disease and its treatments and strong beliefs in the management and even curing of disease should lead to greater beliefs in overall health and well-being."[84] Yet these high levels of education for diabetes and hypertension (instilled in part by the ephemeral visits of these teams) were associated with people feeling more fatalistic and depressed.

The correlation between disease education and increased despair seemed less paradoxical when I thought back on the educational pamphlet that Cresencia read that afternoon. The university team in Vannier's account did not inquire whether local people would have consistent access to the high-quality monitoring tools, therapies, and lifesaving diets they were being educated about needing so badly. Cresencia flipped back to the first page of the stapled packet, which featured a calendar grid with small boxes for each day of the week. Meant for patients to mark off the number of days they were able to stick to its listed recommendations, the chart in this context instead felt like a checklist of absences: foods that would require considerable money and effort to consistently acquire for five servings a day in Belize. This information about diabetes came from a world where the luxuries of varied foods and infinite patient choices were taken for granted.

One doctor from the U.S. recently stated that during the week he planned to spend in Belize, his mission would be to teach local people that "diabetes is not my doctor's responsibility, it is my responsibility," a mantra that many foreign teams thought it was their purview to impart. Yet Cresencia did not need "to be educated" that her health was her responsibility; from what I could understand, she knew that acutely after the state had given her up for dead. By that time, I thought her central struggle was living with the weight of that knowledge. Perhaps being told, once again, that changing the course of her sickness would be so easy if she just individually complied with a list of impossible demands only underscored the more bitter ironies of her life, because Cresencia again repeated the statement to which I found myself unable to respond: for a second time, she told me that sometimes she wanted to die, just to stop the pain.

Everything I could think of to say in reply felt cheap as she cried. Cresencia gave the educational photocopies back to me and told me she was hungry. She asked if I would buy her a creole bun (a dense Belizean comfort bread made from coconut milk and white flour). "I refer to these white carbs as the 'Great White Hazard,'" read the educational pamphlet in Cresencia's hands. "These foods have a very high glycemic index (GI) which means they are rapidly digested and quickly enter your bloodstream as a surge of glucose (blood sugar)."

In that moment, it felt like the "Great White Hazards" referred not only to the lone available meal options but also to the many white foreigners shaping this story: the tourist nurse whose educational packet brought Cresencia face-to-face with a world of life-giving choices unavailable to her; all the fragmented and ephemeral diabetes education that in the end could not offer her livable solutions; the colonial machinations that had carved Belize into a tiny nation completely dependent on imported foods in the first place; the long history of political dispossession in Sagoun, in which tourism often felt like the latest permutation and which came from a world I too was so uncomfortably and obviously a part of. I think Cresencia sensed my hesitation because she added: "Please, I'll be able to sleep if I eat creole bread or honey bun." She looked down. "My body calls for it. Something sweet." Without effective medicine, sugar itself had become her palliative care.

HEALTHY LIVING MADE FUN AND EASY!

By the time Cresencia handed the paper back to me, it felt like a responsibility. So one day, I brought "Healthy Living Made Fun and Easy!" to the open-air weekend market and adjacent grocery complex in town. I wanted to document precisely how much it would cost to actually follow the pamphlet's outlined advice in southern Belize. By that point, it was no surprise to chart its many misfits. For example, some of the fresh vegetables and produce that the packet recommended only came in cans in Dangriga or did not exist in Belize at all: asparagus could be purchased for eleven dollars a Del Monte can, but cherries were not available for any price—they do not grow locally and are not imported. Cassava and other root crops were sold everywhere in market stalls, but the pamphlet omitted these crucial staples of local diets from its advice entirely.

Of the recommended fruits and vegetables that I did find for sale in the Dangriga market, many were imported from Mexico. But there were also bags of insecticide-clouded red grapes still bearing "Made in the U.S.A." stickers that sourced them from California, as well as tiny green apples labeled as grown in Canada. Such produce was thus being sold in the Belize market at North American prices or higher to make up for the shipping costs—not to mention the issue of the carbon footprint of these food miles, or the irony that the produce was most likely being picked by Central Americans who had immigrated to California for work, only to be sold back to such laborers' home countries for sale.[85] I made a chart of the basic arithmetic. It cost nearly three times as much per item to buy food from the diabetes nutrition pamphlet's "recommended items" list as it did from the "forbidden foods" list.[86]

This situation is challenging for institutions as well as individuals. I remember talking with Cresencia in the hospital one day when she was served a plate of white rice and a banana for lunch. "You told me not to eat bananas or white rice," Cresencia said to the nurse who handed her the tray. But that was what the hospital—like many households— could afford that day on an overstretched budget. "Try to only eat two spoons, love," the nurse said gently.

The day after returning from Mexico, I saw Igemeri on the bus, dressed head to toe in a transcendental shade of white. He asked how Cresencia was doing, so I related the news she had told us to share from Chetumal: The doctor believed that her diabetes was probably triggered only as a secondary complication or chronic comorbidity, which likely masked some more serious pathology with its easily discernible symptoms of high blood sugar.

"Sounds like Artelio was onto something," Igemeri said casually.

Ever since our return from Mexico, Cresencia had begun preparing in a curious way for her trip to the United States to get the diagnostic tests that the doctor said she needed. With her savings gone and her relatives living in different U.S. cities unwilling or unable to send money, Cresencia had no way to actually get there. While her Aunt Lisa focused on writing letters to Ministry of Health officials asking for assistance to get the unaffordable tests locally subsidized, Cresencia had begun the process of packing. She bought a few pieces of clothing in Dangriga, a yellow T-shirt and several pairs of new socks, since she reasoned that it might be too cold wherever she was sent to wear "slippers" (the Belizean term for flip-flops), as was her habit. Although her preparations were concrete, the whole thing increasingly unsettled me—a reminder that whether or not it was to the United States, she would be traveling somewhere soon.

So during the last month of my research, I helped Cresencia prepare an application file through a local regional hospital to leave Belize for medical help abroad. It was a terribly uneasy role. A local nurse had first mentioned the group, a small NGO that chooses certain emergency cases from Belize for intervention. Their group usually first tried to support local caregivers by providing consultation with U.S. specialists through a Skype-style telemedicine interface, but often later brought patients to hospitals in Florida or Texas for treatment. *Application* was Cresencia's own word; local administrators who were involved in selection called the process "preparing her case for presentation," as if this was just an e-version of medical rounds, but Cresencia's term is closer to the truth: the NGO gatekeepers were forced to triage for the limited number of spots, usually giving preference to children and people with more exotic diseases.

I wrote up Cresencia's file in clinical detail, replete with terms of the sort I imagined biomedical doctors favored ("Psycho-Social Factors"), trying to capture the urgency. A local administrator had already warned me that a case of diabetes was not likely to be chosen. Cresencia and I agreed that a focus on the worst she had suffered might be an effective tool for the application, so in the file's overview I described her with words like "wasting" and made many strategic omissions from her complex history of care seeking, focusing on aspects that I thought the reviewing doctors might associate with a "good patient."

Yet once the file was assembled, seeing herself cast in this image seemed to hurt her feelings profoundly; the thought of herself as a helpless object of pity had not previously occurred to her. In our conversations together, Cresencia focused most often on her miraculous healing, which she viewed as a defining moment that showed her ancestors' and community's attentive care for her during a moment of crisis. She was concerned that I had left out this key event, a source of great pride and dignity, from the application description.

Worried that religious healing rituals might brand her as "noncompliant" in the eyes of medical doctors, I instead emphasized only paralyzing resource limitations and the complexity of her disease (while squirming with each narrative choice I made about how our existing asymmetries were getting tangled in the enigmatic domains that Erica Caple James calls "bureaucraft").[87] I think Cresencia became worried that my other descriptions of her life would be written in that pitiable image too, because our relationship never felt quite the same afterward. But quietly, she asked me to submit the application and helped me choose a particularly unflattering photograph of herself to submit with the file ("this ugly one") that showed bald spots where her hair had fallen out in tufts, patches that she normally disguised with zigzag braids. Then there was nothing to do but wait.

"Sorrow wears and uses us but we wear and use it too," Henry James once wrote.[88]

STRADDLING

The following weeks found Cresencia "kicking up dust" again, possessed for a third time by Artelio. "Same old, same old," she told me later with a short laugh. Whenever she felt faint after that point, she bathed in clear rum again and treated her rapidly swelling limbs with Florida water (a spiritual preparation common enough to be purchased at any local grocery store). Although her bottle of Florida water was stamped with a red filigreed image of conquistador Ponce de León, its label made me think instead of the Miami hospitals she still waited to hear back from, and all of globalized medicine's life-giving fountains that seemed to slip continuously in and out of her reach.

Cresencia was not the only one in the village who had attracted the attention of discontented ancestors that summer. Others included a young boy who had abruptly lost his vision, which returned after preliminary placations, as well as a "stiff-necked" old man who did not believe in "that culture thing," for which the spirits had punished him with repeated trance states characterized by loss of speech until bathed with *amuñadahani* cassava water. This series of otherworldly illnesses cumulatively signaled a deeper problem in the extended family line, and so in the late summer a *chugú* was planned, a briefer and smaller-scale version of the famous Garifuna *dügü*. (Joseph Palacio emphasizes the two rituals' shared elements by translating them into English as "feeding the dead" and "feasting the dead," respectively.)[89]

I was surprised that Cresencia was not at the *chugú* when we arrived. I attended that night with Jo instead because she had loaned me a dress for the occasion. The offering spread inside the ancestral temple was mostly an expanded version of other ritual tables I had seen, with a few additions: enormous whole crabs with densely bristled claws and a sacrificed pig with its ears accentuated by charring, the quartered section of its roasted head shining in the light of a Saint Jude votive. Many men were away for work elsewhere, so older women sang the male a cappella offering songs. A few men mulled about outside, but Jo explained to me that most of those present could not assist in singing the male *arumahani* songs, having forgotten the lyrics. They occupied themselves by taking pictures of the ritual's highlights with their iPhones to send to absent relatives. Igemeri translated bits of the songs for me: "This is the debt that has been owed to the ancestors for a very long time," he said. "It is so long overdue." Others resembled refrains I had read in old books:

> Our journey has been sad, my grandchild.
> We have been searching for our grandchildren.
> We have been crossing the deep ocean.
> For our descendants are far away.[90]

The air was filled with the sweet incense of termite nests picked from trees and burned, shrouding the ancestral house in smoke to protect it from unwanted spirits. Later, when the *malí* started, I sat on a bench inside the ancestral temple during the dance that months ago had healed Cresencia. It was true that the drums sounded like a heartbeat.[91] There were swathes of pink and yellow fabric hanging in the corners of the room, which Igemeri told me represented the flags of Saint Vincent, flags of families. A few women started collapsing into the arms of swaying family members, possessed by spirits. Once in a while someone would call out, resisting the spirit who tried to possess them, and their foreheads were smoothed with clear rum. Wearing instruments hanging from their necks, the drummers would pivot at certain points and turn back toward the rows of dancers, and the canon (who was also a noted scholar and Anglican priest) called out the names of the dead from a stapled handwritten list. Afterward the crowd resumed their swaying motion, singing in response and waving white *ahuragülei* "fans" above their heads. In addition to the counterclockwise circles, sometimes the drummers would lead the crowd straight toward one of the four directions, calling on the west, south, east, and north as they continued reading the names of ancestors. During Foster's fieldwork in the seventies, people remembered when a grave-shaped hump of dirt used to be formed in the center of the earthen temple floor.[92] I thought of this when I saw the women's unusual dancing, performed with rhythmic mashing steps. Taylor noted that some did not describe such stamping footsteps as dancing; rather, "they trod down the grave with their feet."[93]

The motion of so many bodies filled the temple with an electric energy that became too intense for me, and I moved back out to the beach. The lagoon had flooded the previous morning, spilling a tide of murky water into the sea—but for some reason, the muddy brown had not mingled with the Caribbean blue in the distance, and the water had separated into two bands of color. People suspected this was due to the real estate developers' latest boom, as outsiders kept trying to build on more precarious land by filling in the adjacent swamp with sand, often further amplifying serious erosion in the course of projects meant to extend the beach for expats' vacation homes. I stared out at the two-colored seawater, by then hidden by night.

Evelyn, whose father with diabetes I had visited until his death the previous winter, approached me on the beach and handed me a calabash of something to drink. I thought of the many afternoons watching her father, Francisco, get his blood glucose checked, and recalled the stereo music and yellow light at his "ninth-night" *beluria* (which Taylor translates more festively as a "farewell party" for the spirit of the dead).[94] "Homemade coffee," Evelyn said as I took a sip of the warm liquid. "Made from burnt rice." But it tasted like sugar.

Sometime after midnight, Cresencia arrived. She looked unwell, and someone set up a folding bed for her close to the water. A while later I approached the tideline where she leaned on a pillow a few yards from the lapping waves, but she seemed tired of talking. I asked her how she was feeling. Cresencia glanced at me with a smile that looked tired and then tilted her chin toward the horizon, as if the answer to my question floated over the sea somewhere, times and places waiting to be invoked again: the many borders that she crossed seeking help; Artelio and all the ancestors who looked on; the disconnected x-ray envelope of drug prescriptions and diagnoses from all the doctors who had tried and failed to help her; Allison, alone now in the home they had shared; the fallow fields once farmed by her ancestors, marked by the hardship they had also borne; the two sons who had died from her; the exposures as present and ghostly as her kin; songs of the women who gathered to meet her ambulance under a mango tree; whosever initials were tattooed on her wrist. Or more likely she was thinking of something else totally, beyond anything she wanted me to guess or know.

In many ways, the form of diabetes that Cresencia struggled with was highly unusual and more complex than an average case because of the apparent underlying cause that always seemed just on the verge of being diagnosed. Yet many of the difficulties and realities she faced seemed to me like exaggerated versions of the issues shared by many of those living with diabetes in Belize. The disease never has a cure, and there was chronic uncertainty in a biomedical system that looked navigable on paper but often felt strained in practice, where one might reach for but could not rely on the ephemeral nature of foreign intervention and medical technologies. With powerful drugs often (but not always) available for ingestion and with little continuity in infrastructure, patients like Cresencia were often left to discern the efficacy and side effects of drugs on their own, risks thoughtfully weighed against the cost of changing the habits that vitally supported them. High-glucose food often serves as the lifeblood that sustains kin ties in Belize; for many Garinagu, this cuts across the worlds of both the living and the dead.

Some say that during such rituals, the rafters of the ancestral temple fill with a range of spirits. There are some that assume capricious shapes, but more concerning are those more attentive and demanding, the dead. That night, I looked up at the smoke curling in the hollows of the high thatched roof. The palmetto rafters of the ancestral temple were hung with pale bands of cotton—"fans" that people had tied there as the night wore on, the last traces of dancing a *malí* like the one that had revived Cresencia under the mango tree. Some knots had come undone in the ocean wind, strips of cloth that fell to the ground. The remaining ties of white fabric flapped like bandages against the rafters.

As Joseph Palacio recently said of the changing economies, emerging tensions, and sale of lands among the Garifuna in Belize: "These are issues that confront any group of people who are caught between two *distinct and disjointed worlds.* For us they are coastal Central America and inner city United States."[95] Cresencia used to make me think of Turner's idea of limen, the figure on the threshold. But whenever I thought she had been "reintegrated" into another collective or category, it seemed that in the next moment I turned around and there she was: back on another threshold. In the end, perhaps Cresencia was less like a chronic limen than someone who embodies the original meaning of the word *diabetes*—"one who straddles." Etymologically, this ancient Greek root comes from the literal stance that people with diabetes often endured from the frequent urination that is a characteristic symptom of their disease.[96] Yet today, this linguistic root still cuts to the quick of the layered meanings at stake for many people with diabetes in Belize who are, in a very real sense, straddling multiple worlds. Many live between scarcity and excess; between phone calls and cardboard barrels sent from New York and Los Angeles, appointments and cities and various medicines; between foreign encroachment and pollution of their lands that continuously displace them anew, and profound ancestral and community ties that bind them back again through the very foods that biomedical advice discourages them from eating. People in this setting live with a disease that is both born of their chronic halfway condition and uneasily managed there: "those who straddle."

As Cresencia stared toward the sea, her eyes looked at once attentive and far away. Boats can also represent coffins in Garifuna symbolism,[97] I recalled in the night. At the time, I was still feeling unsettled by her request a few weeks before when she had suddenly asked if I would take her picture—"a nice one"—as I was halfway out the door. The uncharacteristic invitation had seemed directly linked to her comments about the proximity of death. I felt an emptiness in my chest as I pulled the camera out of my backpack.

The look that passed between us in that moment is hard to describe: the charged exchange of being two young women sitting there in a wooden room with all our asymmetrical life chances so palpable, and yet I couldn't stop what was about to happen to her any more than she could. She had taken several pictures of me earlier with the camera on her flip phone, which rested on a pile of folded laundry. Later I tried to hope that the images we made of each other might be another part of some trace left at the "boundary between absence and presence."[98] But at the time, really I just thought that the only thing more disturbing than taking her picture would have been not taking her picture.

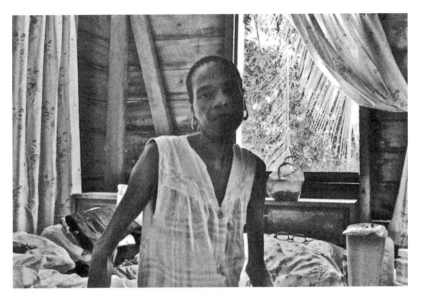

Cresencia (1976–2012).

Through the window, trees faded into glare and ocean. She removed her glasses and looked at me expectantly, her expression calm but posture tense. "I'm ready," she said.

(I wasn't.)

"Take it before I start to smile."

Crónica Two: Insula

Technology, Policy, and Other Units of Jordan's Isolations

Every science has a beginning but no end.
—Anton Chekhov, *Love and Other Stories*

Historian Michael Bliss's *The Discovery of Insulin* moves with the pace of a science adventure story: two young men, Frederick Banting and Charles Best, toiling through a sweltering summer in 1921 in a laboratory at the University of Toronto, incidentally killing dozens of dogs as they removed parts of the animals' organs in complex surgeries focused on the pancreas. They sliced open and stitched up brown-and-white short-haired terriers, stray dogs they found or bought on the street, a few cats and rabbits, surplus organ meats from butcher shops, and calf fetuses from slaughterhouses. The experiments they conducted essentially explored one basic, urgent premise—that something in the pancreatic secretions seemed to control blood sugar.

One dog, Number 92, lived for more than three weeks after Banting and Best gave it severe diabetes by removing its pancreas. A control dog receiving no treatment after this same procedure died quickly from skyrocketing blood sugar, but Number 92 lived beyond all expectations, surviving on improvised injections of an extract from the pancreas's islet cells to control its blood sugar. The dog, a yellow collie, came to be loved as a laboratory pet; they named her Marjorie, and Dr. Banting wept when she died. Best and Banting called the serum that kept her alive for that time *Isletin*.[1]

In 1923, a fellow doctor wrote to a Toronto newspaper to gush about the serum's breakthrough: "No one need die today who is suffering from diabetes."[2]

TYPE WHAT?

I thought about this dramatic narration of insulin's history in 2010, as I stepped off the repurposed school bus in the bright morning. The hospital stood on the edge of Dangriga, far from where the river meets the sea. I jogged across the highway and toward the hospital's entrance as part of my usual interview circuit that year, beginning the research day by asking if any patients with diabetes wanted to talk with me. The hospital's entryway usually smelled of freshly cut grass. It was roughly ninety years after Banting and Best's insulin first kept a patient alive. But in the morning bustle of Belize's regional hospital, that expanse of years and decades since insulin's development—now going on an entire century—seemed swallowed by other numbers.

When we met for the first time, I couldn't decide if Jordan looked stoic or just bored. "Insulin or no insulin . . ." That was one of the first things he said to me. Jordan paused, and I got the feeling he didn't know how to communicate what growing up between those terms was like any more than I knew how to ask. Vaguely: "It costs."

He must have felt at least as strangely audited as I did with all the other patients in the long open room. Their occasional flickering glances conveyed that our hesitant interview was a disappointing replacement for the lack of television. I wrote Jordan's words dutifully in my spiral notebook without really understanding. I hadn't yet learned to read certain bodily signs that a doctor would have recognized immediately—suggesting the particular erosions etched on a person by discontinuous or missing insulin. Jordan was wearing a diaper. His bloated ankles and feet indicated that his kidneys were unable to regulate fluid levels. He was nearly blind at age twenty-one, signaling microvascular capillaries worn out by years of high blood sugar. I saw but didn't fully understand Jordan's sunken collarbone planes, or the diabetic ulcers along his gaunt legs. It appeared his hair had fallen out only recently, with a full shape kept by the few tufts that remained.

Before insulin was discovered, doctors called a slow, shriveling-up death from severe diabetes "inanition"—to become inanimate, a process somewhere between atrophying and ossifying. Seeing it happen over time, you could understand why someone might think the condition required its own verb.

Yet while diabetes seemed to be freezing Jordan's body, our first conversation was mostly about the mechanics of motion. He wanted to become a pilot and had worked at a garage—cars being the next best things to airplanes—while going to technical school for specialized training in engine repair. This energetic tinkering with broken systems seemed an obvious extension of his bodily and existential struggle. Yet as we spoke about such used vehicles—and the garage job Jordan had lost when no longer able to hide that he was going blind and becoming too weak to lift tools or tires—his voice kept slipping between registers and tenses, the alternating ambitions and frustrations of someone who has dreams but suspects they will not come to pass.

Was that why he wanted to talk with a stranger like me? Jordan said that he hoped our conversation that day would be the first in a series of visits. Yet it often felt like I was asking the wrong questions. For example, at one point I had blundered and asked whether Jordan had an insulin pump, coming as I did from a country where this is a basic option for many people with type 1. The majority of people with type 1 who wear these devices, sometimes referred to as "pumpers," can expect to live a long and full life. Such machines connect the wearer's body with a beeper-like box holding insulin in a reservoir. Small enough to be clipped on a belt or tucked in a pocket, they are connected to the blood through a vein-like plastic tube called a cannula, which is inserted under the skin for continuous subcutaneous insulin injection. In countries where pumping is prevalent, these pumps can be programmed to deliver doses in tailored intervals—in calibrated bursts or in slow, steady drips—depending on habits, blood sugar, and foods eaten. New models often come equipped with features such as micro-dose calculators and computer interfaces with blood sugar levels in real time. Some even have the ability to automatically deliver insulin based on the results and custom alarms from continuous blood glucose monitors. But Jordan explained that he didn't have an insulin pump or continuous glucose monitoring because you couldn't get either device in Belize. Only people able to travel out of the country might have access to the larger infrastructures necessary to set up and maintain such intricate machines.

I felt ashamed for making him explain this out loud and groped for a question that would not elicit such terrible patience.

"So, what kind of diabetes do you have?" I asked, to fill a lull. It was a kind of placeholder question—one I thought we both already knew the answer to, but that might open into a more interesting discussion. Yet Jordan surprised me again.

"I don't know," he said.

ISLANDS AND EMPIRE

The word *insulin* comes from the Latin *insula,* meaning "island." This crucial hormone is produced in the human body by archipelagos of cells in the pancreas, floating among other cells that produce digestive enzymes. The unique clusters are named for a nineteenth-century German medical student, Paul Langerhans, who described in his dissertation the microscopic cell groups that came to be known as islands of Langerhans. Medical textbooks now more often label this part of the pancreas as the islets of Langerhans, *islet* sounding suitably technoanatomical but still meaning "tiny island." These islands contain four kinds of cells—alpha, beta, delta, and c, which talk to each other—though beta cells are the most plentiful.

Type 1 diabetes occurs when the islets' beta cells stop producing insulin—the peptide hormone that allows glucose to enter cells, thereby regulating and stabilizing levels of sugar in the blood. No one fully understands the genesis of damages that cause the islet cells to malfunction this way, though there are abundant puzzle-piece insights and theories of exposure: viral triggers, various stressors, genetic inheritance, pollution, and climate, among others. But anyone with type 1 needs insulin injections several times a day, every day of their lives, to survive. This form of diabetes is an autoimmune condition that sets in quickly, classically manifesting during childhood or adolescence. Like other autoimmune diseases, rates of type 1 diabetes are now skyrocketing worldwide.[3]

Type 2 diabetes takes longer to set in. It occurs when someone's pancreas used to produce enough insulin, but this function has slowly tapered off due to cellular stressors that accumulate from insulin resistance. A pattern of consuming high-carbohydrate food is the best-understood factor that can cause this effect, linking type 2 to industrial food systems and imbalanced nutrition, among other factors and exposures. Depending on long-term treatment and circumstances in type 2, the body's ability to produce insulin might become so impaired that pills and diet aren't enough, and insulin injections eventually become necessary.

It had taken me awhile to memorize diabetes's multiple variations before beginning this work, and at first I was puzzled when people like Jordan told me that they did not know what kind of diabetes they had. Some patients would answer readily when I asked about type 1 or type 2—but a significant number of people like Jordan also raised their eyebrows in impatience or confusion at the question or would clarify "sugar diabetes" when pressed on the question of "what kind." Even doctors at times have difficulty distinguishing the difference between type 1 and type 2 as they appear in the clinic[4]—like Cresencia, who lived for years not knowing which type she had.

Anthropologist Melanie Rock has critiqued the politics inherent in hammering down the many diseases that diabetes can represent into two neat types, terming the whole classification process "commensurating bodies of unequal experience."[5] But I faced her questions of categorization from the opposite direction. I had intended to focus on type 2 diabetes, but local realities made me face the meaningful loosening of these labels at the level of actual lives: sugar diabetes, type unknown. Where did this dissolution of diabetes typologies come from, and how was it being inhabited?

Jordan told me that his mother had also lived with diabetes, dying from it in her thirties. Given this fact and his very young age at onset, I felt reasonably sure that Jordan had type 1. (Perhaps it was MODY, the rare variation most likely to be passed genetically? Did it even matter?) Yet over time, I came to see the lived murkiness between type 1 and type 2 in Belize as itself an ethnographic finding with meaningful implications. International media and public policy framings of diabetes writ large often implicitly draw on assumptions and imaginations about type 2. This includes forms of shaming (emphasizing that individuals with diabetes were simply personally responsible for their own health outcomes) that often fit poorly enough with type 2 but can be bizarrely incongruent when applied to type 1—as if patients and their families alone were morally and practically responsible for their own conditions and treatment. People with type 1 in Belize—by definition depending on treatment each day to survive—relied on technology in a way that only amplified broader struggles to reckon accountability amid medical shortages. Yet these negotiations were, in truth, part of managing *any* diabetes on the margins of an overstretched care system, and difficulty consistently accessing insulin regimens and glucometers day in and day out was also part of type 2 for many people. These kinds of struggles show how, as Claire Wendland argues, "technologies can be potent actors even when they are materially absent."[6]

But how do you research the anthropology of an absence—whether of a partially missing treatment regimen or the absent lives it can imply? Stereotypes about diabetes often come alive in the blanks of missing knowledge, eclipsing actual patients with caricatures: the type 2 obese noncompliant patient; or the unfortunate type 1 child who can be saved by science, able to manage with enough hard work. In Belize, these oversimplified tropes at times seemed animated in reality by social expectations of them, as patients moved in and out of various preset roles amid a complex cast of local characters. Nurse Norma often managed to acquire NovoLog insulin pens from a relative with diabetes in the United States (she disliked the messiness of syringes). Sometimes she arranged for Jordan to stay an extra day if there was a free bed in the hospital, which meant he could get an extra meal when he was hungry. There was no practicing endocrinologist in the public system during that time, so the homesick Cuban doctors on rotation learned more than they probably ever wanted to know about diabetes, simply from the sheer concentration of patients they tended. Many doctors focused on inspirational moments, recounting over and over such stories as the loving father who bought insulin by the crate for his three kids blind from type 1, or the diabetes camps for type 1 patients that had started being held in Belize City, where children were taught to use needles and families thickened their support networks.

In this, I saw hopeful stories move across the horizon and circuits of family care taking shape around childhood diabetes in Belize. But I also observed how the fragility of these forms excluded someone like Jordan, without a savvy parent to advocate for him. His story dramatizes the worst that patients are up against. (Happily, most children in Belize today have a much easier time managing than he had—in addition to the Ministry of Health's ongoing efforts, a group called Insulin4Life has now partnered with the Belize Diabetes Association to try to enable fuller access.) But as a marginal figure in childhood awkwardly coming into adulthood, Jordan's experiences at this system's edges also show the spectrum of unequal global realities in which limits are lived out.

In 2010, the in-patient wards were well cared for, but not new. Its corridors reminded me of a story I'd read where "the hospital seemed both futuristic and worn-out, like an old starship."[7] One afternoon I returned to the hospital and found Jordan's usual spot in the room occupied by another patient. He was a banana plantation manager, young and recently revived from a coma. I wondered where Jordan had gone but chatted politely for awhile with his successor, who had just found out that morning he had type 1 diabetes. He was nervous to tell his wife.

On the way out, I saw a row of patients waiting in the hallway for appointments with a team visiting from Texas that specialized in eye surgery to correct diabetic retinopathy. Some patients even had their diabetes diagnosed by the eye care program, which was mixed news: it meant the eye care program provided a strong safety net, but it also signaled that primary care had missed detecting these patients' diabetes at some earlier point, before their complications had progressed to blindness.

In the office, a worried-looking hospital administrator dedicated herself to calling around, hoping to find some anesthesia for the day's surgeries. One Jehovah's Witness began to pray loudly, sharing sobering pamphlets illustrated by pools of fire with others waiting on the bench. It was easy to tell who was expecting surgery by the purple Xs drawn in marker over one or both eyelids. Since Jordan was also going blind from lack of insulin, I wondered how the patients waiting on the bench had been selected. I talked with several of the women with diabetes who were waiting for surgery but also watched for Nurse Norma or another staff member passing through who might be able to tell me what had happened to Jordan.

It was weeks before I heard the news of what had unfolded: he had been returned to the hospital again a few weeks after our last interview. It was a March day when he had been brought in for the final time, drifting in and out of a coma. Jordan's stepfamily had come for this last trip to the hospital but not for the dozens or hundreds of visits that had preceded it. This upset the nurses who had been caring for him all along, who viewed it as an unearned closure on a fate that their neglect had played a role in accelerating.

Norma said that on the last day, Jordan was talking to his mother's spirit. He opened his eyes at one point and saw a woman standing by the door. He asked for two glasses of water. Somewhere in them were the last drops that Jordan would ever take into his fluid-swollen body. He died after drinking the two glasses of tap water. A long dying process often ends in aspiration; trying to wrap my mind around it, I imagined something like drowning. But ketoacidosis is actually not characterized by the excess or lack of fluid; it just looks like that from the outside because the swelling signals it's misdistributed—fluid pulled out of organs and into intercellular spaces, and into the blood.

As if searching for some proxy closure, one morning I went to find his grave near the sea: past the bridge over fishing scales and pelicans too heavy for the electric line, shops selling Nollywood DVDs and bright clothes from India, an old man sketching in charcoal sailboats of a kind that no longer exist. The cement archway leading into the cemetery read GARDEN OF GETHSEMANE in gothic script. Sinewy grass grew straight up to the sea. I searched through row after row of aboveground tombs, some brightly painted and adorned with offerings: ceramic mugs or glass bottles holding rum for the dead and wreathes with purple and

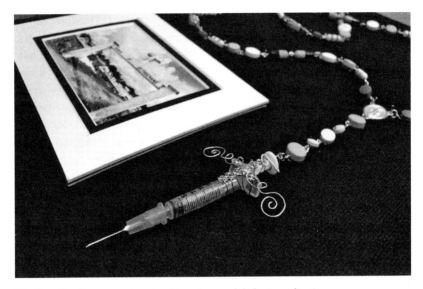

Five Decades. Rosary made of insulin syringe and diabetic medications.

black crepe-paper petals. Jordan's mother was probably interred there too, but I couldn't find her name either. I finally gave up looking and paused under a palm tree with ragged fronds. As a tiny Maya Air prop plane drifted over the sea, I recalled Jordan's dream of becoming a pilot.

I kept wondering to myself how I did not realize that Jordan was about to die, at least not consciously. I knew he was very sick; I knew some people my age or younger died from diabetes. But this person in front of me talking about gearshifts? It just didn't make sense in my mind. I used to think that the platitudes of our strained conversations might fall away in time. But that was all there would be now.

How does a medical cliché at times get sustained, resuscitated, lived out? I slowly and belatedly began paying closer attention to the artifacts that Jordan's life had left behind and the overwhelming complexity of his condition's material culture. Maybe that happens when someone dies: adjacent objects become supercharged with meaning, scraps and partial traces some kind of clues to interactions you never got to have and things you realize you forgot to ask and will never know.

Five years later, I sat paging through files in a New York archive where some of the early exchanges between insulin's discoverers, early prescribing physicians, and its first distributor (Eli Lilly) are stored in boxes. Many of the images have been displayed in museum exhibits, such as the New York Historical Society's 2011 "Breakthrough: The Dramatic Story of the Discovery of Insulin." Banting and Best sold the first insulin patent to the University of Toronto in 1923 for a dollar, in hopes of making it publicly accessible, and Eli Lilly had been granted first pharmaceutical distribution rights in the United States.[8] I leafed through folders of old news headlines and series of before and after images of patients injecting themselves in the thighs. Did Jordan live in the before or in the after of this science?

On colonial maps, the territory of British Honduras was drawn as British *inseln*, even though Belize is part of Central America's mainland. Colonies were already conceptually rendered as islands, in the logics where remote islands have often been central to the formation of "networked empires."[9] Meanwhile, Spanish maps like *Insulae Americana* did not depict Belize at all, drawing its land as open ocean. In this geography, who can say for sure that diabetes is a new issue in the Caribbean? While the history of insulin is canonically told as a history of the white children who received it, it is possible that a large part of this imbalance is because type 1 was primarily diagnosed among this population. No one can provide a global map of type 1 prevalence even today—and certainly not in 1921. As William Julius Wilson observes, imagined geographies of "isolation" can reflect exclusions actively *produced* at the nexus of societal forces—frequently in the very areas deeply interconnected to global markets.[10] With even erasures so often obscured in histories of normalized injury, Derek Walcott once wrote from another corner of the Caribbean: "Every island is an effort of memory."[11]

Insula is also the etymological root of the word *insulate*: to make like an island, to protect something or someone through a layer of substance or distance. This place was an island in more than one sense, I thought as I sat in New York City that day. Certain standards of care had become so normalized in affluent contexts that it was easy to imagine this heartening history of insulin as a global narrative. The museum versions of this history focused heavily on where the story of insulin began but often said little or nothing about where it went globally. People like Jordan fell somewhere far outside this history's purview, missing characters only present as part of "what moves in the margin."[12]

Yet the discovery of insulin changed their lives profoundly as well, because it transformed people's expectations of those living with the condition. Everyone's idea of diabetes suddenly "metamorphosed," as Boston physician Elliot Joslin wrote of insulin's potential: "This limpid liquid injected under the skin twice a day can metamorphose a frail

baby, child, adult, or old man or woman to their nearly normal counterparts."[13] Yet whether the drug that promised this new bodily transformation was actually available twice a day—how, and to whom, and
what the compromises of "*nearly* normal" mean in reality across uneven social and medical geographies—is another question entirely.

Insula also refers to a puzzling bit of our emotional anatomy. Once
"assigned to the brain's netherworld," an article in the *New York Times*
noted: "According to neuroscientists who study it, the insula is a long-
neglected brain region that has emerged as crucial to understanding
what it feels like to be human."

> It helps give rise to moral intuition, empathy and the capacity to respond
> emotionally to music. . . . the insula "lights up" in brain scans when people
> crave drugs, feel pain, anticipate pain, empathize with others, listen to jokes,
> see disgust on someone's face, are shunned in social settings. . . .
>
> It is in the frontal insula . . . that simple body states or sensations [like
> hunger, temperature, touch] are recast as social emotions. . . . Intensely emo-
> tional moments can affect our sense of time. It may stand still, and that may
> be happening in the insula, a crossroads of time and desire. . . .
>
> The frontal insula is where people sense love and hate, gratitude and
> resentment, self-confidence and embarrassment, trust and distrust, empathy
> and contempt, approval and disdain, pride and humiliation, truthfulness and
> deception, atonement and guilt.[14]

These associations are always in the back of my mind when I read
about cutting-edge breakthroughs in diabetes research, coming largely
from North American and European laboratories. There's a steady
stream of headlines: the promise of a bionic pancreas; news of islet
transplants; a variety of insulin marketed for dogs, cats, and rabbits
with diabetes that have fed too long on hyperprocessed American pet
food; cute pancreas-shaped stuffed pillows and necklaces; an amazing
variety of monitoring gadgets, iPhone apps, and care devices being
invented by some with diabetes who call themselves "d-tech heads." I
always feel a mix of emotions when bumping into such news items,
because I am often moved to see how community participation in such
ingenuity can become part of sustaining dignified life with a chronic
condition. But it can be simultaneously unsettling when the ways some
cutting-edge devices get taken up by industries would strike many people in poorer parts of the world as more reminiscent of salubrious toys,
flourishing in the same epoch when many people with diabetes are still
struggling to obtain a century-old drug. Staring at the arrow-straight
time line of diabetes science, I tried to imagine what geometry would be

needed to chart the ways those same discoveries actually reached most of the world.

GLOBAL POLICY GAPS

Since much of the current literature describing the global diabetes epidemic actually focuses on type 2, it is worth pausing to sketch out some basics about the global picture of type 1. Current estimates state that over five hundred million people live with diabetes worldwide, and roughly 5–10 percent of them are thought to have type 1.[15] But these numbers are really all just best guesses. They suggest certain global imbalances: for example, statistics show there are many more people *known* to be living with type 1 diabetes in wealthy countries (like Norway, where an estimated thirty-six per one hundred thousand people are diagnosed each year) than there are in poorer ones (like Peru, where two per one hundred thousand are diagnosed each year).

Yet these broad-stroke portraits themselves raise unsettling questions. It's unclear to what degree this hugely uneven distribution of type 1 is due to humankind's inescapable roulette of genetic and environmental risk factors, or to what extent these uneven counts suggest that children born with type 1 diabetes in poorer nations tend to die before they are ever diagnosed or counted. Many symptoms of seriously untreated diabetes—lethargy, fevers, weight loss, seizures, comas—are easily confused with malaria and other high-profile infectious diseases (the usual targets of multimillion-dollar global health campaigns favored by celebrities and donors), meaning that cryptic deaths in poor regions of the world often get tallied according to the cause du jour.

Such global health policy omissions have a history at least as old as insulin itself. In 1924, almost immediately after mass production of insulin began, the Rockefeller Institute initiated a program in which select hospitals in the United States and Canada offered insulin supplies to patients who otherwise could not afford the new drug. "This is the greatest philanthropic plum of the generation waiting to fall into your hands, and I want you to have the benefit of it," the Rockefeller Foundation's Frederick Gates—who himself lived with type 1—enthused to John D. Rockefeller in support of the program. "New Serum Dooms an Age-Old Curse," read a headline in the *Evening Telegram*.

Yet in the same archival folder as these clippings I encountered a cache of 1920s letters from people around the world—Mexico, Costa Rica, India, Norway, France, Spain, Hungary, Brazil—describing in desperate longhand their symptoms of diabetes or those of loved ones, saying that they had somehow heard about insulin and pleading for access to it. I also found the standard reply to such requests: "[The Rockefeller's insulin provision] activities, however, have not gone beyond this country."[16]

At the time, the dynasty's global health arm—the Rockefeller Foundation, which administered its International Health Division—was aggressively promoting numerous programs in remote corners of the world: malaria, yellow fever, tuberculosis, and its hookworm eradication campaign. Why was insulin deemed worthy of support in North America but not in other countries, when there was clearly demand for it everywhere?

In stark contrast to the pleading letters for insulin pouring in from around the world, the Rockefeller hookworm eradication campaign inspired markedly mixed sentiments—including in the part of Belize where Jordan was later born: "In southern districts, where most of the people are Caribs, it was found almost impossible to get them either to come up for examination or to construct privies," exclaimed one Rockefeller report. Some Belizeans were so resistant to the campaign that the colonial government of British Honduras passed the Hookworm Ordinance, stating that any person "without reasonable excuse" for withholding their excrement from the Rockefeller staff could be detained in jail "as the Court orders until a sample of his feces is obtained."[17] In short, hookworm testing and pharmaceutical treatment were at times being forced on people who actively resisted them, even at the risk of imprisonment. Meanwhile, with diabetes, desperate pleas for insulin therapies were arriving from around the world, without institutional recognition of any medical necessity outside the United States and Canada.

This strand of thinking persists even today. An infectious disease like hookworm is considered a pressing international priority, a "tropical" disease of poor populations and nations. But the global rise of diabetes (even when spreading much faster than infectious diseases like hookworm) has been framed as a different class of disease: a condition of *individual* responsibility—personally tragic but not collectively urgent to address as a society, or under any institution's ethical mandate in particular.

Uneven responses like these are spliced throughout global health archives of the past century, becoming difficult to ignore even when trying to conduct contemporary research on other topics. Just before coming to Belize in 2009, for example, I found myself doing some brief comparative research about guinea worm eradication and diabetes in

Northern Ghana's capital of Tamale—a lively city echoing with prayer calls and dense with bicycles and affable goats, surrounded by expanses of West African red-earth savanna. I will never forget the morning when I started off observing the bustling program office for guinea worm eradication. Inside the office, several dozen campaign staff, Ghanaian Ministry of Health officials on laptops, and Carter Center consultants were debating how best to locate a woman with guinea worm who had run away to avoid treatment. Guinea worm hurts for several days but doesn't kill, though it appears grotesque to foreigners who are not accustomed to seeing three-foot-long parasites. These worms have been the target of major U.S.-driven eradication efforts for several decades. Later that same morning, I traveled a few minutes across town to the public hospital's weekly diabetes clinic for the Northern Region, where more than thirty patients waited outside for hours for a doctor who never arrived.

I waited awkwardly with them on the wooden benches of the hospital courtyard until they were finally sent home for the day. My collaborator in Tamale, Emmanuel, translated from Dagbani, and I took notes as people who wanted to talk approached me to describe their routines living with diabetes in a region where over half the rural population survives on less than a dollar a day. Several people described walking dirt paths by lantern light from their far-flung villages or crossing rivers by canoe to reach a road that would lead to the hospital by dawn. As was clinic policy, the first thirty patients who arrived at the Friday diabetes clinic were handed ticket-like numbers, and the rest were sent home until the following week. "I am number seventeen," offered the young woman next to me. She had arrived by *tro-tro* around 4:00 A.M. to hold a place.

When I met with the government doctor the next week, he explained he had been called away on another emergency. He spoke about the difficulty of being the only doctor assigned to treat diabetes in a region of 1.8 million people, and only on Friday mornings. "I am one man," he said. "It is just me." He told me the weekly clinic felt much different than when it first opened; many of their original patients had already died.

Outside his office door, a man with no legs was being carried toward us on the shoulders of two young men in lieu of a wheelchair. "We used to have dozens of children with type 1 diabetes here," the physician said, but there were frequent interruptions in the region's insulin supply. The emotional labor of triaging insulin often fell to pharmacists, who had to decide which of the prescriptions they would actually fill with the very limited supply. Children first. "They used to come every

Friday. But many of them lived in the villages. We lost them; they died, one by one. They are all gone now."

"What about the Salifu girl?" asked his assistant, an attentive man in a long robe who had worked at the diabetes clinic since it first opened years ago. "We haven't heard anything since she went back to Kampong." The doctor nodded and smiled faintly in recognition. "That's right, we do have one left. Her name was Safia."

Neglected tropical disease philanthropy and global health aid become a different picture when thinking of these comparative scenes (the same city's gutted public diabetes clinic versus its bustling guinea worm eradication program office, and countless other places like them) as *coterminous realities*, drawing from the same limited pool of healthcare workers and monies spliced into vertical programs.

An ocean away, these encounters nonetheless helped me understand that what I was seeing in Belize was part of a longtime worldwide problem. Patients, families, and other caregivers alike were struggling to achieve diabetes treatment regimens in overstrained health systems where neither type 1 nor type 2 diabetes has historically been considered high priority by foreign institutions or international communities. As is the case in most postcolonial countries, Belize's health system has been deeply contoured by an "alphabet soup" of acronyms belonging to foreign NGOs, where piecemeal funding over the past century has inevitably come with certain priorities and strings attached.

But during the second year of my fieldwork, I saw part of a major effort to change this storyline: the rollout of a new National Health Insurance program to three of the country's six districts, Belize's aim to extend primary health services and a basic drug formulary to people in half the country—including insulin for those with diabetes. The hope was that this would be the pilot phase leading to an extension of the program to the entire country. But funding has been strained (largely due to Belize's struggles with serious international debt, following structural adjustment).[18] Some said it was possible the national insurance program may even scale back in the future rather than expand. When I last visited Belize in 2019, the local hospital was again out of insulin.

As in many countries, receiving a diagnosis of diabetes in Belize does not automatically translate into inclusion in national statistics. In Belize, there was no statistical information available on the prevalence of type 1 diabetes at the time of my research and no specialized state program or policy yet to support children with the condition. When I interviewed the charismatic president of the Belize Diabetes Association in 2010, he spoke about his dream of building programs to bring together local families dealing with type 1. "They are usually okay if their parents are involved," he said carefully, when I asked. "But it would be good to have some support. We could at least get a registry of their names, of the children who have it. So we will know."

OTHER ORPHANS

"AIDS orphan" is a well-known category of vulnerability in bureaucracy and activism, but there is no such thing as a "diabetes orphan" on paper or in global health policy. So when Jordan's mother died from diabetes shortly after he turned three, that left him living in a role that lacked a recognized name.

Social scientists write a lot about the power of labels:[19] the reductions and politics that they inevitably entail and what it's like for people to inhabit them. In Belize I met several young adults like Jordan who had grown up without one or both parents (the flexible definition often used to classify AIDS orphans), and I found myself wrestling with questions of how their life experiences were shaped by nonexistent techno-bureaucratic categories. Yet there was Jordan, and his stories.

His mother's name was Tessa. She'd risked a lot to have him: "The ultimate complication of type 1 diabetes in combination with pregnancy is maternal death."[20] It was once considered essentially fatal for women with type 1 diabetes to have children. Even today, having diabetes prior to pregnancy is still "a major risk factor for spontaneous abortions and congenital malformations"[21]—although this risk to the fetus drops to very low in a context where excellent blood sugar control is maintained by using insulin analogs (such as lispro and aspart, more often called Humalog and Novolog).[22] Neonatal growth often occurs during intense bursts, causing unexpected dips and spikes in the mother's sugar, part of why one study found that "the mortality of type 1 diabetic mothers was 109 times greater than in the general population."[23]

Analog treatments, now standard care in some places, were not easily available through the public system in southern Belize, where simply keeping a mother with diabetes supplied with basic insulin injections or access to a working glucometer constituted a meaningful accomplishment. Many experts recommend that pregnant women with diabetes follow an involved regimen: "Pre-conception counseling, carbohydrate counting, use of insulin analogues, continuous subcutaneous insulin infusion (insulin pump) therapy and real-time continuous glucose monitoring with alarms for low glucose values."[24] I imagine that this list would make most caregivers working in small towns or rural villages in Central America want to toss up their hands and laugh helplessly even today, let alone back in the 1980s, when Tessa was pregnant with Jordan.

The dangers of type 1 during pregnancy are greatly increased by not having access to tools like glucometers. Maternal death can be caused by ketoacidosis in cases where high blood sugar goes untreated—but in contexts of partial medical availability, maternal death is more often caused by blood sugar that crashes too low to sustain life. This puts mothers in a double bind, since "tight metabolic control of diabetes during pregnancy that is mandatory for the normal development of the fetus may expose the mother to life-threatening hypoglycemia"[25]—in other words, the more carefully a mother tries to control her blood sugar for the sake of her baby, the more she puts herself at risk for a potentially fatal hypoglycemic episode, particularly while sleeping. This risk peaks at night and can result in so-called dead-in-bed syndrome, which researchers estimate accounts for 6 percent of deaths in people with type 1 under the age of forty.[26]

Despite severe diabetes complications and incomplete medical resources, Tessa managed to survive pregnancy and give birth to Jordan. She lived for several years afterward. What it took for her to manage this double feat, I can only guess. Yet given all the mother-to-child risks that scientists are now examining during mothers' deliveries, it is striking how childbirth with diabetes contrasts with HIV/AIDS.

Obviously, as a classic infectious disease, HIV/AIDS transmission works through very different biological mechanisms than diabetes risk. But medical care during pregnancy is crucial for both conditions. Antiretroviral drugs (ARVs) are now provided nearly worldwide for both parents and children with HIV/AIDS—however imperfectly such a program might function, even extremely poor countries at least have one. Yet there has not been analogous global consciousness or policy supporting diabetes. I struggled to understand why providing ARVs to a pregnant mother or recent orphan with HIV/AIDS is perceived as an automatic "ethical imperative," but ensuring drug provisions for a mother or child who will die without insulin is not.

In *The Republic of Therapy*, anthropologist Vinh-Kim Nguyen describes the advent of new HIV/AIDS drugs (known as HAART, or highly active antiretroviral therapy) with an analogy that perhaps accidentally underscores this comparison: "HAART marked the advent of a therapeutic revolution akin to the discovery of insulin for the treatment of diabetes. An illness that was previously fatal, in most cases, within a few years of diagnosis, is now treatable and has been transformed as a result into a chronic condition."[27] Yet perplexingly, these drugs to treat HIV/AIDS have quickly become more accessible in many poor countries than the consistent supplies of insulin they have been likened to—even though the suite of HAART drugs only began development in the 1990s, and insulin therapy will soon celebrate its centennial birthday.

Something besides pharmacological breakthroughs alone shapes the drastic differences in global availability of seemingly comparable therapies, returning us to the imaginations driving "political will" and social movements in global health politics.

However interventions are prioritized on paper—often with an emphasis on AIDS, malaria, and tuberculosis, contagious conditions often referred to as the "Big Three"—coexisting conditions can rarely be so neatly pulled apart in practice. For example, the immunological toll of having any kind of diabetes can make patients nearly twice as susceptible to malaria and three times as likely to acquire TB. Patients who have diabetes are often less responsive to TB treatment drugs, which (like many pharmaceutical treatments for infectious conditions) can wreak havoc on blood sugar for people with diabetes.[28] Likewise, drugs to treat HIV/AIDS can actually *cause* insulin resistance and diabetes in up to 25 percent of patients—a poorly understood side effect now creating painful iatrogenic ricochets in many countries where AIDS medications are finally accessible. The availability of ARVs is due in large part to major international relief efforts. But these same programs do not supply insulin to HIV/AIDS patients who develop diabetes from their ARVs. "We are getting to the point now that more and more of our AIDS patients actually die of diabetes," one doctor told me.

I met several patients who lived with both AIDS and diabetes in Belize. One man named Raul said he thought his diabetes first started after he resorted to taking expired ARVs when no other regimen was available. Another man with both AIDS and diabetes named Sammy asked me to return the following day for an interview because he was having trouble breathing at the time. I returned the next day to hear the numbing news that Sammy had died unexpectedly during the night, wearing a pair of pajamas that said over and over in tiny font *Who wears the pants?* He was thirty-six years old. It was the first time I had met somebody on the day they died, and I felt unnerved by the Cuban doctor's exhausted laughter as he told me that his patient's cause of death was "unknown" and that he was having trouble filling out the paperwork. Comorbid diseases and treatments might be separated into vertical treatment programs, but people live and die in their unparsed entanglements.

The story of comorbidities can be dizzyingly untrackable even within an individual patient body, but their details become even more complicated when trying to understand how coexisting infectious and chronic conditions interface within families. I began thinking about these relational knots during conversations with a bubbly young AIDS patient named Sadie, who was also in her twenties then, just a few years older than me. She had an easy laugh and impeccable cursive handwriting with tiny spheres dotting each *i,* honed during her time spent on a 4-H scholarship program in Belmopan. As we got to know each other, she began writing little essays to give to me, explaining that she hoped I might be a conduit to people elsewhere who might find them interesting. She filled an entire notebook with longhand letters and word games and had her aunt bring it to me before I went home. Sadie called this being "pen pals" with me, although we lived just minutes apart at the time. It strikes me only now that this is the first time I am writing back.

Sadie was unable to get a steady job—in part because she couldn't breathe some days, in part because of the stigma shadowing *Aidsi* (the Garifuna term for HIV/AIDS) there—and she survived largely through the generosity of her aunts, who often shared food with her. Yet this left Sadie in a perpetual state of indebtedness that had to be delicately managed, an obligation that weighed on her mind. She owned no stove or refrigerator, so in order to prepare food, she had to make use of her aunts' kitchen. Eking by on a few coins' worth of personal groceries each day therefore became impossible because if you want to prepare a meal on another person's stove, using their fuel, in their kitchen, after they had many times shared food with you, then you had to make enough to offer the whole household—eight or nine people in all. So oftentimes Sadie would skip meals because she couldn't cook for herself if she wasn't able to share. Other times she would save enough to buy the cheapest foods she could to stretch for a large group, 1-2-3 oil with white flour or white rice bought by the pound.

"But my sugar is good," Sadie would reassure me with a smile. She liked to have it checked, though casually sticking her finger to draw blood at home (the way many around the world use a glucometer at home, without gloves or biohazard supplies) was not advisable with AIDS. She often asked about my diabetes research; Sadie's mother underwent a harrowing leg amputation because of diabetes and afterward had "given up" Sadie because she felt unable to care for her children. Because it had taken her mother out of the picture (leaving Sadie with the sense of being a partial orphan when she left home alone at a young age, she said), diabetes loomed large in her mind alongside the work of living with AIDS. Sadie wrote in a note dated July 2010:

> The other illness killing much faster than H.I.V./A.I.D.S. [are] illness like Diabetes, Cancer, Heart Disease and Asthma . . . illnesses that all bring weight loss, and also living questions with unsure answers.
>
> That is why I not only consider H.I.V./A.I.D.S. as Human Immune Virus Acquired Immune Deficiency Syndrome, I also consider it as being
>
> H uman—what we all are
> I ntimacy—closeness with our loved ones and society
> V ouch—giving assurance or guarantee
>
> A biogenist—believing in the spontaneous generation of life
> I ntercede—to plead on behalf of another
> D efensive—resistant to criticism
> S urvivor—to remain alive or in existence

Sadie had become accustomed to being branded in hospitals with acronyms that she found somewhat alienating, such as PLWA (an abbreviation that amused us both for being the same number of syllables as just saying "person living with AIDS"). I found her fascination with acrostics oddly meaningful, as if opening back up what Stanley Cavell once called the "non-speak or moon talk of acronyms."[29] Sadie was inventing alternative definitions, spinning the acronyms' rows of capital initials into something less like predetermined labels and more like algebra, equations full of unfixed variables. And *where*, I wondered, did she come up with *Abiogenist* as a substitution for the *A* in AIDS? I was not paying enough attention on the day she gave this text to me, and the enigmatic replacement slipped my notice until much later when I was back home reading her work more closely. It was only then that I finally noticed the wild-card term but barely recalled its meaning myself. The defunct theory of spontaneous generation stirred only vague memories for me of being a teenager in science class and learning about experiments in seventeenth-century glass jars; or biopoiesis theories, about how life sparked at the beginning of the world. But what did being an "Abiogenist" actually mean to Sadie, as she recast her condition in this spontaneous paradigm? Is that what it feels like sometimes to be any sort of orphan, trying to spark life from an interrupted generation? Did abiogenesis resonate with the feeling of trying to produce daily existence

An acrostic from Sadie's book,
"Don't Feel It to Know It."

(let alone hope) against the dead matter of a chronic illness? Or was she evoking something else entirely? She wrote:

G rief you'll leave behind and all its
R esponsibilities and
A nger—that being
V iolence among our family instead of
E quality

Like Jordan, Sadie's words cryptically shuttled back and forth across the dense constellations (whether recognized in policy or not) between parents and children, as well as between diabetes and other coexisting conditions like AIDS. "Don't Feel It to Know It," Sadie wrote elegantly on her notebook's title page. Its handwritten pages were filled with terms nested with other terms in blue and black ink, her work of redefining and making legible the weight of things between lines, and page after page of acrostics that read like puzzles she could decipher but not resolve.

The end that Sadie foresaw when she wrote the acrostic pictured above did not occur for another three years, during the months of winter wind that people call "kite season," while she was imprisoned for an alleged drug possession charge. She called me before she went to prison and told me that she was going to die in there; at a total loss to respond, I found myself returning that night to her notebook. Yet her constant reworking of death's terms had extended deliberately beyond its pages.

She explained to me that one morning, when she was pregnant in the hospital, her roommate died in the bed next to her. Sadie recalled seeing the young woman's spirit fly out the window, and this made her think. When her son was born shortly afterward, she learned that he was HIV negative and decided to name him Wasani, a Garifuna word meaning "our child." Its plural possessive, alive with love and pain, mapped a plan that signaled an intimate sacrifice Sadie would make, as she tied her baby immediately to a larger family collective. He was taken by caring aunts to be raised in Belize City, over a hundred miles away from the place where Sadie and I later spent afternoons talking in her lonely shack. The tiny structure was rickety and stiflingly hot, with no electricity or water. When I returned in 2014 several months after Sadie's death, it had not been converted into a new dwelling place, but instead got refashioned as a kiosk where passing tourists could stop to rent flippers and snorkels.

But during the time when she made that small place her home, Sadie spoke about her kids constantly. She was extravagantly proud from afar and wished—sometimes on the verge of tears—that she could visit them more often. It was in turn both comforting and excruciating to observe her children beginning to view other kin as their mothers. But she wanted to somehow keep distant enough to protect her kids from being irreparably shattered by her death, which she correctly understood was soon coming. Sadie was twenty-nine years old when she told me that she had designed things this way by inventing a different category of chance for her son, as if reworking the misrecognitions of bureaucracy by trying out a new label of the most intimate sort. "Our child" had never really been *hers*. Therefore, he could never be orphaned.

UNSTEADY UNITS

A "unit" of insulin began as an odd measurement: it was the precise liquid dose that would induce low blood sugar in a fasting rabbit.[30] This invented metric caused significant confusion in the early days of drug development because there were sizable differences between the plump four-pound bunnies used for insulin testing in 1920s Toronto (where the Canadian team that discovered insulin was based) and the lean two-pound rabbits in the laboratories in Indianapolis (where Eli Lilly, the U.S. pharmaceutical company licensed to mass-produce insulin, was headquartered).[31]

Establishing a uniform international rabbit size was only the first step on the road to standardizing marketable insulin, which at first could vary dangerously from batch to batch. The whole process was particularly complex because each drop of insulin injected into someone's stomach or thigh first had to be literally extracted from the pancreas of another creature. Until scientists figured out how to synthesize insulin in laboratories in the early 1960s, the drug companies manufacturing insulin inevitably created their products from vats of bloody animal pancreases in their factories' production lines, requiring over two tons of pig parts to extract eight ounces of insulin.[32]

Not just farms but also oceans are teaming with insulin, although it is inconveniently located inside the pancreases of swimming fish. John Macleod, the seasoned Scottish professor who would controversially come to share the Nobel Prize for insulin's discovery with Banting, envisioned harvesting the necessary islets from monkfish and stingray-like skates. One summer, his students paid a team of children to travel on an Atlantic trawler with the National Fish Company for the purpose of bottling the fish's pancreatic tissue, but they soon "learned that it was impossible to gather islets of Langerhans as fast as the fisherman gutted one catch of cod and washed the mess overboard."[33] For a brief time before World War II, Japanese scientists also extracted insulin from whales. Various other animal sources in vogue in their day have included pigs, clams, and water buffalo. Sensitivities to these animals could thus cause welts and other allergic reactions; for instance, Nurse Norma once recounted to me the experience of going into a coma in Belize from pork insulin, which was how she first learned she was allergic to pigs and switched back to beef-derived injections.

Another of the top experts of the 1920s, Bert Collip, contributed tremendously to stabilizing insulin's preliminary formula by adding alcohol, becoming part of the history-making Canadian team alongside doctors Banting, Best, and Macleod. But Collip later tarnished the brilliant reputation he had earned as part of Banting's team by erroneously announcing in *Nature* that he had discovered an insulin-like substance in green onions and potato peels.[34] These scientists' extensive searches for sources of insulin throughout nature's diversity of plants and animals also contributed to refining its formulas and mechanisms—such as when it was discovered that insulin's action could be slowed down and made "long-acting" by mixing it with fish sperm, regulating the absorption of its proteins.

"Insulin, which is both a hormone and protein, is a balled-up string of chemicals called amino acids."[35] Each batch is made by living organisms—which is what makes insulin a "biologic"—one of the few major modern drugs that cannot be made into a pill (though many attempts remain underway). Its amino acid chains break down in the human digestive system, which is why insulin is useless if swallowed and still must be injected by needle or intravenously under the skin to be effective. The entire history of insulin extraction therefore would not have been possible if another milestone in medical history had not preceded it—the hypodermic syringe, dating back to the 1850s but constantly evolving, from heavy glass and stainless steel to plastic and rubber varieties like today's specialized insulin syringes, standardized in 1949 to be uniquely marked in units of one-hundredth of one milliliter. Most insulin syringes today are disposable, made for one-time use, but they get reused constantly in homes across the world (including in Belize). Insulin syringes' highly specialized units could also create confusion of their own: I once observed a home visit where someone had acquired a syringe marked in centiliters and almost used its numbers to administer the prescribed insulin units to her father, which would have resulted in a potentially lethal overdose. From time to time, pharmaceutical companies have also tried to market an inhalable kind of insulin, misting through a plastic-tubing apparatus that resembles some component of a college sophomore's novelty bong. Relying on perfectly healthy lungs, it is known for uneven dosing.

A basic difficulty in calibrating doses comes from the body's constant and intricate flux in its oscillating methods for delivering insulin, so pharmaceutical replication of the process requires an elaborate variety of offerings. In 1951, a molecular biologist finally discerned the structure of bovine insulin (just three amino acid residues different from human insulin), and the gene that made insulin was later located at the top of chromosome 11. The subsequent research breakthroughs that followed meant that each dose no longer needed to be extracted from an animal; soon, various formulas of synthetic human insulin could be made in the laboratory. By the late seventies, researchers announced they had managed to produce human insulin by splicing a rat gene into E. coli bacteria. Within five years, Eli Lilly brought genetically engineered insulin to market.

This paved the way for later biosynthetic recombinant insulin brands that have since become the norm. The production of Humulin, for instance, involves thawing a tube of E. coli from a "master cell bank" that was frozen in the 1980s, feeding the bacteria sugar and antibiotics as it doubles every twenty minutes in enormous tanks called fermenters, and then triggering the bacteria to produce insulin that soon gets harvested in a many-staged process (including being purified in electrified columns and getting turned into stable crystallized powder).[36] Other biotech fields have dabbled with experimental techniques such as biofarming, in which human genes are spliced into yellow-blossoming safflower plants and grown in fields as "prairie insulin."

Today, the average pharmacy in the U.S. will carry at least a dozen insulin varieties, each with its own peaks and valleys of efficacy: fast-acting bolus insulin to be taken with meals; slow and steady basal insulin to provide healthy background levels of glucose management; cloudy "intermediate-acting" NPH insulin, invented by European biochemists at Nordisk who toyed with crystalline zinc molecules in existing formulas; and a growing multiplicity of premixed bolus and basal blends such as Novolin 70/30 or Humalog 75/25, which require less finely calibrated precision and provide built-in convenience in the form of fewer injections. Some insulins (including Humalog) have a smell reminiscent of scotch and Band-Aids because of the cresol that helps preserve their stability. This scent was almost undetectable to me but was pungent with memory for some everyday injectors.[37]

In practice, even the most basic taxonomy of insulin often gets very loosely adapted in poorer countries. Some private pharmacies in Belize chose not to stock insulin at all because it was easy to fatally overdose if people did not have proper access to glucometers, and they did not want to risk the responsibility. Government posts, meanwhile, prescribed insulin widely—but at times had to change patients' regimens from visit to visit, depending in part on what was in stock at the time.

Some patients learned to be flexible and creative in taking the kinds of insulin available to them. For example, some days only Novolin would be found locally. Maybe you would forget the name of the exact type of insulin you usually take (something I observed frequently), and no one would be able to locate its paper trail, especially if you had gotten it from another clinic or country or mission group. Or perhaps that kind wouldn't be available at a new place where you were receiving care or wouldn't be familiar to the caregiver there—situations that were usually negotiated by the doctor prescribing a 70/30 insulin formula, reckoned the safest bet. But all the numbers could be hard to keep track of—at times, people went home confused at the differing doses prescribed to them from various places as types of insulin changed, bringing new doses to memorize and daily regimens to reshuffle.

Yet beyond issues of differing units, the number attached to insulin that concerned Jordan most of all was its price. This began to change toward the end of his life, but when he was growing up there was no state program to provide affordable insulin to children with diabetes.

Family members occasionally bought him a vial out of pocket, or he might receive one sporadically from a nurse at the hospital or through someone's kindness, but this did not amount to anything like a constant supply. Jordan—and, I suspect, many other people like him living with type 1 diabetes in the world's margins—followed no consistent medical protocol over time. He took the insulin he could access as it became available to him, a regimen patched together from mismatched bolus and basal injections and missing doses. It only cost about ten dollars a bottle when he was a teenager, still often out of reach for a struggling family or entrepreneurial youth.

What I can tell you about Jordan at times feels generic, but the drug that shaped his story still is not. As historian Jeremy Greene and Kevin Riggs explore in their essay "Why Is There No Generic Insulin?"[38] this long series of formula evolutions and updated patents are key factors in the persistent issue of what some have called "insulin sticker shock."[39] Insulin prices vary hugely for people depending on their resident country and insurance plans, and several pharmaceutical companies have made efforts to lower pricing in poor countries, but some prices are actually currently rising for a complex mix of reasons.[40]

Some attribute these price hikes to the fact that key formulas are about to come out of patent, so companies are trying to make what additional profit they can before generics flood the market;[41] others say that corporations rely on insulin as their "golden goose" during times when other drugs fail to create their anticipated market splash and have coordinated "shadow pricing" schemes to raise prices in unison, techniques that Jose Gomez-Marquez charts in "Insulinomics."[42] In 2019, the price of insulin in U.S. contexts reached costs for some people of more than one thousand dollars per vial, leaving a growing number of patients also unable to afford basic access.[43] Grieving family members placed cardboard tombstones on the steps in front of the U.S. drug companies that make insulin, as tributes to loved ones who have died without it. When I saw the photos, I found myself imagining a version of their cardboard cemetery that captured the scale and duration of how widely "Living with Type 1 Diabetes When You Can't Afford Insulin"[44] has been happening in the world. Of the countries included in a recent survey, insulin cost the most (in relation to average incomes) for patients in Zambia.[45]

The social relations inflected by insulin's highly variable costs generate different personal expectations and legal norms: for example, California courts once ruled that U.S. parents whose child died from insufficient insulin treatment were accountable for second-degree murder.[46]

More recently, some are trying to sue companies over unaffordable insulin, dramatizing a global issue of pricing. A study in India tracked the actual cost to families for treating type 1 diabetes in a context of poverty. It found that the cost of treatment for a single type 1 patient was 16–23 percent of a family's total income, depending on whether or not the child had to be hospitalized. In lower-income groups in India, this figure was significantly higher: it cost 59 percent of an entire family's annual income to buy insulin for a single type 1 outpatient[47]— *more than half* a struggling household's money for food, rent, and clothes for the entire family. Although these figures obviously shift a bit from country to country, they begin to show the impossible choices that many poor families face. Such quandaries raise the question of how family units—like insulin units and hospital units—collide and compound.

Trying to understand how these numerous elements had come together and inflected each other in Jordan's specific trajectory, one day I took a bus to his village.

Jordan had described to me, in almost obsessive detail, the stretch of road that led there. Sometimes he couldn't tell whether his blood sugar was very high or too low, but he could sense the feeling of disequilibrium that signaled he urgently needed to go to the hospital—dizzy, sweaty, itchy, thirsty, nauseous, and shaky, with flickering vision that could signal he was beginning to hallucinate—and Jordan knew that if he was unlucky, the trip might take more than a day on foot. I can only picture him as I knew him later, walking along the side of the road time and again over the years, with determined steps and uneven gait, wearing an ill-fitting polo shirt billowing on his thin frame.

He recalled counting things to make the time go faster as he walked along the sun-scorched highway trying to hitchhike: the number of cars that passed him as he walked or the exact tally of buses that might or might not allow him a free lift to the hospital out of charity on days when his former school principal (who had often dipped into her own pockets to help him) wasn't able to give him a few dollars for the fare.

Myself, I traveled Jordan's well-tread route in fast-forward, on board the public line of a repurposed American elementary school bus with the *S* and the *H* scratched off its original labeling (the "COOL BUS"). The driver told me that we had reached Zericote village, and I stepped down onto the highway near a stretch of empty-looking fields. I thought uneasily of the women who had been attacked or killed in recent years along this road: a Guatemalan mother; a British medical student; a woman from the United States riding a bicycle; the Belizean woman whose body Nurse Suzanne was recently called to tend to after her son was found holding her in the high grasses, unable to speak after witnessing her rape and murder. The same kindly principal who had helped Jordan became his stopgap caregiver, too. My heartbeat quickened as I walked through weeds toward the low buildings far ahead, which I hoped and doubted made it appear that I knew what I was doing there.

The wooden houses on stilts on the edge of the village looked like sinking ships or tiny arcs in a permanent state of readiness for the next storm. I knew Jordan was not there but kept thinking I saw him anyway. As I walked deeper into the community's center, there were also active signs of construction: piles of cement blocks, metal rods jutting out of concrete foundations—meaning that many houses contained both an actual architecture and a phantom rebar superstructure outlining the contours of what someone hoped it might grow to be.

Zericote's land also had a reputation for swarming with yellow-specked "doctor flies," so named for their painful needle-sharp bite, which feels like getting an injection. I stopped at a tiny grocery shop with an old rocking chair on the porch. They sold flour, rice, brown sugar, and white sugar from four round trash cans next to an old-fashioned double scale. The prices were listed on a black slate board hanging from the ceiling, along with the chalked prices for a few other staples sold by the pound: lard, pigtail, beans, salt, onions, and butter (lard cost only half as much as butter). When I left the store, some young children outside said they would show me where to go.

We walked past very old women playing bingo under a tree, arranging scallop-edged Belizean pennies on their boards; past a home with peeling paint and a battered sign that said POST OFFICE. Men called "Spanish" by local Kriol residents (mostly from Guatemala and Honduras) rode past in the back of packed trucks, headed to nearby citrus plantations—where fruits were grown and then quickly boiled down to concentrate for exported juices, making the air smell sweetly of grapefruit and oranges.

Walking through the unfamiliar terrain, I felt anxious at the thought of meeting the people who somehow both had and hadn't been Jordan's family—unsure what I was really looking for, but hoping that another perspective might help fill out some larger story that was already missing too many pieces. "Is this their house?" I asked the child leading me along when we paused in front of a shack on the dirt road, but the little girl with seashells looped into her hair only giggled.

The children who led me there scattered at the sounds of footsteps across floorboards. I was alone on the porch when the door swung open.

MANY MACHINES

Somewhere in Belize, the electronic glucometer that Jordan once received must still exist in some form—perhaps used each morning to measure another teenager's blood sugar; or forgotten on a kitchen shelf, awaiting a replacement batch of digital test strips; or reduced to a charred lump of microchip-studded plastic buried in the region's land-fill, which perpetually smoldered on the edge of the highway, emitting uncannily colored flames and chemical-smelling smoke.

By the time I interviewed people years later, no one could remember the exact make or model of Jordan's first glucose machine—some said it was an Accu-Chek, others a OneTouch. But everyone remembered the woman who gave it to him, his mother's friend. "I call her mom," Jordan told me of Lorel, who by then was working in Chicago. But at first, I knew Lorel only through the medical artifacts she had provided, particularly the glucometer.

Glucometers are integral to this story because they play a vital role in carefully dosing insulin. Since proper doses depend in part on how high or low blood sugar is to begin with, it matters to have relatively consistent ways to gauge that starting point. This was particularly important in a context where many people didn't have access to other common blood sugar tests, such as hemoglobin A1c measures, which gauge a person's three-month average glucose level to give a sense of how stable things look over time. Another missing gauge is continuous glucose monitoring, which consists of a filament inserted into bodily fluids under the skin, the sensor kept in place with a medical-grade adhesive sticker, often on the stomach or upper arms. It communicates information about the wearer's blood sugar levels to a monitoring unit, via radio waves. This creates metrics that will sound an alarm about highs or lows (the main reason users wear them), but in turn must be calibrated against a glucometer's finger-stick measures twice a day. While the circulation of glucose meters anywhere inevitably involves the meaningful rituals of people learning to measure and monitor their own bodies, there was also something more than textbook "biomedicalization" logic at play in the unruly ways these technologies mattered and moved. The machines' own chemistry became part of what structured their users' stories.

Early glucometers like the 1972 Eyetone had to be carried in what resembled a suitcase and plugged into the wall. From what I am able to reconstruct, most struggling patients in the era of Jordan's mother would not have had access to this first generation of machines in domestic settings at all—for a huge variety of reasons, including the fact that most villages in southern Belize were not connected to the electrical grid until several decades afterward. These bulky machines detected glucose levels in blood using reflected light, captured by a photoelectric cell that translated shades of blue color into a numerical readout using a swinging needle. Engineer Anton "Tom" Clemens at Ames Company (now part of Bayer) developed the first model that worked this way, which hit markets in 1970. Clemens later recalled the way most physicians initially balked at the idea that patients could safely perform blood testing at home, believing these machines required the expertise of a doctor's office or emergency room. According to a long trail of wary publications over the ensuing decade, North American and European medical establishments at the time heartily opposed the idea of patients self-monitoring their own blood glucose. Many considered it risky amateurship and "a dangerous practice."[48]

But the increasingly popular meters became more and more user-friendly over the years, and soon there was a flooded market filled with competing technologies spanning North America, Europe, and Asia. Corporate one-upmanship in the quest for new patents made machines increasingly easier to read, less expensive, smaller in size, and more accurate to use at home. Requiring larger drops of blood at first, many worked with a menacing-looking finger-stick apparatus, recalled by some patients as "the guillotine." One odd generation of meters, such as Boehringer Mannheim's Reflomax, sold in the harvest-orange hue that characterized many other fashionable appliances in the seventies, had a dial covered with tick marks like the padlock on an old gym locker. In 1980, the Dextrometer had the first digital display. A later generation of models instead had small screens and buttons, resembling credit card swipe machines used at cash registers (including the Reflolux, which later became the popular Accu-Chek series). Interestingly, Glucometer was originally the name for another model that Ames introduced in collaboration with a Japanese company called Kyoto Daiichi; but the easy-to-use machine's catchy name became so popular over time that it is now often used as a generic term for any glucose meter.[49]

Although they share the same general name, each glucometer can use only the strips specifically designed not just for the brand but for the model—meaning that you must pay attention not only to whether your device is made by Abbott or Bayer or Nova or Sanofi-Aventis but also to additional micro-specifications. For example, if you acquired an Accu-Chek glucose meter (made by Roche), is it an Accu-Chek Aviva or an Accu-Chek Nano or an Accu-Chek Compact? A Compact or a Compact Plus? Missing any of these details could mean your savings are spent on a jar of strips that will not work.[50]

Glucometers' role today in frontline diagnosis also hinges on a painful irony: such measures help to make visible an enormous population of people living with diabetes in contexts of poverty, many of whom cannot consistently access the same meters vital for day-to-day care. In Belize in 2010, glucometers—some purchased at grocery stores or local clinics, others acquired from visiting care groups or sent by relatives in the United States or elsewhere abroad—were priced around fifty to one hundred dollars. Some corporations even provided the devices for free if you bought enough test strips, which are the truly expensive component of this system. Prices for the test strips are declining today, but in 2010 they went for around fifty to seventy dollars per jar of fifty strips (which would last less than a month for someone testing twice a day, but were often stretched much further by people trying to make supplies last). A thriving gray market flourishes around them even in the national contexts they *are* specifically designed for,[51] a problem reflected in suspect website sales or signboards like CASH FOR DIABETIC TEST STRIPS posted along U.S. roadways.[52] According to a CNN report, in 2012 diabetes test strips became the number one most frequently stolen item in the United States, surpassing alcohol and cigarettes—and raising disturbing questions about the systems in place when a top target of criminalized theft is entwined with health-seeking behavior.[53]

I saw countless machines that were unusable or broken. For those who could acquire them, these devices commonly indexed the generosity of relatives abroad or served as artifacts of transient philanthropic interventions—networks difficult to sustain day in and out. I encountered malfunctioning meters with elaborate features such as Bluetooth compatibility, on the shelves of homes without electricity, artifacts of vast gaps between the contexts these machines' designers envisioned and the places where they have become necessary. Patients stored their devices on kitchen shelves or carried them in weathered plastic bags, looking for ways to repair them. People's bodies and devices often seemed to be wearing out together.

Although glucometers can seem like the closest thing there is to a "solution in a box" for global diabetes management,[54] their upkeep entails engaging a transnational supply line of expensive, complex parts. While portable, these devices require intricate socio-technical networks of specific components to maintain: codes and calibrating fluid; lancets to draw blood from fingertips (some people substituted safety pins or sewing needles); and lithium and other specialized imported batteries, shaped like small coins.

Managing these messy assemblages often became a family affair. Certain models left people "recoding" their machine's time stamp, which might allow recently expired strips to come back into circulation. Many said a jar that expired a day or two ago could still work just as well, but no one knew exactly when a strip was too far expired to be worth consulting: a month? a year? Of course, drawing such lines returns to much larger questions about glucose meters: How bad is less than ideal care—and how are people navigating its risks against the dangers of no care? I wasn't sure what the ethics of expiry backdating were in practice, but saw many cases when refusing to fiddle with a meter would have meant no way to test at all.

But even when a glucose meter wasn't working, people often kept these little machines in prominent places. Signifying more than fragmentation alone, such devices inevitably are also (as Sherry Turkle writes) "things we think with"[55]—reflecting logics of the places where they originated, to be sure, but also shaping what social interactions and ethical exchanges were possible between people on the ground. They were artifacts of care and intentions over time, perhaps waiting to be replenished by a new visitor or returning intervention. Sometimes people were able to have relatives use their own health insurance to cover the test strips and send them by mail, although this strategy was just as likely to result in a new machine. Through these networks, even poorer households might accumulate one or two unusable glucometers. These circulated in intimate economies of their own, traded and loaned. Strips might also be resold or scavenged for the slivers of gold and precious metals their electrodes contain, part of what makes them so expensive. Or so I had believed, until I read a *New York Times* article about glucometer gray markets

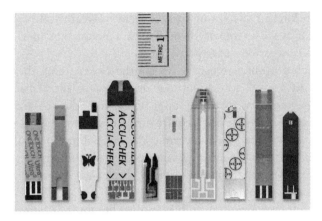

Testing strips for a variety of glucometer models.

in 2019 estimating that they only cost around ten cents each to print.[56]

I heard a story, perhaps an aspirational fiction, about the early days of diabetic test strips: There were two major competing companies shaping design when the first glucometer machines came out, one in England and another in Germany. A top employee of the British company described a proposal for an open machine that would read either company's strip. He called their German counterpart with a proposal to coordinate. According to his recollections, the German company turned down the idea and did not want their strips read by any but their own machines.[57] Hundreds of incompatible strips circulate today in this multibillion-dollar global industry.

While this structural premise has persisted over many decades, the machines themselves have changed constantly. Today, many meters' digital memory banks function like little computers and are designed to graph the glucose highs and lows of their owners—programming that by default assumes the machine's user is one individual person, who has a laptop or iPhone to collect and centralize the glucometer's data. Some machines like the Contour Didget even synchronize with Nintendo video game consoles.

But in Belize, many glucose meters had no parent devices to report back to for data collating. If readings could be downloaded to a base station somewhere, their graphs would often compile something different than a single person's fluctuating blood sugar over time. There would instead be the stop-and-start counts of barters and home visits, frequently charting not individual biologies but other kinds of exchanges and bodies: survey routes, mobile clinics, or sharing among families and neighbors.

Instead of a linear time line of breakthroughs, perhaps glucometers in that context could be better said to occupy a horizon where "things jump into relation but remain unglued."[58] Some scenes from Belize I remember like still-life images: The man who cut his test strips in half with a fishing knife, hoping to stretch the expensive jar twice as far, not realizing he was irreparably mangling the computerized microchips he had saved for a month to buy. A well-heeled couple in Dangriga who invited me over before breakfast one day to see how they test each other every morning: tissues pressed to their bleeding fingertips, him pouring grapefruit juice afterward as she laughed, still wearing her nightgown. They had enough savings and connections to acquire four different brands of glucose meters and could usually find matching strips available for at least one of them in Belize at any given time. One Maya shrimp farmer had received a FreeStyle machine from a "mission trip" medical group from Arkansas during their visit to Belize and could not acquire replacement strips for the meter anywhere in Belize or Guatemala. I hesitantly agreed to bring a replacement vial during one trip back to Pennsylvania—unavailable at CVS but finally located at Walgreen's. They sold for seventy dollars, which felt both too expensive not to strain our relationship and completely insufficient (since it was only a thirty-day supply anyway, thus perpetuating her initial problem). But the dilemma turned out to be moot: it ended up that she had a FreeStyle Lite, not an original FreeStyle, so even after I made the long trip down miles of dusty backcountry roads in a borrowed pickup truck, the butterfly-embossed strips didn't work on her machine. Another woman's glucose meter had been mailed from a donor in England, its replacement blood test strips sent as gifts but subject to heavy taxes at the post office. She had since become uncannily adept at multiplying any number by eighteen—the factor necessary to convert a European machine's readings (in mmol/l) to units of the Americas (in mg/dL) favored in Belize, an equation specific to the molecular weight of glucose.

Looking back, I wished I had counted all the broken mechanisms for counting. The devices showed how people with diabetes were living with fragments of care, and the labor it took to transform these incoming devices into something besides a nonsystem. They indexed much more than blood sugar. The stakes could be low or high: at its most extreme, not being able to test one's glucose could lead to miscalculating a dose of insulin. The comas caused by this so-called bottoming out could strongly resemble stroke symptoms and were common enough in Belize that one nurse I knew refused to prescribe insulin for type 2 at all, after seeing it cause numerous overdose "hypos" and deaths. In this way, glucometers at times also become part of charged mediations that occur whenever caregivers try to determine which patients could safely manage insulin.

Though glucometers at times reproduced global fragmentation, they could also become part of unlikely communication—such as the time no one could talk with an older patient with diabetes who had come to the hospital alone, speaking only Kekchi Maya. He wanted to leave and could not understand the Cuban doctor who was trying to convey in Spanish and then English that lab reports showed his sugar was still high. Finally, a Nigerian nurse was summoned to stick the Kekchi patient's finger and squeeze out a drop of blood onto the glucometer strip, so the screen could be held for him to see his count in context. As framed by the machine (the only translator available), his glucose was a language we could all understand. The patient nodded solemnly when he saw the number and lay back in bed.

Or consider what glucometer checks meant for Nancy, whose diabetes led to a doctor missing her renal cancer for several years, until it was badly metastasized. A mother in her fifties, Nancy's comorbidity with diabetes made her treatment particularly difficult—both chemo and kidney damage superadded to diabetes meant her blood sugar was constantly spiking, and her body was suddenly responding to her usual diabetes pills in unpredictable ways. On the day we had arranged for an interview at the country's first cancer center, which happened to be her birthday (her family surprised her with cake a day early to make sure she could keep it down), Nancy went into terrifying convulsions during chemo—perhaps some drug interaction with her diabetes pharmaceuticals, she would later speculate. She stopped breathing, her whole body jerking in wide arcs of motion. Following terse directions that the nurse called out, I sprinted from an adjacent building with an oxygen tank and pushed it with shaking legs down a seemingly endless hallway. The nurse grabbed the oxygen from me in the doorway of the room and expertly tended to Nancy until she stopped rocking wildly back and forth in the chemo chair, steadily smoothing her hair when it was over.

Rattled, I thought it might be better to postpone our exchange, but Nancy summoned me later and said she wanted to talk. During the interview it was hard not to think of the image of her seizing in the very same chair, everything fine again but crisis hovering just offstage. But maybe that was part of why she wanted to talk right then and pass the time on that slow drip; she never looked over at the needle taped in her arm, so I tried not to look at it either. Most of our conversation sidestepped cancer and the tests and the other doctors who had missed it for all those years, focusing instead on her doting family and her glucometer. She had a OneTouch that came with a little stapled workbook, lined with calendars, to write down five glucose counts each day. It was the only such book that I ever saw in Belize, filled out fastidiously with printed numbers in pencil and pen. Unlike malignancy, when it came to blood sugar, Nancy and her husband could follow along, incremental tallies indexing each step of her body's gains and losses. Nancy called the worn glucometer pamphlet her "little book of history," as if keeping herself in time.

Nancy had stage four cancer; Jordan would have had stage four diabetes by the time we met, if that had existed (no matter how serious complications become, it isn't biomedically recognized practice to label "stages" of diabetes). It was another uninvented category of person that Jordan could not be. So there was no palliation toward the end of his life, despite the serious pain, only basic diabetes treatments that continued moving in and out of his reach. His meters circulated in intimate exchanges and leaking economies: pawned for food, only to be bought back; once stolen by an aunt, allegedly in exchange for unpaid rent; later replenished by Lorel, who promised to send replacement parts from Chicago. The machine's metrics also gauged her present absence.

One night, shortly after I had contacted Lorel's sister in Dangriga and left my phone number, I received a call on my Belize cell phone from an unfamiliar U.S. area code. It was Lorel, calling me from Chicago. I barely had time to explain my project and go through my rehearsed request for a phone interview before she began talking, as if the story had been pent up and waiting to pour out. "Let me tell you something," she said. "This was a case of pure neglect." She described seeing Jordan one afternoon in front of a game room by the river in Dangriga years ago. For some reason, the gangly teenager looked familiar to her. He had been born with an ear tucked in on one side, perhaps due to the effects of sugar in the womb. "To me, I know this child from somewhere," Lorel said. Following her instinct, she stopped to ask his name and learned he was the son of her best friend, Tessa, who had died over a decade earlier. Lorel asked if he needed anything. "Jordan told me, 'I'm hungry.'"

Lorel's voice started to break over the phone. "He was shivering, like in snow."

Suddenly, there was a new character on the scene—offering last-ditch love, trying to undo neglect, buying time. Lorel reported that at first she had tried talking to Jordan's stepfamily, even offering them money for a time and paying a high rent for Jordan's little shack in Zericote.

"His aunt promised to take care of him, then sold his diabetes machine," Lorel said of the glucometer she had bought for Jordan. "I tried to get him back." Alongside hospital appointments, she had taken him to a private clinic in Dangriga run by a charismatic Nigerian physician, who combined evangelical prayer with his medical practice. "With the diabetes, he was so far gone. When I found Jordan he was skin and bones," Lorel recalled. By then, the glucometer that she gave him was only precisely quantifying damages that they didn't know how to stop.

Increasing numbers of people share these struggles. The global explosion of type 1 diabetes (now on the rise nearly as fast as type 2) raises questions about the factors contributing to its increased prevalence. The good news is that this increase might be partially attributed to the heartening fact that more people with type 1 are living healthily into adulthood and having children themselves. However, studies show that the children of people with diabetes—even in resource-rich medical systems—may have a slightly increased chance of getting the disease (a 2 percent risk, higher than the general population's risk of 1 percent).

What do these figures look like in more unevenly resourced contexts? There is virtually no real data on this topic. But it is known that when a mother receives incomplete medical care during her pregnancy and experiences badly fluctuating blood sugar over those crucial months or during delivery, it significantly increases the chance her child will also later develop diabetes, making intergenerational risk much steeper than it needs to be. Stretched-thin primary care, in other words, is not just treating type 1 in poverty—it is also a key contributor to its rising manifestations. And similar to type 2, an abundance of population studies suggest that the uptick in type 1 is also exacerbated by exposure to pesticide runoff from agriculture and other synthetic chemicals and pollution in our food, air, and waterways. In light of these escalating risk factors, the name "diabetes machine" that Lorel used for Jordan's glucose meter made me think back to Sarah's words and about how much of the world seems to be becoming a "sugar machine," requiring many other machines to survive.

Yet the minute I started to wax philosophical, Lorel pulled me back to the minutiae of daily care, where the routine struggles of Jordan's life had been borne out. "Sometimes I would go on my bicycle to take him some oatmeal," she said. "He was my baby." She felt torn that she had to return to Chicago for work. The money she earned from home nursing in U.S. eldercare was the reason she was able to support Jordan, but distance fractures too. "If I didn't have to go back to the States, maybe he would still be alive today," she said, her voice growing soft. "I tried to leave everything for Jordan. I bought him all this food before I go. And new sneakers."

"In your documentary," Lorel repeated, "it was a case of pure neglect, you have to put that. But . . ." her voice wavered. "Maybe you could go see the barrel of groceries I send for him. My sister Jessica has it in Dangriga." For some reason, that image of the cardboard barrel with nowhere to be delivered made us both break down. Never before or since have I had the experience of being on the phone with an absolute stranger and both of us bursting into tears, which says something about how few places existed for Lorel to channel mourning for a death like Jordan's. Her absence as she worked in Chicago "to save something" to send home for him was simultaneously a tie and a disconnect, a caring relation and a break in care. In the United States, dialysis and kidney transplants—treatment options unavailable to Jordan in Belize but flat-out necessary to continue his life—have been legally provided by the federal government since 1972, as part of Medicare.[59] But the products Lorel purchased in Chicago to fill the barrel for Jordan (a new Accu-Chek machine, matching test strips, and diapers) were the only pieces of the healthcare infrastructure it was possible to export.

The ancient Greeks once considered diabetes to be "a melting down of the flesh and limbs into urine," according to third-century medical chronicler Aretaeus the Cappadocian. He described the humiliating dilemmas often caused by diabetes's kidney damage and resulting urination issues: *"How can shame become more potent than pain?"* For a young man struggling with self-consciousness of all kinds, the loss of urinary control is perhaps the most anxiety-producing aspect of living with advanced complications of diabetes. Lorel explained that for years, Jordan tried to avoid the daily embarrassment of wearing bulky diapers. This usually made his condition less immediately noticeable but also introduced new fallibilities. Once, he could not hold it on a taxi ride home from the hospital, and the taxi driver jeered at Jordan with a string of emasculating insults when he saw the vehicle's wet upholstery.

Lorel found Jordan crying at home in humiliated silence, unable to hide his shame. Furious, Lorel got on her bicycle and searched the streets of Dangriga until she found the taxi driver. "I yelled at him. 'Have compassion,' I said. 'Don't you *see?*'"

Since talking with Lorel across the odd telephone reversal of me in her country and her in mine, I have often thought of the question she posed. What does it take to *see?* To make sense of what we are seeing? To know what can't be seen?

When glucose is high, a person's urine can leave behind a subtly visible powder of sugar, like a crystalline white dust. In fact, earlier glucose tests had been based on precisely such traces. Some of the first known technoscientific testing for diabetes was conducted with urine and bits of sheep's wool dipped in stannous chloride chemicals, which turned black to indicate the presence of sugar. Urine tests using paper steeped in alkaline indigo carmine were in vogue by 1883, when *Bedside Urine Testing* was published in England. The messy material culture of boiling your own urine was finally replaced in the 1940s by an Ames urine dipstick test for sugar, the Clinitest. Based on the major breakthroughs of dry-reagent chemistry (the technology behind litmus paper), this new type of urine testing later helped to inspire Dextrostix, the first blood glucose testing strips.

These older urine dipstick tests are now part of a new global controversy. Today's blood glucose machines are far more accurate than urine tests because they provide real-time blood glucose levels, whereas urine (by the time it's expelled) reflects the body's state several hours before. This, along with other limits in precision, now makes blood glucose meters a basic standard of care for home testing in affluent contexts. But in recognition that maintaining a working glucometer at home remains utterly out of reach for many patients in huge areas of the world, one of the International Diabetes Federation's (IDF) important policy and patient advocacy steps was to issue a position statement on glucose testing access. It boldly supported the use of urine testing at home for people with diabetes who cannot afford personal blood glucose meters. This official position statement on urine glucose testing was publicly issued by the IDF in 2005. The three-page document reads, in part:

> Before the advent of blood glucose monitoring in the 1970s, urine glucose monitoring was universally used, with many people able to maintain good control. Blood glucose monitoring has now replaced urine monitoring in resource-rich settings. However, insistence on blood glucose monitoring

in economically disadvantaged settings could result in no monitoring at all. . . .

- Urine glucose monitoring should continue to be available throughout the world.
- Education about its role and appropriate use should be part of essential education about diabetes for healthcare professionals and governments.
- It can be used separately to, or in conjunction with, blood glucose monitoring in particular circumstances and settings.
- It should continue to be included on the World Health Organization Essential Drugs List.
- The major promotion by industry of blood glucose monitoring should not result in the appropriate role of urine glucose monitoring being underestimated.
- As long as results are interpreted correctly, and limitations understood, it provides valuable information in persons with type 2 diabetes treated by diet or diet and tablets, in people with type 2 who use insulin, and in people with type 1 diabetes who cannot afford blood glucose testing. . . .
- Because it is significantly cheaper than blood glucose monitoring, it has a very important role to play in settings where blood glucose monitoring is not accessible due to cost, or where blood glucose monitoring can only be done relatively infrequently. This occurs in some situations in both developing and developed countries.
- Its use should be determined by the individual healthcare professional in conjunction with the person with diabetes, taking into account all circumstances.[60]

The IDF confirmed to me in 2017 that they had not updated this statement, though it is not widely publicized. Perhaps this relates to diplomatic negotiations with glucometer manufacturers, key players in diabetes policy arenas today. Yet controversies about digital glucometer machines versus urine testing are also tangled up in much larger debates in global health ethics: When is outdated basic technology a stopgap measure for pragmatically addressing inequality in the meantime, and when does it risk normalizing complacency with unequal standards of care? When can the donor visions at work in the name of corporate social responsibility become a mutually beneficial situation, even if vested interests do not easily align? Are there even any other options left for shifting the current system except from the inside? We are all caught amid so many machines.

Ultimately, in Belize at least, health workers I knew did not recommend urine dipstick tests for diabetes homecare because they weren't considered best practice. But the stark reality persisted: poorer patients often had no way to test their sugar at home at all. Once, at a local clinic, I asked how they dealt with this quandary and was surprised to find out that this simple alternative glucose test—costing pennies instead of dollars and requiring no machine—had been right there on the clinic shelves all along. It turned out that the same urine dipsticks used to check for infections measured not only leukocytes but also a row of other indicators, including nitrates, albumin protein, bilirubin, uro-bilinogen, pH levels, and—most important for people with diabetes—glucose and ketones, present in urine only when the body is off-balance. There were numerous cardboard boxes filled with urine test strip jars in storage, a visiting nurse added; it was one of the few things they easily kept in stock. She invited me to take a look. For a moment it felt like some sort of clue to alterative indices, which I suppose I was searching for at the time, trying to find a plot through the senselessness and pre-dictability of Jordan's fate. "Intended for use in the U.S.A.," read the bottle's evasive label.

What would it have meant for Jordan to have had these outmoded (but actually available) urine tests at home every day during the many years he was growing up without a glucometer? I pried off the jar's plastic lid and examined its contents, but they yielded no easy answers either; just little strips of rainbow-colored patches, paper bands expiring in a jar.

THE LIFE OF MUERTE

"Jordan made history," his stepmother, Agnes, told me with a smile.

I had not expected the woman who answered the door and found me on the porch that day in Zericote to extend such hospitality, but to my surprise she readily agreed to participate in an interview for my research, saying that Jordan had told her about working with me. She led me past her outdoor fire hearth and a hand-crank press for making coconut oil and up the wooden steps of another raised plank-board house. I found myself sitting next to Agnes in a small kitchen belonging to a wiry old woman, who told me to call her Aunt Lil. The kitchen's plywood shelves were lined with repurposed jars. Its bright wooden shutters were tied back with string, revealing jackfruit and tamarind trees. The two women spoke about Jordan with no detectable sense of tragedy, in a tone more like the mythic flavor of a tall tale. This made it at once very easy and very difficult to talk with them.

"Once, his blood sugar was over 1,000, and he was walking around. The doctors told us, we don't know how this was possible. He made history, *fi true.*" Lil laughed in assent, nodding at the memory. They handed me a copy of the paper from Jordan's funeral, which Lorel had sent money from Chicago to pay for. "Jordan (aka Muerte), 1989–2010," the program read. That was how I first learned that everyone had called Jordan by the nickname Muerte since he was a young teenager. In a place where Spanish was the third language, this was perhaps several degrees more polite than just calling him Death or Dead.[61]

"He is now flying God's Plane in Heaven," the paper said, next to a reading from Ecclesiastes 11. I looked it up later: *Rejoice, O young man, in thy youth; and let thy heart cheer thee in the days of thy youth, and walk in the ways of thine heart, and in the sight of thine eyes: but know thou, that for all these things God will bring thee into judgment.* The Xerox featured a blurry close-up photo. In the image, Jordan's gaze is level, his eyebrows slightly raised. It is difficult to say whether his expression is stoic, skeptical, or some other countenance of waiting.

"Jordan was not careful," Agnes repeated as I held the photocopy—never careful about what he ate, even when he didn't have medication to cover it. Before insulin's discovery, a so-called starvation diet was considered the best possible treatment to prolong life for children and teenagers with type 1 diabetes who otherwise would be poisoned by the carbohydrates in their food. It seemed this was related to what Agnes alluded to, in suggesting that Jordan was not "careful" by eating during times he did not have insulin coverage. "He take insulin sometimes," she added, the present tense of Kriol verbs haunting the stories of foreclosures they animated. She reported that Jordan continuously ate all the worst things: "He would save his coins to get biscuit, even mango." Depending on their location, fruits from some of the region's plentiful mango trees were at times considered common property—but this readily shared and accessible source of filling food was very high in sugar.[62] Lil and Agnes both affirmed that by the time he became a teenager, Jordan was constantly passing out from the increasing complications of his uncontrolled diabetes.

Studying the "enculturation" of another chronic condition, anthropologist Duana Fullwiley "found that people's ability to make-do with scant biomedical palliatives functionally filled a resource gap."[63] In the face of lacking technologies, Fullwiley observed how sickle cell patients in Senegal "find ways to get by with its chronic reality," manipulating bodily thresholds with a wide range of substances that come to stand in as medications, such as coffee, sugar, and water.[64] Sidney Mintz likewise emphasized the potential for using energy-giving substances for intervention when he reframed sugar, chocolate, and caffeine as "soft drugs."[65] During the years that Jordan spent stretching his insulin doses—or trying to survive until another dose could be obtained—cheap foods also became for him a way of "manipulating bodily thresholds."

"Jordan is always buying Ideal," Agnes told me of the dirt-cheap freezer pops, locally made of bright-colored frozen sugar water in a plastic tube or sandwich bag. Zericote village had several grocery shops with freezer and refrigeration chests. These community grocery shops are incidentally the very places where Partners in Health recommends that people with diabetes like Jordan, too poor to own a refrigerator at home, might consider storing their insulin alongside the ubiquitous cans of soda—bottled sugars and the bottled hormones needed to metabolize them chilled side by side. At around five U.S. cents, Ideals are perhaps the cheapest food available at an average grocery store. Because the liquid is frozen solid, it feels like eating food. Although adults with diabetes living in poverty were more likely to endure skipped meals by drinking sweetened coffee, Jordan became sick with diabetes as a young child. His "soft drug" of choice was popsicles.

People with uncontrolled diabetes sometimes told me that I could not understand what their cravings for sugar felt like. "Like you need it. You can't think, you can't think about other things." "Your body calls for the sweet." "Like you can't keep going if you can't find it." Yet these sensations are not necessarily correlated with diabetes if it's being managed; such extreme cravings are associated with *untreated* forms of the disease. Insulin (the hormone that people with type 1 diabetes cannot produce) is what allows the body's cells to actually use the glucose you ingest. This means that without insulin, your cells are starving for sugar, no matter how much food you have already eaten—the body has no way to access it.

Without glucose, cells in the body face death.[66] The brain receives signals that something must be eaten immediately, and concentrated "simple sugars" require the least processing time for the body to access in a state of crisis. Taking this into consideration, perhaps Jordan's habit of eating sweet, cheap food begins to appear less like a self-destructive paradox and more like twin faces of a single coin tossed up to fate: sugar as deadly risk; sugar as attempted release, in the absence of other medicine.

As they related fragments of all this to me, Agnes and Lil were not the callous people I had imagined from my conversations with Jordan.

They joked with me, fed me fruit, handed me babies to hold in rooms bustling with young children, and generally seemed to care more than I thought they would—enough to talk with a stranger about Jordan, as if they had been waiting to say out loud just what had happened. Yet at the same time, their focus on Jordan's noncompliance with specialized diets and inaccessible medication was so pronounced that I found myself grappling with what that plotline meant to them. João Biehl has described how "the overburdened family" is today "increasingly the medical agent of the state. Illness becomes the ground on which experimentation and breaks in intimate household relations can occur. Families can dispose of their unwanted and unproductive members, sometimes without sanction, on the basis of individuals' noncompliance with their treatment protocols."[67] In Zericote, Jordan's young age when he lived among this fragile network of stepkin almost caricatures the problem with the notion of "noncompliance"— as if a child's choices were his alone, rather than shaped at the nexus of many state, global, and family structures.

Yet the unstable texture of Lil's and Agnes's comments constantly seemed to escape the framework of false consciousness that many scholars turn to in interpreting moments of family tension—most famously in Nancy Scheper-Hughes's explanation of ruptures in family care and letting die among "angel babies" in Brazil. For all her powerful ethnography, this particular interpretive tag has never felt fully convincing to me. The Marxist diagnosis of false consciousness can seem to imply a kind of moral vacating instead of conflicted micro-practices entailed in making relations go numb, sometimes only to later be revived. Sitting in stifling kitchens as I visited Zericote numerous times throughout that year, I found myself considering the kinds of storytelling and uneasy choices within these breaks from a different direction, grappling with how Jordan's "living death" took constant labor to normalize in this world.

Disregard also requires maintenance. Rather than a "suspension of the ethical,"[68] the deferrals that Agnes and Lil kept narrating were more like the innermost capillaries of some overstrained system in which participants grappled all too accurately with how lives were valued by external markets. Their accounts suggested how finite stores of care had slowly been hollowed out or replenished over time.

Instead of Engels's master switch of false consciousness, then, I found myself returning instead to Edward Evans-Pritchard's famous ethnographic questions stemming from divergent theories of causality:[69] How did different actors tell stories of cause and effect not by narrating *how* a thing happened but *why?* Could these various starting points help to better unfurl distinct social logics and ethical fabrics, which might be better reckoned without starting from the premise that they were false? After all, everyone agreed that Jordan died from complications of his diabetes—that he had eaten foods he should not have eaten, that he did not have a regular supply of insulin. But *why* those things happened—that was the question up for grabs, and it inflected the moments we narrated to each other with undertones of responsibility and deflection.

Before I left that day, Agnes gestured toward one last place where Jordan had been found unconscious, in an adjacent wooden house. That time, she said, it was the middle of the afternoon when they found him. He had fallen still clutching a package of crackers, and there was a putrid-sweet alcoholic scent on his breath. "Drunk," she said, sounding angry now. He must have friends and money they did not know about, she added, and gone out drinking rum with them. Lil agreed, shaking her head in disapproval: the smell on his breath was strong.

I suppose it's not impossible that Jordan was drunk; I have no way to know for sure. But certainly, there are other probable explanations for these symptoms. In diabetes, one of the body's most acute states of emergency is called ketoacidosis. It can cause coma and death. This state is the leading cause of injuries and mortalities among young people with diabetes. It shares many possible symptoms with other conditions—semiconsciousness, nausea and vomiting, difficult breathing—but has one unique telltale sign: a sweet, alcohol-like scent on the breath, a smell reminiscent of rotten fruit or cheap schnapps. In contexts of poverty, ketoacidosis is most often caused by missing doses of insulin.

This life-threatening state occurs in conjunction with extremely high blood sugar. Yet it signals cells starving for sugar, unable to use the glucose already consumed due to insulin deficiency. Searching for other sources of energy to keep its cells from dying, the body instead begins breaking down muscle tissues and taking apart the carbon skeletons of the amino acids they contain, in order to release the emergency energy stores they hold. This is one face of *catabolic* metabolism, or catabolism—the breakdown. Some of these amino acids are glucogenic, meaning they can be converted to glucose and allow the body to keep going. Yet catabolizing a muscle means releasing all of the chemicals it contains, including those that aren't useful. Some amino acids are ketogenic, meaning they turn into ketones, which can be toxic at high levels. In biochemistry, this energy-or-poison difference is known as each amino acid's "metabolic fate."

Instead of life-sustaining glucose, the ketogenic amino acids yield harsh acetyl compounds (related to acetone, the nail-polish removing solvent). This causes the fruity alcohol smell of "acetone breath" during ketoacidosis. The major causes of death from diabetic ketoacidosis include collapse of the circulatory system, erratic potassium levels, infection, and swelling in the brain—potentially causing major organ damage for patients who survive, including neuron injuries and mental deficits. Though a relatively minor pathway, each amino acid's distinct role in this molecular breakdown has been charted, which I found in one text labeled like a chemist's dramatic poem: "The Fate of Carbon Skeletons."[70]

When it was time to catch the bus back, Agnes offered to walk me to the highway. "It's like Jordan is in Dangriga. That's how I feel," she said. A tall man approached on a child's bicycle to ask her who I was. Agnes introduced me as Jordan's girlfriend. There was some unkindness in this joke, I thought as they laughed, but also an eerie intimacy: according to what Agnes told me as we continued down the dirt path, I was the first "girlfriend" Jordan ever had.

I stood there wondering whether Jordan's last coma felt different than all the other times he had slipped into unconsciousness. Maybe it felt like familiar dark, or he dreamed of flying an airplane. I have heard you can learn to sink into a ketoacidosis sugar high, a feeling I imagined like the creepy sensorium of Sixto Rodriguez's seventies song "Sugar Man": *You're the answer that makes my question disappear.*

White ashes drifted down from the sky. Probably someone burning cardboard boxes, Agnes said. The disintegrating flakes looked surreally like snow falling through the heat.

I often think back to conversations with Jordan in 2010: both partly still kids in our twenties, talking about continuous glucose monitors and insulin pumps that existed in other places—never even mentioning the colossally warped inequalities behind the realities we compared, only their results surfacing in the details of the highly different technologies available in our respective worlds. But our tone during those interviews was almost absurdly casual, and so much lurked behind what was about to happen to him: global health bureaucracies that somehow blotted out the medical support and political advocacy available for other diseases; broken instruments of counting that linked together missing categories and metrics of various sorts; a local community's precarious labor of sustaining his social death; the hope that Jordan and his adoptive mothers held out of undoing it; and the highly specific technologies and machines that were part of extending (one measure at a time) the life that was left.

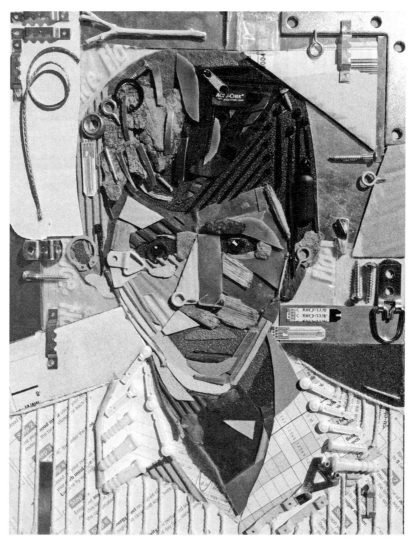

Portrait of Jordan as a Teenager, in Broken Glucometer Parts, by James Young.

From this perspective, the history of insulin or glucometers—like any other science—was not just one of breakthroughs; there were many kinds of breaks. Amid interfacing stories—specters of his lost mother, Tessa; phone calls from faraway Lorel and edgy interviews with his stepfamily; and all the persistent comorbidities and fleeting characters and distant technological inventions bound up in his fate—I realize that

Jordan himself was a person I would never know that well. Really, I only knew him in islets, little archipelagos of connection. But maybe that is not so uncommon between people in the world.

DESIGN ARCHIPELAGOS

At a 2010 meeting of the Belize National Diabetes Association in Belize City, I counted cardboard boxes on a folding table, with compartments inside for nesting fragile things. The boxes held rows of glucometers. I made the trip from Dangriga to learn what was happening in the central branch of the country's most active patient support group. The glucose machines being distributed for free that day were donated by the Miami branch of the Belize Diabetes Association, and strips for them—more expensive than the machines themselves—had been donated by the Belizean Diabetes Association of New York. Its members knew how such objects at times become remote outposts of care, across the uneven terrains some anthropologists have called "medical archipelagos."[71]

Since 2010, the cost of glucometers has finally decreased significantly. But the larger design quandaries remain: norms of "black box" design make delivery-oriented collaborations unnecessarily costly and prone to breakdowns. Historians of science commonly point to the way a tense politics of assigning responsibility gets materialized "between value-neutral technologies and the value-laden choices that determine how they are used."[72] These divisions develop sharper edges when set in global perspective: Observing devices being used in places where they broke down in such predictable ways, one had to ask: Were these technologies really so "value neutral"? From the lack of generic insulin persisting nearly a century after its discovery, to the built-in complexity and high price of glucose meter strips that could only be used with brand-matched machines, it often felt like inequalities were built right into these therapeutics. What might it look like if diabetes care technologies were *designed,* as well as distributed, with contexts like Jordan's in mind—for example, a method of blood sugar management engineered specifically to be functional and repairable in the parts of the world where most people with diabetes actually live today?[73]

Some scholars have envisioned a productive "open source anarchy" at work in arenas of global health governance—hoping that private organizations and public institutions alike would collaboratively contribute to building health networks and catalyzing competition to drive technological innovation.[74] But the case of brand-matched strips and proprietary glucometer parts for global diabetes care seems more representative of what Ruha Benjamin calls "discriminatory design," technologies with foreseeable injustices built in.[75] And like many forms of discrimination, taken-for-granted norms and complacencies that exclude certain populations from access can produce worrisome effects without being deliberately unjust.

What is "best care" for whom? From whose perspective do we assess what a "better" technology is?[76] The glucometer's historical emergence in high-income contexts sets the stage for certain kinds of innovation being constrained around industrial players' concerns with retaining control of lucrative markets. It is an uncomfortable truth that global access to decades-old standards of basic care for diabetes treatment remains fragile enough to become life-threatening for many patients like Jordan—not just despite ongoing advances in diabetes technologies, but at least partially *because* of them.

As Madeleine Akrich observes in her classic essay "The De-Scription of Technical Objects," it is often "only in the confrontation between the real user and the projected user [that] the importance of . . . the difference between the two [comes] to light," taking ethnographic work to "follow the device as it moves into countries that are culturally or historically distant from its place of origin."[77] But when unequal design problems are identified, what happens next?

Glucose meters stand out as a boundary case example of technological design that has not been transformed by recent enthusiasm around other point-of-care diagnostics.[78] Why have affordable, portable tests been developed and manufactured for human African trypanosomiasis but not for blood glucose? What would it take to think about tinkering on the level of equitable design—crafting technologies to maximize robust access that include the majority of people who now need them to survive? As Akrich notes, when lived histories and "processes involved in building up the technical objects are concealed," it can easily short-circuit our imaginations of devices' alternative forms. "The causal links they establish are naturalized. There was, or so it seems, never any possibility that it could have been otherwise."[79]

COUNTING

Trying to give a thicker historical context to the social and medical puzzles I observed kept leading back through the infinity loops of interlacing questions that so many observers have faced: What "counts," and how are various scales of counting and accounting bound up with each other?[80] In Belize, glucose machines were just one nexus where metrics were electrified. Counting on the molecular level when meters measured light or electrochemical charges in blood became part of what shaped statistical currents on an epidemiological level and even helped animate the forms of moral accounting taking place in a hospital unit's triage or a stepfamily's rural home. These different modes of counting and accounting were each interconnected without being reducible to each other, numerologies bound up with global flows of medicine.

Even with better global numbers of diabetes cases now becoming visible, the issue often continues to be profoundly misrecognized. I once heard an Ivy League economist suggest that a particularly promising policy approach to the world's diabetes epidemic would be raising the price of glucose test strips (via higher taxes) so that poor people with diabetes "thought more carefully first" about what they were eating, knowing it would be difficult to test their sugar afterward. We had all just listened to a public health talk about death counts from diabetes escalating in contexts of scarcity. At the time, I was too taken aback to speak. The weight of our privileged surroundings in that moment seared itself into my mind: a well-appointed U.S. conference room full of white social scientists, using database statistics to discuss the assumed behavioral responses of imaginary nonwhite (and eminently misbehavior-prone) poor people to hypothetical policy scenarios. Everyone sat around the climate-controlled room over an opulent lunch platter arrayed with roasted vegetables—as if the entire world looked like this, covered with catered plates of organic grilled vegetables! And I thought of Lorel's question to the taxi driver: Don't you *see*?

In the future, some researchers predict, people will be able to wear glucometers like watches. Equipped with tiny microneedles and infrared sensors, they could tell us our blood sugar the way clocks tell time. I thought about this when I found an old glucometer in a storage box from my fieldwork. A Belizean nurse had given it to me when their clinic switched brands. Like most machines, it automatically stores hundreds of readings in its digital memory, even if they have nowhere to be downloaded. Dated now, the machine tells times already past, like some relic or last vessel.

I flipped through, wondering if one of the counts might be Jordan's reading. Amid dozens of numbers, each indexing some day and real person, a clinical encounter ending in anxiety or relief, there was also the familiar sight of scattered letters—*Err* for error or *Hi* for dangerously high sugars over 600—and I thought of Cresencia's little joke to herself. She's long gone now, interred in a family tomb labeled with only her mother's name. Her cousin Sadie, whose birthday would have been tomorrow on the day I type this sentence, was the one who told me the news, and then she died in her thirties too. Both made it over a decade longer than Jordan, whose grave I still couldn't find the last time I went back with a handful of red bells that wilted later on the dashboard.

But I felt closer to them bumping into the old meter than I did at the edge of the cemetery where they were unlocatable—perhaps the glucometer remembered Jordan too. I was not even sure whose blood was once measured through the electrical current of the machine in my hands, but found myself handling it like the planchette of an Ouija board. It was also a fragile archive of sorts, both anonymous and personal—one that required contextualization, but told a very different story of diabetes science than the one cataloged in North American history of medicine archives or European museum exhibits. For a moment, the monitor's digital screen even read like the remainders of a message, as if we might squeeze a few final words into a conversation that ended without answers.

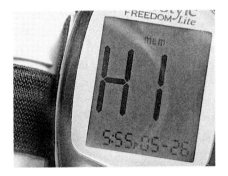

Hello.

Crónica Three: Generations

Approaching "Biologies of History"
with Arreini and Guillerma

Did I know anything about diabetes? Not much, I replied,
but my maternal grandfather had died of diabetes. . . .

Hearing this, the *commendatore* became more attentive
and his eyes smaller: I realized later that, since the tendency
to diabetes is hereditary, it would not have displeased him to
have at his disposal an authentic diabetic, of a basically
human race, on whom he could test certain of his ideas and
preparations.

—Primo Levi, *Periodic Table*

"He said, how are you still alive?" Arreini's expression was both amused
and proud as she recounted to me the doctor's words when he first diagnosed her condition. Her blood sugar that day had been "six change,"
over 600. "But I survive," she smiled mysteriously. The threadbare silk
purse in her hands was filled with old prescriptions and forgotten pills,
her own archive of illnesses and healings gone by. Arreini shuffled
through expired packets, pointing out the baggies of medicines she was
currently taking: metformin and glyburide for diabetes, captopril for
hypertension. There were new pills in a small brown paper sack from
her most recent trip to the regional hospital, when she had gone to seek
treatment for the diabetic ulcer on her foot: a tiny ziplock bag of white
pills called piriton, a foil card of acetaminophen tablets for the pain,
and a large box of antibiotic pills called tro-amoxiclav, too large to
swallow without first cutting each in half with a fishing knife.

But weeks had already turned into months, and the pills had not been
enough: the wound on Arreini's foot continued seeping and "jamming,"

her name for the most intense pulsations of pain. She had tried every medicine she knew, techniques learned in a lifetime spent healing others. Now more than eighty years old, Arreini had lived her entire life as a legendary healer and certified midwife. Yet in her plastic pail filled with bundled leaves, bark, and clusters of herbal medicines—cloves in a withered but fragrant plastic baggie, Billy Webb bitters, balsamo, a bottle of blackened seedpods purchased in Guatemala, coiled bits of contribu vine she picked herself, a shaker of oregano manufactured by McCormick's—there was nothing that could mend the hurt skin. She had tried a topical oil treatment like her mother had once used on her grandmother's feet back in Honduras; it had helped, but not enough.

Likewise with the boiled guava leaves to control the infection (helpful but not fully curative, like the hospital's antibiotics) and an experimental mixture of herbs that she had prepared in a base of rum, stored in a cherry juice bottle. "My mother didn't have this disease," she said by way of explanation for her rare uncertainty about treatments. Nearly all of Arreini's medical practices had been learned from her mother, who had also been a midwife and nurse. As a condition that only emerged as an epidemic within her generation, diabetes fits uneasily into a Garifuna system of herbal knowledge passed through generations.

Seven years ago, Arreini told me, she had been able to contain a similar ulcer by creating an herbal medicine and injecting it into her foot with a syringe. All the skin had peeled off, and afterward she was healed. "But now this diabetes has come," she said. "Now, this foot. It's black again." I could tell she was expecting some reaction from me, but I wasn't sure what.

"Did you hear me? It's *black*."

I looked up from where I was kneeling on the beach, trying to light the fire she had asked me to start, with the familiar feeling that Arreini was trying to tell me something I did not really understand. She doused the dried coconut husks in the fire pile with more kerosene from an old plastic water bottle and waited with sharp eyes for me to try again. But I have always moved gingerly when handling matches, and I struck the box too cautiously for the flame to hold against the wind from the sea. She grabbed the packet of matches out of my hands and muttered in frustration, a characteristic rebuke that was both her trademark gruffness and the hard-won right of very old women. But it still upset me that night because it was the end of a long day, among many. The night before, I had fallen asleep facedown on my keyboard while trying to type notes. At the time, I was spending full days observing at clinics or visiting people at home, then coming back to sit around eating dinner and doing errands until long after dark with this renowned village midwife. Those evenings that passed talking with Arreini were perhaps my favorite moments of fieldwork, but decoding her cryptic references and free-wheeling English was not easy, especially when her temper ran short.

Maybe Arreini realized that her sharp tone had hit a nerve, because after the coconut husks began smoldering and her day's trash of peels and crumpled papers were going up in flames on the sand, she patted the bench next to her. "And thing done," she said soothingly. No matter what language she had been speaking, this was the English refrain that usually marked the end of a tense moment, all absolved. "Come, my beloved." I got up from where I was kneeling and joined her, stepping carefully past her foot. We sat together in the shadows under her stilted house and watched it get dark over the sea. She pulled a cigar and a kitchen knife wrapped in masking tape from her apron, slicing off a stub of tobacco to light in her pipe. "Time is passing, my darling." She asked me to bring gauze so that she could bandage the ulcer without dedicating mornings to the careful midwife's art of sterilizing her own cotton.

Like Arreini, the majority of her family now had diabetes: her husband, who for decades had lived in the United States, and some seven of the thirteen children she had raised between his sporadic visits home. Even a number of her grandchildren now had diabetes, the disease seeming to advance at younger and younger ages.

In an interview I had conducted at the hospital, one of the Cuban doctors voiced his theory of why Garifuna patients were statistically at greater risk for diabetes: "Did you know they are Black *and* [American] Indian? Double risk." I heard similar explanations countless times during my research. Such "ethnic" labels draw on the sort of naturalized categorizations that have been forcefully critiqued by anthropologists as part of the "genetic reinscription of race"[1] in diabetes research.[2] Yet "there is at present no consistent evidence to suggest that minority populations are especially genetically susceptible" to type 2 diabetes.[3] For more than fifty years, genetic research searching for a race-linked "cause" of diabetes has been unable to conclusively identify such an inherent gene.[4] Instead, diabetes has become emblematic of the more troubling "racializing narratives"[5] in genetic research. Such repackaging of race, Anthony Ryan Hatch cautions, can "revive naturalist thinking about racial groups, and ultimately obscure our vision about how racism transforms and seeks to profit from bodies."[6] It also can resurrect forms of "biological determinism"[7] embedded deep in the interpretive problems of how historical time can go unexamined in genetic medicine, as historian Keith Wailoo and colleagues suggest with their title *Genetics and the Unsettled Past.*[8]

I saw my work with Arreini as an alternate way of attending to the emergence of diabetes from an "unsettled past." In her practices and accounting, Arreini kept calling attention to dimensions of uneven risk that genetics and other bodily sciences leave out, citing family and community histories across deep time as fundamental to understanding and treating diabetic injuries. The margins of survival made possible by these therapeutic techniques were sourced in the collective forces of the ancestors, places, and materials that she summoned across generations.

Between family and science, the term *generations* holds causalities and origins in tension: it can imply newly produced energy, or a long perpetuation with histories past and ahead.[9] It comes from the Latin root *generare*—from genus, meaning race. And like the kin Arreini kept evoking across the centuries, notions of race also have potent afterlives.

SCIENTIFIC RACISM: LINEAGES

The species of "spontaneous" sugarcane pictured in this chapter was classified and mounted by the legendary botanist Carl Linnaeus. He named it *Saccharum spontaneum,* in distinction to *officinarum,* the species of cultivated sugar quickly spreading throughout the Caribbean at the time he was becoming known for his taxonomies. Linnaeus had affixed the sugar plant with glue made from the scales of a Carolina bowfish, now a preserved holotype I once uneasily held in a basement vault within the Linnean Society of London. Founded in 1788, it is the oldest biological society in the world.

Sugarcane's scientific classification had unfolded alongside—even conjoined with—the historical records that I had traveled to the Linnean Society archives to study. In the late 1700s, scientists whose work would be assembled there had also become interested in studying and delineating "Black" from "Yellow" Caribs on Saint Vincent, the lost ancestral home of Garifuna people like Arreini—which is how colonial documents administering the Garifuna exile from their homeland came to be housed in the Linnean Society building. Samples of sugar "types" like these were among the crops grown on the British plantations into which Garifuna ancestral territory was divvied, after the scientific labeling of human racial "types" helped to rationalize this colonial plunder.

Anthropologist Jonathan Marks noted of Linnaeus "what is probably his most significant contribution to modern life: the idea that groups of people can be regarded as naturally distinct taxonomic entities, or sub-species, in the same fashion as species, genera and higher categories."[10] In *Systema Naturae*, Linnaeus infamously classified four subspecies of humans. He characterized white Europeans (*Europaeus albus*) as a spe-cies that was optimistic, ruddy, muscular, gentle, inventive, and gov-erned by laws. They were "sanguine"—with the healthiest humors and balanced red blood. Everyone else, he theorized, had imbalanced blood and disordered bodily fluids. He labeled each "type": Red Americans (*Americanus rubescens*) he described as choleric, stubborn, and free, with an excess of bile. Brown and Yellow Asians (*Asiaticus fuscus* and *Asiaticus luridus*) were classified by Linnaeus as stiff, severe, and prone to strong opinions. Meanwhile, Linnaeus invented the label Black Afri-cans (*Africanus niger*) to classify the group he deemed indolent and gov-erned by caprice, casting this supposed subtype of human as prone to excess phlegm and known for women producing too much breast milk.[11]

Today, Linnaeus's taxonomy proposing that skin colors mark differ-ent human subgroups is remembered by many people as a profoundly troubling example of scientific racism. It further codified colonial notions of race that fed into atrocities and violence of all kinds. And yet, searching for biologically inherent differences linked to bodily fluid and categories of race is still a primary way that metabolic disorders are often studied today.

Historian Dorothy Roberts explores how "the racial concept of dis-ease" actually long preceded ideas of genes and genetic determinism.[12] She traces the warped medical theories of influential physicians such as Dr. Samuel Cartwright (b. 1793), who argued that due to the inborn disordered biologies of African constitutions, the daily exercise pro-vided by slavery held important health benefits for African people. His research attributed sluggish blood circulation and reduced organ capac-ities to people with dark skin, providing a bolstering scientific and moral rationale for imputing that enslaved people naturally needed less food and physically required the exertions of plantation labor. This cast slavery as a corrective medical solution.[13] In a sense, the New World's racial orders were partly built and sustained by such rationalizing theo-ries of what later came to be called cardiometabolic disorders.

Biological concepts from various eras, however misguided, profoundly shape the material components of our present.[14] This is a key insight offered by historian of science Hannah Landecker, who argues for focusing

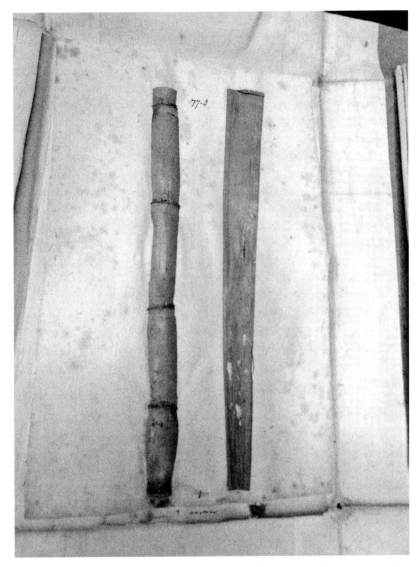

Specimen of wild sugar, mounted and classified by Carl Linnaeus as the separate species *Saccharum spontaneum* (spontaneous sugar) in his taxonomy.

not only on the history of biology but also on the "biology of history": the way actual biologies become altered by ongoing practices and interventions over time, which were in turn shaped by past theories of biology.

This framework suggests a series of disturbing questions in the aftermath of past biological labels, when it comes to reading blood sugar "beside itself."[15] Colonial sciences and medical explanations helped to produce and rationalize terrible histories of dispossession, often premised on theories of racial difference that framed certain populations as inherently dysfunctional. These events caused trauma of many kinds, in systems and psyches as well as bodies.

Today, new sciences have come into being to study the bodily implications of stress and trauma in relation to uneven risk for chronic conditions like diabetes. Yet this is one of the deepest paradoxes of "the biology of history"—its material effects are mostly only legible through more biology, still being produced in today's history and its blindspots. New and old paradigms of biosciences thus need to be carefully considered in relation to each other, Roberts adds, if new biosocial research projects are to avoid reproducing the inequalities that this work aims to describe or even redress: "Without this scrutiny of its assumptions, methods, and indeed, its values, the new biosocial science—like the old—risks reinforcing, rather than contesting, today's unjust social order."[16]

While anthropologists' traditional work once focused on understanding "etic" versus "emic" perspectives, I found myself struggling most of all to keep up with the "omic." From epigenomics to metabolomics and from the "methylome" to the "exposome," a raft of biological news and scientific controversy was coming to light during the time of my research. Some of it promised to perhaps reconfigure how diabetes risk is understood—laboratory perspectives that triangulated my ethnographic observations into different constellations of meaning. I scrambled to keep up with these critical debates as they exploded onto the scene of diabetes research, and at times reopened the realities I observed in everyday life to fresh multidimensional interpretations.

These medical and scientific studies often expanded the concepts I was thinking with in Belize, but they just as frequently perplexed me as critical objects unto themselves. They suggested incredible stories of injured molecules and new ways of tracing bodily strains and recoveries across generations—yet laboratory biology theorized into social models can also quickly animate its own abstractions. In particular, the very data that promised to persuasively provide evidence for the possible bodily tolls of inequalities were often taking place in laboratories totally removed from what those inequalities might actually look like in real life. This placed such social contexts (ostensibly, the very point of this research) at once squarely at the center of these debates and largely outside the thinkable scope of intervention, which became molecularized in turn as a search for therapy and drug targets.

Learning from Arreini and her family kept reminding me of all that gets muted when researchers focus on cells and molecules alone. In addition to places of knowledge production and clinical care like laboratories and hospitals, there were material traces of bygone biological theories in the living worlds around us. Thinking of these interstitial spaces as also part of "biologies of history," I started to see how life forms rearranged by past sciences remained legible, touched by historical events and still present far beyond genetic and epigenetic lenses alone: in rearranged plants and seeds and food systems, access to both synthetic and herbal medicines, changing weather patterns, dispossessed lands, and lost family members, as well as in the travails of bodies and families trying to heal against histories of violence and their legacies today.

Social and medical scientists have unwanted ancestors in such colonial stories. In 1785, a Scottish medical surgeon named Alexander Anderson was dispatched to Saint Vincent to observe and record the people and landscape. "What renders the natural history of Saint Vincent more interesting and curious than that of any other West India island," he wrote from what was then the Garifuna homeland, "is its being long the residence of a singular tribe of men nowhere else known (the Black Carribs [sic]), whose history, manner of gaining possession of greater part of the country, modes of life and manners are at this time but little known in Great Britain."[17]

A natural historian in the days before social sciences and biological sciences were framed as separate fields, Anderson's taxonomies destined for the Linnean Society at times became a double classificatory schema— in some cases he would note both the species of plant being cataloged, and his designation for the type of human from whom he had learned that herbal knowledge. Anderson's post as director of the hospital botanical garden on the British-controlled edge of Saint Vincent may sound relatively innocuous at first, but the outside envelopes of his correspondence from the Crown stated his position more bluntly: he was there under the aegis of the War Office.

After most of the Native inhabitants of Saint Vincent whom the Europeans had labeled "Yellow Caribs" had been killed or displaced, British administration declared they had once been the "original and lawful owners of the land."[18] They argued that the Black Caribs, in contrast, were by their reckoning not Indigenous enough to qualify for land rights—an attempt to put into question their ancestral claim to their homeland.

There was thus a heavy political undercurrent to any human taxonomies created in this context, as Julie Chun Kim explains: "Anderson worked to subject the Saint Vincent Caribs to regimes of classification that would render them into two completely distinct races." He sought biological samples from Carib bodies as part of this project, searching for examples of the "Craniums of the Yellow Caribs, or Aborigenes." The collection endeavor was complicated by the fact, he wrote, that "Caribs considered 'any attempt to disturb the ashes of their Ancestors . . . as the greatest of crimes,'" though "Anderson went forward with the violation of their burial sites."[19]

Anderson would write later that his goal in such collection projects and his efforts to systemize a natural history of the island's Black Caribs had a motivating aim: "to exculpate the English inhabitants from inhumanity or tyranny . . . as to ordering [Garifuna people's] total expulsion from the island . . . and to do away with similar charges against His Majesty's ministers in sanctioning their extermination."[20]

Given histories of science and medicine like these, it is little wonder that some descendants from harmed groups remain cautious of certain science and medicine made around sugar these many generations later—even when its treatments become necessary for survival. Navigating this tension is one way to think about Arreini's care work in what follows.

HOUSEKEEPING

When I arrived one morning with the gauze she had requested, Arreini's yard was filled with people I did not recognize. It was Good Friday. A procession walked down the road, led by a man in sneakers and a fishing cap carrying a cross over one shoulder, enacting the Stations of the Cross. Several dozen people followed behind, singing hymns, dressed in the funeral colors of black and white. Arreini, who was soaking beans in a bucket and grating coconut, disapproved that more of the village was not in attendance: "What are they doing, this young generation?" Her grandson Sheldon looked up from where he was tinkering with the oven in the corner of her kitchen, repairing the aged appliance so that Arreini could bake a cake. He wiped his forehead with a hammer in his hand.

"They are just living," he said.

As we sat on the porch I began speaking with Guillerma, one of Arreini's daughters. She looked much younger than fifty-eight. Carefully

adjusting the gold and red turban wrapped high around her head, Guillerma stretched in the hammock and said that she wanted to walk in the
Easter procession but felt too sick because of her diabetes. "My stomach
is hurting me. I feel better after I vomit," she said. "But I hate to throw
up." She had ten children and some thirty grandchildren, a few of whom
she pointed out to me in the bustling yard below: a girl on the beach,
another plaiting the hair of her grandson Kevin. "They are cooking for
me now, early," Guillerma said, gesturing toward the women slicing
chicken and pressing biscuits with forks. "Because of my diabetes, they
know that when I have to eat, I can't wait."

Guillerma told me that she lived in "the city" now (there was no need
to specify *which* city because Belize City is the only city in Belize). When
Arreini had visited there to receive IV antibiotics at the hospital, a
young teenager had been shot on the street in front of their house:
"Muerto upon Muerto," Arreini said. "Fock!" Guillerma's husband
tragically died there too, around the time she was pregnant with their
tenth child. "The sugar started," she said, not long after, and never went
away. Guillerma said that her main memory of that time was trying to
answer her littlest children's questions. Arreini came right away and
lived with them for a long while. Guillerma recalled, "The kids keep
asking when he is coming home. We just have to hold them. Cherish
them and show them love . . . a whole lot of love."

As the years went on, Guillerma said she tried everything for her
sugar—pills, insulin, diet—but bodily wear accrued, especially during
the time she spent working long hours as a home caregiver to the elderly
in Chicago. The cold winds became unbearable as she grew sicker. She
missed her kids. After more than a decade away, Guillerma came home
to Belize City. But the cost of dialysis in Belize was far outside the realm
of possibility for most, 680 U.S. dollars for one week of three sessions.
Guillerma looked so full of vitality that it took time for what she was
telling me to sink in. As long as dialysis remained impossible, she said
the doctors didn't think she had much longer.

I stayed until after dark to help with the baking: creole buns, two of
which I was given to take home in a plastic bag fogged with warmth,
and the cassava cake, which I was not invited to taste. Arreini asked me
to come back in the morning, "so you can see how we do things." The
next day was Holy Saturday; I heard humming when approaching her
kitchen and saw the family holding hands in a circle through an open
door in the distance. "She's been dreaming," one grandson's girlfriend
told me. From bits of our conversation that day, I pieced together that

Arreini had been having dreams of her mother and that this ritual was an offering for her *áfurugu*—a person's spirit double, which can travel and be hungry or thirsty both during life and after death. These are said to be light or heavy. In matters of the spirit world, it is much better to be *heavy,* which is more like strong energy or bandwidth than corpulence. The food for her would be buried in the sand.

Since the girlfriends of family members were not in the back house, I waited with them for an invitation. Kevin tapped me on the shoulder after awhile and brought me back to the "thatch kitchen," which stood adjacent to her cement kitchen and looked like a smaller version of an ancestral house. Inside was a living museum of family artifacts and furniture: long serpentine cassava strainers threaded through the rafters, a cracked machete sheath, old blackened pots and metal bowls. Arreini had me sit on one of three plastic chairs near the door. There was a small altar in the middle of the room, with heaping plates of food: rice and beans with plantains, the cassava cake, and huge pieces of creole bread. Lined up in front of the altar sat an array of plastic or glass bottles, each partially full, with caps unscrewed but a small tuft of cotton stuffed in the top. Some younger spirits now request Coca-Cola or processed foods in the rituals honoring them, reflecting the tastes they favored in life, but the older generation of spirits still prefer homemade beverages. Arreini instructed various grandchildren to sip from a carved wooden bowl of cassava wine as they helped to clean up and bring in two huge drums. Her grandson picked up the wax pooled into the sand, and Arreini turned to me. "Everything is okay now, thank God." She nodded. "Thanksgiving for my mom. The candle burn[ed] good. The smoke went like this." She twirled her index finger. "She is happy."

Kevin and Arreini played drums together for awhile, hers in the lead. There were three pieces of wire stretched across the top of the drum's tight peccary skin that had a tune of their own, and Arreini played the metal strings like a separate instrument. "Gran raised me since I was four," her grandson told me as he kept a *segunda* bass rhythm. "My mother brought me into this world and then she was gone. I love her like my mom. She's my mom," he repeated of Arreini. A small cluster of family gathered as they played. Guillerma leaned against the altar, picking up her grandmother's old pipe in her hand, and then as her mother sang she stood to do a dance that looked like a slow strut, her elbows lifted high. She started singing too, shaking her voice like her mother's, and knew all the words—an *abaimahani* song usually composed in dreams, often about sickness and death, at times becoming "verbal memorials"[21] passed down in families. Her health too tenuous to dance for very long, soon Guillerma handed the pipe back to her mother. Arreini told me that she would light the pipe later and leave it in the sand for her mom. "Everything is okay," Arreini repeated later, draping a pair of denim pants over the drum. I understood the offerings for her mother as the strengthening of kin ties for the family's protection in general, with a petition for Guillerma specifically—"a patience for the possible,"[22] trying to stretch time at the limits of care until another way might open. Arreini picked up an ancient-looking cauldron filled with burned leaves, their carbonized shapes intact in the ash. "Herbs for my mom," she explained—at the edge of death, offering to the dead. She knew what medicine they needed.

There was a bottle of anise rum, her mother's favorite drink, at the base of the altar, next to a Sprite bottle filled with holy water. I was surprised when Arreini poured me a tall glass of the strong, clear rum. "Come, let's finish it off," she said. Its taste reminded me of a harsh sambuca. There were two spirals of silver hair sticking out from under her old fishing hat, which looked like it had once been repaired with white string only to unravel again, its sutures now stretching decoratively across gaping holes. She wore a red bandana tied tightly under the hat, patterned with paisley and tiny white skulls. Everyone in the stream of visitors trickling in for the Easter holiday weekend called her "mom" so often that I lost all track of when this was literal. Arreini was close to many of her "grans" and "great-grans." Another woman whom Arreini and her mother had raised together also came to visit and recalled her mom's words: "After I'm dead, I'll come for you." They laughed together, the threat revealing great intimacy.

Instead of her ubiquitous fictive kin term of "my daughter," Arreini sometimes called me "my husband." I was unsettled by the playfully serious term, which in her case implied intervals of great disconnection and distance. But it was true that after being around every night for a short while, sharing meals and spending time with her, like her husband I would leave the village and go away for years on end.

Arreini lit her mother's pipe again, and its smoke filled the night air. It was probably because I felt drunk after splitting the bottle of her mother's anise rum, but I was distracted by how much the droplets actually looked like tears as she blotted her foot with a tissue. I did not realize until many years later that Arreini's condition had a very particular name: Charcot foot, one of the most complicated of all diabetic foot conditions, requiring treatment so intricate that entire multidisciplinary textbooks are dedicated to its care. Charcot involves nearly every bodily system, and hence the likelihood of keeping a limb increases when specialists from each subfield work together, including hematology, orthopedics, endocrinology, podiatry, and vascular surgery. Before ulceration with Charcot, something called "rocker bottom" and associated breakdown and dislocation of the bone structure happens first. If this is not treated, it can lead to a situation like Arreini's known as a "volcanic crater," mottled at the edges but with many deeper changes inside. A general practitioner in many places across the Caribbean facing such a wound alone often would recommend amputation. This was indeed the course of treatment that one physician had suggested for Arreini. "Not yet," she had told him.

Sometimes our bodies recall things that we don't. This is the premise behind studies in "metabolic memory"—a technical term for the lasting effects on the vascular system when treatment arrives late, making recovery from an ulcer or other diabetic complications more difficult.[23] It describes how blood capillaries previously worn by sugar contain forms of cellular memory about strains, its mechanisms only partly legible to science. This idea of metabolic memory felt larger than its strict definition as I sat with Arreini.

There were careful patches covering everything in Arreini's house: holes in shirts repaired with pretty bits of fruit-patterned fabric, red-and-white checkered dish towels of the sort most people would simply have thrown away rather than painstakingly mend, slivers of various materials between flowers on her kitchen tablecloth, the repeatedly patched and repatched pockets of her bulging apron, in which she kept certain medical and kitchen supplies. There was a sense in which Arreini lived her life as a patch on a larger health system, working in the holes of care. She had never lost a baby in all her years as a midwife, she often repeated, and was famous for her expertise in listening for infant pulmonary infections (which she referred to the national hospital upon detecting: "You have that certificate of human life. You have to *take care*"). Against this backdrop, the day's gathering and the scrap of gauze she applied to the ulcer on her foot both looked like swathes of her careful preventative work.

It would be easy to think of mundane scenes like this—daily care for maintenance—as occurring somewhere far from metabolic science. Hannah Landecker argues that such assumptions are an additional part of how key metabolic mechanisms went so long without being acknowledged by most experts. In cellular biology, just as in social life, she notes, "the (extremely gendered) separation of the 'housekeeping' from the 'executive' functions of the cell" was part of why DNA was viewed for so long as the only important part of human genetics, while the crucial regulatory function by epigenetic processes was overlooked. In her view, such a gendered conception of work "probably has something to do with the difficulty of seeing metabolic activities as complex gene regulatory activities."[24] This represents a major divergence from DNA-centered paradigms of biology, to the point that some scientists had difficulty believing their own evidence at first. Moshe Szyf, the well-known molecular biologist and geneticist who conducted some notable laboratory experiments in this area of epigenetics in the early 1990s, would later remember his breakthrough conversation with collaborators like this: "The longer we talked, the more I realized that maternal care just might be capable of causing changes in DNA methylation, as crazy as that sounded." Szyf would later recall of their early research on how senses of safety get embodied: "It sounded like voodoo at first."[25]

TRANS-PLANTATION

One of the pasts evoked by Arreini's ritual was not a person but a place: Saint Vincent, the dispossessed Garifuna stronghold where spirits like her mother's were said to reside in eternity. I turned to archival records to read more about this land that kept being called into memory and its present absence in this "biology of history."

By the late eighteenth century, most of the Caribbean islands were said to appear "polished smooth" with sugar plantations, since nearly all forests had been burned to clear cane fields and to supply fuel for distilling the cane.[26] Against this backdrop, the Garifuna's verdant homeland presented a sharp contrast: "a picturesque and fertile island, and very healthy," with the towering volcano Mount Soufriere visible for miles. "The ground seems overloaded with plants, which have barely room enough for their development. The trunks of the older trees are everywhere covered with a thick drapery of ferns, mosses, and orchideous plants. . . . rivulets of the purest water urge their meandering course through the brushwood,"[27] wrote one colonial observer of Saint Vincent's forests.

Key parts of the island had early been protected by what colonial forces called its Indigenous inhabitants' "poison arrow curtain," volleys of blades hewn from sharpened tortoise shell and the spines of predator fish, tipped in local toxins so potent that European forces began collecting them for pharmaceutical scrutiny. In fact, useful plants were key among the valuable materials driving colonial collection and expansion at this time. A century later, nearly a quarter of the plants published in the *British Pharmacopoeia* originated from herbs in the Americas, Abena Osseo-Asare notes.[28]

Dr. Anderson had been obsessed with transplantation from the time of his first arrival in 1785. The island's Botanical Station that he had been dispatched to run was originally founded by General Robert Melville, descended from the same Scottish family line as *Moby Dick* author Herman Melville (and, more distantly, the musician Moby).[29] "Great was the interest taken in this garden, which promised to be a source of much profit to the colonies, and of commerce to the mother country," he wrote of Saint Vincent.[30]

The garden was designed in part to capture the island's unique concentration of herbal knowledge that drew not only from a healthy forest, but also from its residents' botanical expertise spanning Africa and the Americas. The governing general instructed the hospital's surgeon in 1766 to try to "get as much information as possibly you can from all quarters relative to the indigenous medicines. . . . physical practitioners of the country, natives of experience, and even old Caribs and slaves who have dealt in cures might be worth taking notice of, and if at any time you should think that a secret may be got at . . . I shall readily pay for it."[31]

Though geographically remote, Saint Vincent at this time was deeply connected to global networks of empire and the material worlds that they rearranged. British planters on their edge of the island maintained strong ties with their counterparts in Barbados and drew from the region's thriving commerce with the newly named United States. Once Anderson arrived on Saint Vincent after serving on the losing side of the U.S. Revolutionary War, one of his key projects was an attempt "to propagate the Cochineal insect" and the nopal cactuses they fed on.[32] Appropriated from Nahua people in Central Mexico, the crushed insects' bright red dye was in high demand because it was crucial for the bold red stripes of the new U.S. flag, as well as most colonial military uniforms.

These materials were linked to the region's human trade with the United States, as well as Europe. Those enslaved on the Barbados sugar plantations included a population of "recalcitrant Indians . . . occasionally shipped from New England,"[33] most likely enslaved Pequot and Wampanoag speakers, who arrived in the Caribbean not long before an influx of Cherokee captured in the Carolinas. Tituba, star witness of the Salem witch trials, was traded in the opposite direction to Massachusetts from a sugar plantation on Barbados. Some records describe Tituba as Black, others as Indigenous, others as both. She may have descended from those captured in the first wave of Arawak families who signed two-year labor contracts to teach British planters to grow crops in Barbados, before the British later declared them enslaved and broke apart their families for sale.

Saint Vincent's Black Carib population, meanwhile, forged their own networks. They traveled freely by canoe through trade networks in mainland South America, returning with Amazon greenstones, caiman teeth, and a particular metal alloy that Europeans did not know how to meld. Anderson wrote about them with a mix of admiration and disgust, referring to the population as the island's "infernal bandetti," yet he was intrigued with their deep pharmacological knowledge. He had once been kidnapped in Suriname, and knew from that experience that many of the medicinal plants on Saint Vincent seemed to have been transplanted by Caribs from mainland South America. When he identified a new species of *Cinchona* plant, Anderson hoped it might offer an English alternative to the crucial antimalarial drug *Cinchona officinalis*, which he called Spanish quinine (though it was also an appropriation, from Inca Peru). By describing these transplants, one historian notes, "Anderson found himself confronting issues of indigeneity in a different, botanical register, and his study of plants forced him to recognize the contradictions inherent in his attempts to classify the Caribs."[34]

At a point in history when the surrounding Windward Islands had already been subjugated by the British for nearly 150 years, this mixed group that came to be labeled by colonial authorities as Black Caribs managed to defend their land through adept diplomacy with the French—"the beginnings of what we might call a foreign policy," Nancie Gonzalez writes[35]—and, later, by sheer military strategy. By 1770 the group had received official backing from the governor of Martinique, as well as funding from the French radical author Victor Hugo.

They held off the British colonial forces in multiple Carib Wars—an amazing series of victories spanning many decades. After their upset victory in the first of three wars, the revered Garifuna leader Satuye (also known in history books as Joseph Chatoyer)[36] was among those who signed a treaty with the British in 1773 that spelled out Garifuna legal ownership of land on Saint Vincent.

The British broke the treaty by degrees. "The Mode of Carrying on the War has been changed," one colonial observer reported by 1796.

Unable to win against the Garifuna in battle, the British decided instead to secretly attack their food supplies. "By this means it is expected that the Savages will be starved into Compliance."[37] The British rounded up five thousand enslaved men from Martinique, armed them with cutlasses, and brought the force to Saint Vincent as a troop of "negro rangers" focused on finding and destroying provision grounds. It was a classic case of divide and conquer—still bitterly remembered today by Garifuna people, who recall that the rangers found their paths and burned their food supplies with much more skill than the British had ever possessed. English observers applauded the brutal "scorched earth" policy they had engineered, and then wrote in amused tones that the rangers had seemed to expect a material thanks or even freedom after this destruction of food supplies. But instead, they were thrown back into slavery on the sugar plantations of Martinique afterward.[38]

Food sovereignty, thus, became a key fulcrum in an otherwise unwinnable war. When one British-backed party went searching for food supplies to attack and also found the longhouses containing the wives and children of the Garifuna warriors waiting on the battle lines, they burned everything and everyone inside. "Posterity will hardly believe the number of lives lost on these islands," one British officer wrote from Saint Vincent.[39] Even with their food supplies decimated, Garifuna warriors fought on long after being abandoned by their allies, the French soldiers who had fled the island shortly after eating their mules.

EPIDEMIOLOGICAL TRANSITION

Nearly the entire surviving Garifuna population was eventually captured and imprisoned on a tiny island called Balliceaux, just off the coast of Saint Vincent, while the British administration waited for ships to deport them further. Over five thousand Garinagu held on there for nine months, "starving and destitute,"[40] taken from their own farms after the war and subjected to desperately insufficient rations by their captors. The sick were provided with rations of sugar and rice. The British general in charge attributed the epidemic to, in his words, "the sudden change of Diet and Situation."[41]

A much smaller number of surviving Garifuna families also managed to escape undetected in the forest. When the last known group emerged years later, the British administrator expressed astonishment that "their last position where they raised their Vegetables of every description,

was in the gorge of a Mountain within three miles and half of a flourishing plantation from whence they were never discovered."[42]

Archaeological traces provide windows into what Indigenous farms
across the Caribbean might have looked like before conquest, including the farms of the Garifuna people's Kalinago ancestors. Their "settlements were often located along the eastern shore, facing the Atlantic
Ocean, and in proximity to rivers. Kitchen gardens were located near
houses, and larger horticultural gardens were located in the mountains."[43] In addition to the crucial staple of cassava, including many
varieties of bitter and sweet manioc (yucca), farms also featured small
mounds of beans, squash, and peanuts. Yams and sweet potatoes had
leaves that could be eaten like spinach. *Canna* blossomed orange with
nutritious edible flowers and starchy roots that could be cooked. The
yautia cocoyam yielded flowering edible vegetables. *Yampee* roots
grew purple and black, and they could be baked or ground to make
bread. The heart of young *allouia* shoots could be cooked like arti-
chokes, while its leaves and sap were used for flavoring and medicines.
Water-chestnut-textured *Lleren* was packed with protein, crispy when
cooked, and could be ground into flour. Arrowroot starch provided
medical ingredients and martial poisons, and yielded a flour rich in
potassium, iron, and vitamins that could be blended with coco or cassava or used to thicken soups and complement sweet potatoes.

British plantation owners often did not recognize Indigenous farms *as*
farms at all. To European eyes, they often resembled wild forest, subtly
dispersed and largely worked by women. This was in stark contrast
to British planting methods, which by the late 1700s had caused soil
erosion, deforestation, and changing cloud and rainfall patterns. Their
methods had also dried up several rivers, which caused the desiccated
land on the British-controlled edges of Saint Vincent to crack open, creating gullies so wide that they could not be crossed with a wagon.[44]

Yet misrecognizing Indigenous food systems was more than an innocent error: There was an ominous implication to the inaccurate British
argument that Garifuna people were not farming. One earlier botanical garden custodian on Saint Vincent had written that the Caribs
barely seemed to acknowledge Vattel's *Law of Nations*, which held
that people "who having fertile countries, distain to cultivate the earth"
had "no reason to complain if another nations more laborious . . .
come to possess a part" of their land. In fact, the *Law of Nations*
argued, any such people "*deserve to be exterminated as savage and
pernicious beasts.*"[45]

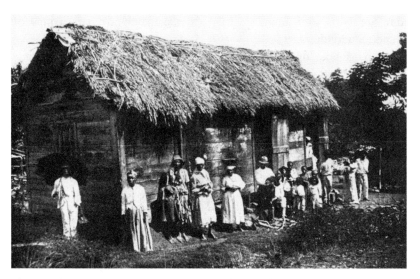

Plantation house on Saint Vincent, one century after Garifuna exile.

On the island prison of Balliceaux there was no water and few trees. Before its soil was exhausted, the land there had been used as a cotton plantation. The majority of the Garifuna prisoners had already died of starvation and disease by the time the British ships finally arrived in March 1797;[46] it is estimated that only 2,248 were still alive to be sent into exile. E. Roy Cayetano has described this historical moment as "an exercise in genocide." Most of the survivors were boarded onto a fleet of ships, hundreds more dying in their holds on the way to Central America.[47] Colonial records at the time comment on the emaciated state of the survivors by the time they reached Roatán off the coast of Honduras. During this two-year period, some 77 percent of Garifuna people died.[48]

It did not take long for Garifuna lands back on Saint Vincent to be turned into British plantations. The first year that one expelled leader's former farmland was planted, it produced 78,400 pounds of sugarcane and 1,977 gallons of molasses.[49]

Some seventeen hundred miles away on Roatán, the British officer in charge of overseeing what colonial administrators called the Garifuna "transition" noted that the amount of food being supplied to them was "very inadequate."[50] It was uncertain if crops would grow; Roatán's soil was not like Saint Vincent's. It was described as an island "on which, it was said, not even iguanas easily survived."[51] The British forces left Garinagu there with packages of flour, biscuits, sugar, saltfish, salted beef, and rum. Survivors soon managed to reach the mainland Spanish port of Trujillo in Honduras.

It did not take long before the British were criticized for their extreme brutality on Balliceaux. The governor at the time defended himself by claiming that Garifuna people had not actually been starved by the British administration, because they did not require as much food as other humans: "Referring to 'the Carib,' he wrote, 'I am told it is incredible how small a portion of food will serve him.'"[52] As historian Christopher Taylor details: "The colony's leading figures were later forced to deny claims that they had not provided sufficient food for the captives. Indeed, the authorities said that if anything they were guilty of providing too much for the Caribs to eat."

Although other records emphasize that the Garifuna captives were hungry, Dr. Anderson also became a key proponent of the "too much food" theory, saying he had no "hesitation in ascribing the death of so many of them to the overabundance of food during their stay."[53]

Reading this, I thought back to the memorably upsetting headline from *The Economist*, "Eating Themselves to Death," published 212 years after Anderson's account.

HUNGER AND DIABETES

The seemingly opposite attributions of a population either eating too much or being malnourished, it turns out, have a long history of confused linkage in debates about diabetes—also raising questions for colonial histories. In 1955, a doctor tracking several hundred people with diabetes in Jamaica noted that 13 percent of these patients seemed to present with a strange form of diabetes characterized not by obesity but by severe malnutrition, appearing to fall between classic type 1 and type 2. He proposed calling this atypical form of the disease "J-Type Diabetes" (the *J* was for Jamaica).[54]

Later the same year, a Dr. Zuidema in Indonesia described poor patients who had a strange form of diabetes characterized by emaciation and pancreatic calcification,[55] which he labeled "Z-Type Diabetes" (after his own last name). Sizable burdens of malnutrition-related diabetes were subsequently reported in Nigeria[56] and Uganda,[57] followed by a scattered cascade of malnutrition-related cases around the world: in Bangladesh, Brazil, Cameroon, the Democratic Republic of the Congo, Ethiopia, Fiji, Ghana, India, Indonesia, Kenya, Madagascar,

Malawi, New Guinea, Pakistan, South Africa, Sri Lanka, Tanzania, Thailand, Zaire, Zambia, and Zimbabwe.[58]

Yet as more and more reports of "tropical diabetes" trickled in, they seemed to complicate rather than clarify a clinical picture of the diagnosis. After a publication from Ethiopia linked diabetes to the poorest sectors of the population, it was hypothesized that the new form of diabetes might be a variation of the glucose intolerance commonly seen in starving kwashiorkor patients.[59] Meanwhile, other reports investigated the interplay of immunological factors (including polluting toxics and parasites) found in certain ecologies.[60] Pancreatic calcifications linked to protein deficiency were frequently reported but not always present as an infallible diagnostic.[61]

Today, evidence for biological mechanisms underlying a form of "atypical" diabetes remains debated.[62] Clinical reports documenting heterogeneous and even contradictory indicators have trickled in from around the world for more than fifty years, and the biological differences they document have led to a bewildering array of proposed names for this alternate form of diabetes, often overlapping but not quite synonymous: J-type diabetes, Z-type diabetes, tropical diabetes, protein-deficient diabetes, pancreatic diabetes, African diabetes, ketosis-resistant diabetes of the young, type 1b diabetes, types 3, 4, and 5 diabetes, and malnutrition-related diabetes. One Nigerian team suggested using "tropical diabetes" as an imperfect placeholder to refer to such cases until more is understood, since "the syndrome known as tropical diabetes seems to be distinct from the two main types common in developed countries" despite the unknown impact of malnutrition and wide "clinical and biochemical variants."[63]

Many medical experts now no longer believe that tropical diabetes should be distinguished as a separate diagnosis. The World Health Organization added malnutrition-related diabetes mellitus as a new category of diabetes in 1985, but then deleted it again in 1999. Now only type 1 and type 2 are recognized, with malnutrition-modulated diabetes considered a poorly understood subtype operating between the two.[64] Meanwhile, another atypical subtype proposed as African ketosis-prone diabetes has recently been theorized, again blurring the presentation signs of types 1 and 2 and thought to be characterized by an emergency state of ketoacidosis at the time of diagnosis.[65] But since the condition of ketoacidosis represents the pinnacle of medical crisis for anyone with diabetes—a potential complication that can lead to heart attack, kidney failure, coma, and death—this raises the disturbing question of whether this characteristic of "African diabetes" is actually a unique syndrome acting through specific immunological mechanisms at all. Its manifestation may instead be an example of the life-threatening end point of treatment access so unequal along racialized lines that people with diabetes in many parts of the world experience complications severe enough to make their symptoms appear as a clinically distinct disease.[66]

That question haunts varied diabetes manifestations and racialized social inequalities the world over, not just in countries that some call the "Global South." Another name by which ketoacidosis-prone type 2 diabetes became popularly known in medical literature in the 1990s was "Flatbush diabetes"—so named by concerned New York City physicians who noticed patterns of ketoacidosis crises afflicting patients from the East Flatbush area of Brooklyn, a precinct known for New York's highest violence rates and lowest income levels.[67] "Basically, these are Type 2 diabetics who look like Type 1," one of the physicians who identified this pattern explained in 1999.[68] The label "Flatbush diabetes" is still used by some worldwide. (In Belize, the phenomenon was widespread enough that I hadn't even realized it was supposed to be named as an extreme anomaly when people with type 2 go into ketoacidosis.)

Yet the underlying confusion—of not only bodily safety and nutritional issues, but also treatment access inequalities—was built all along into the fabric of historical attempts to define "tropical diabetes." As early as 1961, a follow-up study to the original 1955 identification in Jamaica suggested that J-type diabetes was not a unique disease after all, but rather a divergent clinical picture that resulted from the complications of very poor treatment of type 2 diabetes in a context of poverty and bodily insecurity.[69]

While many unknowns remain, the long debate about tropical diabetes might be read as a catalog of how "situated biologies"[70] shape different *versions* in which diabetes manifests (and is unevenly treated) across uneven political economies and different "eco-social" contexts. This implies a need to better understand the relationship between bodily insecurities, malnutrition, historical trauma, deferred treatment, and *any* form of diabetes.

WHAT IS THE "EPI" IN EPIGENETICS?

Epigenetic theories of uneven diabetes rates are gaining attention today; to understand why, it helps to know about the explanatory paradigms that this science is proposing to debunk. Over half a century ago, geneticist James Neel proposed the notion of a "thrifty genotype"[71] that puts certain ethnicities or racial groups inherently at risk for diabetes. This concept came to popularize the idea that Indigenous societies that engaged in hunting and gathering food systems (rather than permanent agriculture) must have frequently experienced famine and evolved slow-metabolizing "thrifty genes" via processes over millennia to cope with the presumed material insufficiency of their lives before European contact. It was hypothesized to explain the astronomically high rates of diabetes among many Indigenous groups, African descendants, and other nonwhite people. This theory thus implied that people who descended from those populations would carry this inheritable thrifty gene as a natural consequence of their ancestors' unenviable existence outside an industrial system.

Neel's theory caught fire; his 1962 article has been cited thousands of times, and continues to be evoked by public figures such as Jared Diamond.[72] This "thrifty gene" theory was the version of unequal diabetes risk attributions that I grew up hearing, for example, and for many years never thought to question. It wasn't until I read more closely that I learned about social historians' observations that during many ensuing decades of DNA-combing research, no one has been able to actually identify any such elusive gene that could explain the vastly unequal distributions of diabetes. As the widely popular theory gradually became more closely scrutinized, anthropologists were key players in arguing that the thrifty gene model relied on several problematic assumptions. Most prominently, these researchers showed that the supposedly massive and ongoing precontact famines did not exist—in fact, if anything, famines and food shortages actually grow *more* common as societies move toward industrialized agriculture.[73]

Pima tribal members living on the Gila River reservation, who have diabetes rates among the highest in the world, became a constantly invoked statistical case in these ongoing debates about the thrifty gene. Scientists like Neel argued that this group's unequal risk was because of their ancestors' legacy as a seminomadic foraging people. Yet others have pointed out that this theory does not make much sense when one considers that there are Pima peoples living on both sides of the border; populations on the Mexico side were geographically buffered from U.S. imperial policy in the early twentieth century and did not develop higher than average diabetes during that era. Meanwhile, Pima on the U.S. side of the border were relocated to a small barren strip of land, and shortly afterward the U.S. government diverted the river that fed it, causing their remaining crops to die. Many would argue that "innate" diabetes risk on the U.S. side of the border would be better investigated in relation to the subsequent violent events recorded in news headlines like "Indians Starving to Death—Six Thousand Perishing on the Gila Reservation in Arizona Because of Failure of Crops."[74]

How do bodies cope with hunger? In 2011, a group of scientists published on a "cure" for type 2 diabetes: starvation. Their study found that the disease could actually be reversed—possibly even permanently—*not* by a reasonable, healthy diet but by an extreme starvation diet of fewer than six hundred calories a day. The pancreas's insulin-producing beta cells, which are typically understood to be in a state of irreversible failure with diabetes, suddenly normalized themselves, leading the team to conclude that the "abnormalities underlying type 2 diabetes are reversible" with a drastically insufficient nutritional intake.[75] This "cure" underpins growing trends, though labeled as periods of fasting instead of starvation to "prevent and reverse type 2 diabetes."[76]

Evidence is also growing that maternal hunger and neonatal malnutrition play a fundamental role in the later development of diabetes. Rather than arguing for linkage to some racial or ethnic gene, more recent research suggests that nutritional stressors during *any* mother's pregnancy can potentially later contribute to her baby's risk of insulin resistance—a plasticity activated during fetal life or infancy to help a child survive in the context of scarcity or hardship, which in adulthood increases the risk of diabetes up to threefold.[77] Various biological mechanisms have been hypothesized to explain such intrauterine or childhood nutritional risk factors for diabetes, an etiological puzzle that spans both maternal and fetal undernutrition[78] and exposure to malnutrition during infancy and early childhood.[79]

On top of all this, a mother having any form of diabetes—including gestational diabetes, which can emerge abruptly during pregnancy and typically dissipates after the child is born—highly increases a baby's chance of erratic blood sugar during birth and of developing diabetes later in life. This is especially true if blood sugar is irregularly controlled during pregnancy, as is so often the case in contexts of difficulty or poverty.[80] Some public health frameworks estimate that up to 30 percent of the burden of type 2 diabetes may emerge from gestational diabetes alone, especially when mothers are lacking adequate treatment access and nutritional support during pregnancy.[81] The cellular alchemy that produces these risks holds many unknowns. But collectively, these clues suggest a picture of diabetes as part of a complex developmental system that interrelates maternal and childhood malnutrition with erratic blood sugar levels and later insulin resistance and likelihood of diabetes, with implications across generations.

Some milestone studies in this area of research include a famous data-set analysis showing that the Dutch Hunger Winter left descendants of starvation survivors particularly prone to metabolic disorders.[82] Similar findings were also reported from wide-ranging data sets, including the descendants of Holocaust survivors.[83] Meanwhile, laboratory experiments have shown that pregnant mice exposed to starvation can continue passing on the programming for metabolic conservation for at least three (and possibly up to seven) generations after the initial metabolic shock occurred. Obviously, that must mean something hugely different—both biologically and socially—for human beings. But these preliminary lab studies shed light on the possibilities of continuously changeable mechanisms that many biologists previously thought to be implausible.

Among countless potential pathways, scientists have pinpointed a few notable mechanisms at work as part of reversible imprinting meant to help the body survive in harsh environments. One of these is the epigenetic process of methylation,[84] which—to make an incredibly long and extremely intricate story short—plays a role in regulating RNA transcription and protein expression. Instead of a mutation within the alleles, such a process can influence the way the chromatin structure is controlled and genes *expressed,* without actually changing the DNA's underlying sequence.[85] If diabetes appears more often in certain families or neighborhoods, looking at the issue with an epigenetic lens focused on processes like methylation would suggest that this is true not because of Neel's racialized geocontinental thrifty gene—but rather because historical and ongoing atrocities and persistent inequalities may have material effects on ever-changing human biology, even at a cellular level.

These theories of risk might also be read against histories of violence. Historical anthropologist Jerome Handler conducted archaeological excavations on one former Barbados sugar plantation. He was joined by physical anthropologist Robert Corruccini, whose area of specialty is dental specimens. By examining individuals' teeth, they found patterns of childhood "metabolic shock" and "nutritional trauma"[86] that resulted in a wildly disproportionate number of young deaths, traceable in large part to "highly improper foods."

The particular sign they examined in these enslaved individuals' teeth is called *hypoplasia,* the "pitting, mottling, and bands and lines on teeth where enamel deposition stopped suddenly during a tooth's growth in its crypt."[87] It signals chronic malnutrition or epidemic disease. Hypoplasia can also appear in fainter bands such as "fever lines," but the archaeologists found that "extreme or severe hypoplasia was by far the most common type" among slaves of Barbados, revealed by "deeply indented horizontal depressions running completely around the tooth. These growth arrest lines are generally considered indicative of extreme dietary deficiency or starvation."[88] Although the authors note how closely chronic malnutrition and disease "are interrelated," they repeat that the particular "periodicity" in these patterns of damage firmly suggests "severe metabolic crisis during childhood."[89] In this group of over one hundred people, this signature of "metabolic shock" was recorded in 98 percent of the population.[90]

The Dutch Hunger Winter studies that broke open this field of epigenetic research described the trans-generational effects of an event that took place in 1944–45. Yet any attempt to consider the implications of this World War II study for another kind of trauma runs up against an uneasy difference—what scholars point to with the reminder that settler colonialism is "a structure, not an event."[91] An account of the traumatic factors potentially at play in a story about Garifuna dispossession, for instance, would be distorted if it focused on the 1796 starvation episode alone. That is one traumatic event within a structure that additionally includes many other forces: impacts of lost land and foodways, the unequal strains of endurance in the face of ongoing violence, and ecological injustices that are still being faced anew by each generation.

Perhaps the fact that a risk for diabetes could be mistaken as somehow inherent to categories like "African" or "Native American" DNA instead signals how chronically these same constructs of race have been deployed in the "terror of history."[92] This science suggests that metabolic *re*programming for healthy metabolism occurs through the same mechanisms of biological plasticity that made changes possible in the first place—even within a single lifetime—once the body is alerted that it is in a secure ecology over time. Epigenetic mechanisms "do not involve changes to the DNA sequence," so "unlike sequence changes, they can be reset or undone."[93]

If bodies at times continue to bear scars at the molecular level, a lack of "reset" does not suggest a problem inside people, but rather signals larger structures still recreating harms in need of institutional redress. In this light, uneven risk for diabetes might be iconic of Didier Fassin's truism: "The epidemic thus invents nothing; it uncovers."[94]

PREVENTION

When Arreini and I were both around the village, we had dinner together almost every night. It was an unofficial arrangement, but it felt like I learned more about food from meals shared with her than would have been possible from a hundred "food recall" surveys—the traditional tool of quantitative measurement for social scientists studying diabetes (although the affective meanings of eating have little to do with paperwork, and people are well known to lie or misremember on such forms). Sometimes I would help Arreini a little with the cooking, shaping flour tortillas with the empty rum bottle she used as a rolling pin while she flipped them with a fork over the stove.

Other times she would send me to a Chinese grocery in the village for certain store-bought items: tins of Guaymex sardines (my least favorite meal, although it helped that they were served in ketchup and paired with Belikin Stouts); wheat bread with spreadable Happy Cow cheese; or pigtails, which I had expected to look curly and did not know enough about to choose carefully from their bucket of brine. Arreini promptly sent me "back to the Chinese," this time escorted by an amused grandson to help me select ones with less marbled fat. Such sources of protein were central in Belize's colonial rations, although they represented a cut of meat I had not previously realized was edible, preserved in such a saline state that (in Arreini's method of preparation, at least) they had to be soaked in fresh water for a day before cooking. We ate the unevenly textured meat with pinto beans and a tandasha mango, the last of the season to ripen.

Once Arreini made a delicious shark *serre,* which was my favorite of all her soups because I could enjoy the flavors of the legendary Garifuna coconut milk soup base without worrying about choking on delicate fish bones. *Serre* was best when eaten with labor-intensive *hudut* dumplings, and on a few occasions, I took turns inexpertly pounding the green plantains in a large *mata* (*hudut* literally means "it is pounded"), the grooved wooden bowl that she cleaned fastidiously afterward with the rounded edge of a nail. More commonly though, Arreini prepared simple whole fish, usually fried with all their fins on in Malher chicken bouillon, doused in vinegar and a squeeze of lime, and served with cooked ripe plantain. "Head fish or tails?" she would ask if we were sharing a larger fish; I preferred the tail, always uncertain what flecks of meat were proper to consume inside a fish's head.

Arreini had a midwife's firm touch. When she kneaded extra flour into the mix for creole buns with her bare hands, it looked like she was giving the dough a massage. Years ago, she had transplanted a clump of fevergrass from her farm to the beach near her house, and sometimes on more relaxed nights, we would go just beyond the place where her laundry was hanging to pick tufts of the plant from a patch of dark sand. From this, she made a savory tea with the aroma of lemons, flavored with the contents of the crusted pink Sweet'N Low packets her doctor had recommended some years ago.

And always, there was the cassava bread. Most people in the village ate it occasionally, but Arreini was one of the few people I knew who was constantly able to keep a steady supply in a clear plastic bag in her kitchen, even with changing economies that made it increasingly difficult to acquire on an everyday basis. The word *Garifuna* literally means "cassava-eating people."[95]

This mainstay food became oddly entangled in the history of diabetes education. For decades, scientists mistakenly theorized that cassava caused a risk for diabetes through the trace amounts of cyanide it contains.[96] Yet later science showed that this was untrue[97]—in fact, certain "clinical use of cassava bread is suggested for diabetic and obese patients"[98] because it is far healthier than white bread or white rice. Yet even today, there is not clear consensus about cassava. Some Garinagu are advised by doctors not to eat it for health reasons. Meanwhile, cassava snacks have begun arriving in U.S. stores like Whole Foods, marketed as nutritious paleo-friendly "real vegetable chips."

Likewise, in the 1980s biomedical research called into question another staple of Garifuna cooking, coconut oil. It was during an era when scientists could tell that coconut oil contained saturated fat but did not yet understand the more subtle points of chemistry this entailed. (Because coconut oil is a medium-chain fatty acid, it is burned more easily by the body, and may speed up metabolism.) Acting on the medical advice they were given by doctors, over time many Garinagu stopped processing oil from the coconuts growing in their yards and started buying cheap gallons of vegetable oil instead, now shown to be less healthy.

This list of errors in the advice of nutritional scientists begins to demonstrate the serious implications of assuming that "ethnic" foods are the main locus of risk for a population's high diabetes rates, a pattern all the more worrisome because people's ordinary diets have often already been harmed by the time mistakes in biomedical advice are recognized. But like diabetes education, eating itself has a moral force. Throughout several decades of doctors advising otherwise, Arreini had persistently continued eating her cassava bread, using coconut oil, and making coconut milk dishes. Noncompliance can have its health benefits too.

As early as 1802, Garifuna people first sailed to Belize in gradual waves of refugees, looking for safety from encroaching violence in Honduras. Arriving in Belize later in this cascading wave of refugees was Arreini's family, although she never spoke of herself in those terms. Arreini told me of the violent events that brought her family from Honduras only in cryptic pronouns and sharp sounds, a flash interlude in hours of conversation: "They kill they. Bam, bam, bam! When we got here, I saw my sister who died waiting on the dock. Clear. She looked like you."

Her family began working a stretch of difficult land that no one else wanted, where her father built a longhouse with his machete. But he died shortly after, and it was her mother whom Arreini talked about constantly. She had learned her healing and midwife techniques from her, and when Arreini was coming of age, she even returned to Honduras with her mother to acquire further training in Garifuna medicine: "It all comes from there." But only once did she speak to me of her mother's death. Their village was poor enough at the time that no one yet had a radio, she said. She looked away from the sea as we spoke, out toward the dark road, and continued: One night, there was a blood-red sunset. That was their warning that the hurricane was coming, although people recognized it as a sign only afterward.

I had heard from many older people that it was a devastating storm, ripping apart homes then made of thatch with walls of palmetto log and cabbage bark while frantic parents tied their children to palm trees in the dark (certain trees, pliable but rooted, are often the only thing left standing as buildings topple). One man described to me his earliest memory: his mother put him and his brothers on their upended kitchen table atop the surge waters and pulled them to dry land—"like Moses," he laughed, recalling how her whole body shook to keep her grip as she pushed them against the water's current. In Sagoun, the destruction was so total that they moved the community before rebuilding, to a place where Arreini's family had already constructed a complex of houses. Most other people had previously used the land there only for farming.

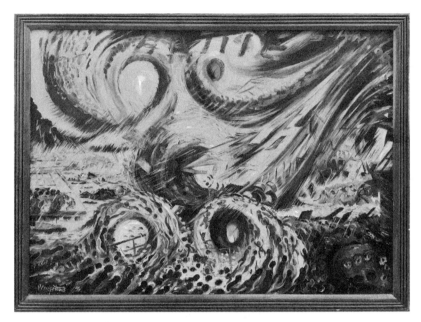

Hurricane Hattie Belize, by Pen Cayetano.

But Arreini's account focused not on the countless details of destruction but on one fact alone: afterward, her mother was gone.

As Arreini paused, I thought of the Pen Cayetano oil painting I had seen in the artist's studio in Dangriga. The image depicted a roiling Hurricane Hattie hitting the Stann Creek coast in 1961, the stormy green waves of the Caribbean foaming with the souls of the dead. It had been a Category 5 hurricane, the most powerful kind.

Her mother had already been missing for days by the time Arreini started dreaming of her. When she woke up the next morning, she followed the scenes envisioned in her dreams, taking seven men and telling them where to dig in the rubble. They found her mother's body quickly. "She was facedown," Arreini said. "There was money coming out of her pockets."

There is a deep human politics behind hurricane responses. Before being exiled from Saint Vincent, Garifuna people's ancestors knew how to read coming tropical storms in the subtle signs of the sea life, trade winds, and atmosphere. They were so famously adept at the prediction of coming hurricanes that British and French populations who occupied neighboring islands would bargain with them to be included in the loop of their knowledge. In the 1700s, one sea captain described the British and French colonial custom at the start of hurricane season "to send in about the Month of *June*, to the Native Caribees of *Dominico* and *St. Vincent*, to know whether there would be any Hurricanes that year: and about Ten or Twelve Days before the Hurricanes came, they did constantly send them Word; and it very rarely seldom failed."[99]

After the British military exiled the inhabitants of Saint Vincent from the living place integral to such science, the region's storms became much harder to predict with adequate notice. Even when colonial meteorological instruments eventually were able to identify coming hurricanes in advance, later English officials in Belize at times chose not to spread the word—such as the notorious unnamed hurricane that hit in 1931. Colonial records show that the government of then British Honduras received news about "the cyclone" a day and a half in advance, but for some reason, the authorities made a decision not to tell the local citizenry,[100] who had been agitating for independence and were considered particularly unruly at the time. The hurricane was followed by a ten-foot tidal wave that killed approximately 15 percent of the city's entire population and "destroy[ed] at least three quarters of the housing."[101] Many say Belize City has never recovered. According to Kriol oral histories, it was Garifuna farmers from southern Belize (rather than the colonial administration) who sent food aid to those in need in Belize City in the aftermath of certain hurricanes.[102]

Some three decades later, major towns had been at least partially evacuated for Hurricane Hattie, but Sagoun apparently received no notice of the coming storm through the national emergency system. Listening to the heavy quiet after she described finding her mother, I thought that it was the most broodingly distant I had ever seen Arreini and waited for her to speak first. She added that she had buried something under the cement house's present location. Straining, I could not understand what she said, but it seemed to have something to do with both her mother's protection and untimely death and the many times she had told me emphatically: "Thing serious. This place is *fixed*." Often she would send me to the cement house to fetch something she had forgotten (usually her Icy-Hot thermos) with a giant ring of keys in hand, hung on bits of string and a sturdy diaper pin shaped like a yellow duckling. Many of the keys were for doors that no longer existed. While fiddling with the difficult lock, I found it unsettling to notice the unusual amount of hair visible under the door's blue paint, like living veins.

Arreini received phone calls constantly. It seemed like she was always fishing around in her apron pockets for the cordless phone. One evening, there was good news and bad news from Belize City: Guillerma had fallen into a diabetic coma, but the hospital was able to bring her back; she had finally gotten one of the limited twenty-one spots in the country for dialysis, but the government could only "help with this one" of the three sessions each week. She hoped for the standard therapy of three sessions per week in order to have the best chance of staying alive, but it would cost several hundred U.S. dollars for each of the remaining two sessions, a total of around 450 U.S. dollars every week. "So she's going to stick with just one," Arreini said of the single subsidized session, and focused approvingly on the good care that Guillerma's children were taking of her. This was the main news of the phone call—not the fact that Guillerma seemed on the precipice of death but that her children were tending to her lovingly there: the girls were sending food every meal, and Sheldon had purchased a used car to drive his mother to the sessions each Tuesday.

"What's that disease she have?" Arreini murmured to herself later. "Dialys," she answered herself, her careful truncation (of the equally truncated sessions) turning it into not only a Garifuna word but also a disease rather than its treatment. "She's in Jesus's hands now," she said and abruptly pulled a rosary from her enormous apron pockets. Arreini said that her rosary prayers and improvised *misas* were most effective in Spanish, her mother's language of interface with the outside world— one more way that Arreini spoke *in* her history, if not always *of* it. That night she first taught me the Prayer of Saint Lucas. *"Aquí tenemos el milagro,"* she recited for Guillerma, and I never knew whether this line—Here we have the miracle—was calling a miracle into being by demanding its materialization or was recognizing the marvel of what already was. "Santos, santos, santos," she prayed, as if reworking the hierarchical trinity into some friends nearby: saints, saints, saints.

Although the thatch kitchen (where the offering for her mother had taken place) was padlocked, Arreini's everyday cement block kitchen actually had *two* locks—one printed with the rusting word GLOBE and a second blue padlock sporting the Pepsi logo. Inside was a meticulous jumble: calabash shells; handmade wooden cassava-grating boards with teeth of jagged white pebbles; handwoven nets storing enamel bowls; hammered tin cups hanging carefully from nails on the rafters, inter-mixed with plastic mugs bearing different scars of heat; and a smatter-ing of shelved groceries. There were empty jars and plastic bottles of every size, a box of cornflakes, a plastic orange strainer that she used for grated coconut, a broom she used to sweep the beach (treating the sand outside as a kitchen floor), a can of Diet Coke on the windowsill, a cardboard box from AccuSure 1cc syringes. These were apparently left over from before she decided to stop the daily insulin therapy that made her feel too sick to function, although she kept a single vial on reserve in her refrigerator. The syringe box was now used as a container to store fruit, avocados,[103] and saved plastic bags.

Once, after a violent illness caused me to lose ten pounds in three days, I nervously broke the news to Arreini that I was going to start drinking only from my own water bottle. I was worried this might interrupt our rhythms of commensality, but to my surprise she locked eyes with me and nodded emphatically, as if I was finally beginning to prove a worthy student. "Now you're like me. I *always* carry my own water," she said, looking at me intently. "You have to take care."

Her attentive protection of the kitchen each night before bed was also part of her daily work of *taking care*. She would begin with the bench under the front house where we most often sat to eat meals, tilting the wooden furniture at a forty-five-degree angle and then resting against it a perpendicular stick of bamboo. Likewise, in the kitchen, each and every opening and surface had to be covered: bowls turned concave-side down, every plastic bucket covered with a wooden board, all food and utensils draped one by one with towels, a black mat (like the kind used to protect automobile carpets) covering the stove top, a rinsed yogurt container to cover the spout of her teakettle. After the door had been closed for the night, she would put in place the Pepsi padlock, the last step in her careful labor of maintaining security. "For protection," she would explain. Once I asked what she meant. "You don't hear me? It is for protection," she repeated with an impatient glance in my direction. I understood her to mean that the world's many poisons could not be separated, and ingestion was one of the primary ways that something might reach you. On one occasion I saw her rebuke one of Guillerma's youngest granddaughters after seeing her carelessly discard leftover scraps and water left in her glass on the beach by the porch steps. "Don't you understand what I teach you?" Because she spoke in English, I thought she was trying to explain to me as well. "You risk death," she said.

Many of the precise details of the events that killed the majority of the world's Garifuna people at the cusp of the nineteenth century have faded from oral history. But there is one exceptional detail: the memory of their food supplies being poisoned. Over time, many Garinagu have firmly maintained that the white flour they were given by the British while captives was poisoned with white lime.[104] (Barreled flour was the main food that their population was supplied with during their "transition.") While malnutrition and disease were both rampant on Balliceaux, it is documented that for some reason "the Carib death rate was 85 percent, compared to a reported rate of only 5 percent for the British slaves and Negro troops, who also suffered from the diseases."[105] An assistant surgeon in the British Navy observed this "malignant pestilential disease" firsthand and, even factoring in the group's severe malnutrition at the time, reported that he was wholly unable to account for the scale of these losses.[106]

Was the poisoned white flour an idiom of mass violence, or a tool of mass violence? Through her attentiveness to obscured forces and insistent dead, Arreini kept bringing me back to the returns of an enigmatic history. In addition to foods' tastes and memories, for her eating also evoked a cryptic need for protection and vigilance, a mindfulness of danger and the daily work of *taking care* to establish one more "interval of security"[107] in a series of chronic stressors. Community and history returned through food too, present in the everyday realities of nutrition and medicine. According to Arreini, the security and insecurity of each generation are interlocking. I thought of Guillerma, being kept alive on a machine now, and wondered what to make of how white flour and violence had reached her too.

BLOOD'S SUGAR

There is a sense in which patterns of death in Belize—sugar and violence—represent gendered stories that remain deeply interconnected. "Without geosocial exception," Herbert Gayle wrote, dead bodies are now becoming for people across Belize "part of their social reality and everyday life."[108] In a study conducted with the government, Gayle's team found startling levels of social violence among school-age children. His research showed that 38.8 percent of Belizean youth had lost a family member to shooting, and another 23.5 percent had lost a family member to stabbing.[109] Over 41 percent of children had witnessed a shooting, while 13 percent of boys and 8 percent of girls had personally been stabbed, and more than 25 percent of youths reported being beaten by police.[110] "This would be equivalent to living in a place where war has been declared,"[111] Gayle writes of the psychic effects of these strains in Belize.

In researching the roles of chronic stressors in relation to diabetes, scientists are earnestly trying to grapple with how felt emotions, losses, and experiences become part of biology. Yet *stress*, like *environment*, is another catchall that could mean so much and so little at the same time. It might include levels of cortisol, but only as a partial measure.

Or at least, I think how the metrics of blood chemistry panels alone would fail to capture the kinds of strains I observed and encountered moving through Belize at times. A huge surge in weapons (mostly circulating from the United States) has accompanied these shifts; today in Belize City, you can rent a gun in certain shops by the day or hour. Belize's underfunded and overburdened legal and social infrastructures contributed to the growth of these illicit economies. Against a backdrop in Belize City where "the biggest single problem identified at 51 of the 59 schools is chronic hunger,"[112] "many gangs extort money to provide children with lunch money on a daily basis."[113] Gayle describes the often-noted paradoxes when a collective known for illicit economies is also a key provider of food and social services in contexts of state neglect, becoming an important neighborhood institution through structures of care as well as violence.[114]

Violence and chronic stressors wear on institutions like hospitals just as they do on other bodies. Gayle also reported on this problem in Belize City, documenting that "gang violence can wipe out over a third of all resources allocated to hospitals, thus retarding the very ability of the state to provide basic health care."[115] There was major unrest among the Cuban physicians stationed throughout Belize after one volunteer in their cohort, a twenty-eight-year-old woman, had her face slashed. This incident prompted the head of Karl Heusner Memorial Hospital— whose brother had been recently murdered by an escaped convict—to write a passionate editorial titled "Violence and the Health of a Nation." He wrote: "Violent crime and accidents often leave the emergency cupboard bare—and expensive medications, instead of going to the sick, end up diverted to the victims of violence . . . [who] take priority over your child who is sick, or you with abdominal pain, or your high blood pressure or diabetes that is out-of-control."[116]

In 2012, all outpatient services at the understaffed Karl Heusner Memorial Hospital (the country's main referral hospital in Belize City) were canceled for several days due to the murder of its critical care unit physician.[117] After he was strangled to death at home, all the specialist clinics at the hospital were suspended: "Somebody has to start something somewhere," one physician told the local press as the hospital staff marched, holding posters about unsolved murders.[118] The previous year, a U.S. doctor had also been murdered in Belize, thrown into his van and doused with gasoline before the vehicle was set on fire. A news story reported of the doctor and his wife: "He often provided free medical care. . . . They were going to be treating diabetes."[119]

In 2010, I went with some nurses to watch the Carnival parade from Belize City's Southside. A guy in his twenties about my age stood next to our cooler, marked in mud and with one-dollar gold coins featuring Queen Victoria resting in each ear. I was about to ask him if it was real *J'ouvert* mud (especially prepared for Carnival by one particular lady) when I saw the revolver in his waistband and looked away. Suzanne handed me her purse to hold for a few minutes, which I handled carelessly only to realize I was now carrying a gun too, a .357 beside her cell phone and tissues. Ratios of guns to people in a given area would be a more useful metric of stress than cortisol. I told Suzanne she should have mentioned it when handing her purse to me, shaken at the thought we had been jostling through the crowd. But she just laughed at my inability to tell whether the safety was on and pointed out the brick building near us on the river where slave ships from the sugar islands used to dock for market. Today the building is a bank, but its basement is lined with rows of shackles, Suzanne said; it was not a historic exhibit, just no one knew how to get them out of the foundations.

Did she mean that as a metaphor, or did I just hear it that way? We watched the Belize Defense Force tank rumble through Southside. The soldiers' sand-colored camo had the opposite effect of most camouflage, since the beige stood out starkly against the bright homes and Carnival parade's stream of exuberant sequins and bright feathered masks. It was a tense anniversary because the city's first grenade explosion in the streets had occurred during Carnival two years before, killing several children. In the hours after we watched the parade, four people were killed in tiny Southside. Among them was an eight-year-old child named Eyannie, struck by stray bullets while sleeping. The thousands attending her funeral overflowed the streets and shut down the city, outnumbering the crowds at Carnival.[120]

Other protests were also fomenting. Chinese shopkeepers were being targeted countrywide in a wave of ethnic violence, a phenomenon bound up with Belize's long history of grocery politics. Every time I went to Belize City, people talked about the latest shop where it happened; there seemed to always be a new picture of foam-sandaled feet next to a dark puddle on a concrete grocery store floor in the newspapers. In August 2010, I came into Dangriga one morning and found the town buzzing yet strangely quiet: all the Chinese businesses across the country had shut down in solidarity and mourning for a fourteen-year-old girl named Hellen Yu, who was shot along with her father in the family's grocery store.[121] This followed shortly after a string of other Chinese murders, including a twenty-seven-year-old woman shot with her baby tied to her back on Mother's Day.[122]

Protests began verging on riot level in 2011, after two Chinese women were shot in separate grocery stores within a two-hour time span. Both women were behind iron bars in the store, so nothing could even possibly be stolen.[123] A two-day nationwide shutdown of Chinese shops followed. Protesters dressed in white gathered around the Belize Supreme Court, carrying coffins that bore the women's photos and chanting "Give me back a life."[124] One of the stores where I used to go food shopping was also targeted; a slight teenager I often saw stocking groceries in his family's store was shot in the aisles, the only student of Chinese descent in a class of 480 attending a Dangriga school. The article in which I read about his death was titled "One More Asian Belizean Murdered."[125]

Still other deaths were barely reported in the papers at all. Once back home again, I wore a pair of earrings I inherited in Belize from an acquaintance named Leanna, seventies-style tarnished silver loops I had imagined hanging under her long auburn hair at some European discotheque in the prime of her beauty. When I learned of her murder in Belize several weeks later, my shock at the surreal news somehow attached itself to the more tangible fact that I had unknowingly worn her earrings out to dinner sometime after the night she was raped and strangled. This felt heavily ominous, and I began dreaming of her, although never a gruesome image of violence. "Why do they break her jaw?" my friend Gia asked me over the phone after seeing her mother's body. Some months before then, it was Gia's son whose body I had been asked to hold while they went upstairs to look for his birth certificate. From movies I had always thought a dead body would be cold and heavy, but he was still warm and felt light in my arms while I sat holding him on the green couch.

The sudden deaths, especially violent ones, of people I knew felt very different to me than the slow medical deaths, and they were distinct from the seemingly small risks of everyday living, but they all compounded for me into a nerve-ridden fog I hadn't experienced before: reeling nightmares, dissociative voids, hyperplanned routes from one place to another, anxieties verging on paranoia. (Yet in her dissertation on mental illness in Belize, Mary Kenyon Bullard notes: "Generally speaking, the idea of baseless paranoid behavior and thought is an alien one to British Hondurans. There is no corresponding local term for it and the concept is a difficult one to explain to the residents. They surely recognize paranoid conduct as an aspect of human existence but they feel that the person is justified in some way and that he or she is laudably realistic and properly cautious, certainly not deluded or insane."[126])

Sometimes I think it was only people's small gestures that kept me from fully losing it. Once Arreini saw me at my lowest point, and although I didn't tell her that I had hallucinated the night before and was frightened, I must have seemed off somehow because she looked at me intently and then, with some flash of patience or pity, told me to sit down. I had always learned that pity can wound, but in that moment I felt only gratitude that someone noticed something was wrong. The list of small chores she usually had waiting for me evaporated for the day without a word, and she prepared an impromptu meal of tea and *ereba*. What she said to me over our makeshift meal was, I later imagined, one of many potential free falls she had preempted in her lifetime. But I still wasn't myself afterward, throwing myself into the routines and relationships of fieldwork with a kind of obsessive attention. When I went back home for a visit, it accentuated all the ledges; I felt miles away from most conversations and remained on high alert, unable to shake a thick, sweet scent that nobody else could smell. Looking back, I see that there is a section of my notes from this time titled *Smell of Death?* I kept dreaming of being followed down a dusty orange road.

Is this anything like what the proximity to violence felt like to others in Belize? I suspect not, although I sometimes imagined I was glimpsing for the first time the mildest edge of a spectrum of bodily awareness in which other people lived out their whole lives. The constant possibility of death was one of its axes, and this triangulated different laws of gravity, like some extra dimension of movement and responsibility I had not known existed, in which the default assumption was not safety but a vigilant social savvy and the specter of loss. I could only gropingly discern its codes but glimpsed for the first time their charge, and when I continued, it was with the queasy sense of knowing that whatever slight threats I faced as a white U.S. American citizen anywhere were laughably miniscule in contrast to what that privilege protected me from. And yet I marveled at how much effort it took just to keep my mind intact, when really the only thing I was facing was not being completely exempt from this. I learned just how quickly a crisis could start, the way something might well up unplanned and move in a kind of oversaturated slow motion replaying in memory. I struggled to learn from the women who somehow brought grace and resolve from the situations of pain or fear that paralyzed and enfeebled me. I watched white doctors from foreign countries lecture these same women about why preventive health was important, seemingly without realizing how entire lives were already being lived in a mode of preventative care.

At the time I couldn't put this vague feeling of complicit anger and dawning awareness into words. But it was only in retrospect that I wondered about how much Coca-Cola I had started consuming at this time. I rarely ever drink soda at home, but in Belize I found myself stopping for a bottle or two each day. Some of the reasons were conscious: it was cheaper than water and cut more crisply through the dust and heat that stuck in your throat; it provided an energy boost in times of exhaustion; and it was a safe bet (in the short term) to avoid getting sick, unlike juices made with tap water.

But over time, I also came to rely on it to stop losing weight. After an upsetting day, when something scary happened or after the kind of interview where what I had just heard was too sad for processing, I often lost my appetite for food, but never for Coke. I loved how the glass bottles could get so cold. In Belize, as in much of Central America, Coke is still made with sugarcane (instead of U.S. corn syrup sweeteners). And buying one gave you a reason to stand around and chat or rest or get oriented for a minute while you drank it before going back into the sun, since the shop proprietor needed the thick bottle back. Behind the small social comforts of such rituals, lab studies have suggested the soothing bodily effects of sugar, both emotionally and physically—mice take twice as long to step off a hot burner when they've been fed sugar water first, and only cry half as much when taken away from their mothers.[127]

And even beyond all pragmatics, later I would wonder if there wasn't also something less functional that was part of its sensory draw. Why did I find real comfort in consuming the product most iconic for contributing to the exact diabetes injuries and deaths that I was nauseous from observing? But somehow it became a toehold in my routine, at a time when each day felt like its own horizon. By my last month in Belize, I got a blood sugar measurement of 128, which technically gets labeled as "prediabetes." Why did the news make me laugh? And why *didn't* it make me stop drinking Coca-Cola every day?

In however profoundly partial a way, as Bartow Elmore describes in *Citizen Coke*, "It seemed I had become trapped in the history I had come to investigate."[128]

QUICKSILVER

If bodies' memories are never solid state, at times people's stories of danger and memory or cause and effect seemed like striking parallels to the implications of biomedical sciences of bodily plasticity. But other times both got messy, pulling things in directions of their own.

For example, I once met a man with diabetes who checked into the Dangriga hospital not because of his usual blood sugar emergencies, but because he couldn't stop hiccupping. Calvin was in his fifties and between hiccups spoke briefly but tenderly about constant visits from his daughters and of working in the local hot sauce factory. Two weeks later, I was invited to a Kriol wake of a friend's uncle and was just handed a Styrofoam plate of rice and beans when I realized that the wooden casket was holding Calvin. People said the hiccups had killed him. It didn't make any sense.

Or consider the fate of Mr. R, an older man with diabetes who came to a local mobile clinic complaining of "wind in his head." He handed the doctor on duty a little ziplock bag with a few yellow pills left in it. An extremely common scene unfolded, which I watched play out dozens of times during my fieldwork: the black marker labeling the bag of pills had worn off to illegible smudges, Mr. R did not remember the name of the medication he had been taking, and the Cuban doctor (both amused and perplexed at how to interpret the symptom of wind in one's head) did not have the time or the means to track down the hospital where they had been prescribed. Mr. R died the following month, in what I took to be at least partially the outcome of these inconsistencies of treatment. But I never really understood what he meant by wind in the head, and everyone made their own attributions. "That man stole pumpkins from my farm once," Arreini told me as we sat under her house, watching people pass by on the road as they gathered for his *beluria*. Her tone in that moment was unforgiving. "If you have a dirty heart, you can't survive long."

But even amid what felt like hazy risk and vaguely ascribed causalities, I also met people who had trouble dying. For a number of months, each week I visited a very old man named Toribio and his wife, Alexandrina, at the request of their daughter, Bea. She took painstaking care of her aging parents, who both had diabetes and lay in side-by-side narrow beds in a sun-filled room near the kitchen. Only once did I see Alexandrina at the kitchen table, eating a bowl of soup. When Toribio died, Alexandrina and Bea put a tattered stuffed animal on his bed's pillow, a little joke. Yet its spindly legs and wide eyes evoked his silent presence with uncanny gravity.

Alexandrina was rumored by some to have quicksilver—a metaphysical substance said to make it difficult to die. She was always bathing her neck in fresh lime juice and usually had a can of Coke and a bottle of Florida water near her bed. It was said that she had spent her life pursued by ancestral spirits, going into fugue states and awaking, for example, in the forest amid a swarm of ants, yet they did not sting her; some said that even though she refused to undertake the official training necessary to become a *buyei,* she was covered and "held" by their good prayers. She had sky-blue eyes and silver hair always twisted into two braids and couldn't take pharmaceuticals because of kidney damage so severe that doctors could never believe she was still alive when they saw the lab results of her urinalysis. But Alexandrina liked to have her sugar and pressure taken anyway—being monitored meant something to her even when no treatment was possible, maybe just for touch. While her glucose was being taken, sometimes Alexandrina would describe the bright images she saw floating through the air: schools of extinct fish, people she had known. One afternoon I was sitting on the floor next to her bed while we talked when suddenly she was looking over my shoulder. She said something in Garifuna that I couldn't understand, squeezing my hand.

"She said she sees her coffin," Bea told me.

When I attended the *rusariu*[129] for Toribio at their home, the front room was crowded with women praying novenas. I fumbled with the glassy purple rosary beads I had borrowed, disoriented by the number of unknown faces in the familiar room. The furniture had been rearranged, the couch moved to clear space for an altar along the west wall. A black fabric cross was pinned to the white sheet on the altar. The altar held lit white candles, two vases of bright orange hibiscus flowers, and a giant gold-framed portrait of Jesus. The room smelled of baking bread, and there were loops of dried palms stuck into the curtains. A maestro stood by the altar, calling out prayers in a mix of Latin and Spanish to the crowd of women. "Dígame," they responded to each of the names in a long list of saints, crossing themselves repeatedly: tell me, *espiritu santu*. Alexandrina lay listening from her bed in the adjacent room, while Bea's daughters rubbed her skin with a lotion of marigold and myrrh to keep her comfortable. The last time I saw Alexandrina, the gold-framed acrylic painting of Jesus had been placed next to her on the bed and she was staring at the portrait with great intensity. I was in Dangriga when I got the call saying she had died at the end of the ninth and final night of Toribio's *beluria,* the festive farewell rites that would send his spirit off to the afterlife. But there was no talk of diabetes at all; everyone just said, "He came for her." It was said they were traveling together now to *Seiri*, an afterworld described to me as connected to cassava gardens on Saint Vincent (before the sugar plantations), going to the homeland that had been lost generations before they were born. In death, it was a love story.

I was not surprised, some years later, to hear rumors that Arreini also had quicksilver. Its protection meant you could drink poison and it would not kill you; you could be shot and survive; you could have diabetes and live on and on. But the translation of *quicksilver* into English is especially perplexing because its Garifuna equivalent, *likornia*, comes from the French *licorne*, for "unicorn." It seems the substance originated somehow in the materia medica of Saint Vincent during the time when the Garinagu formed an uneasy alliance with the French to ward off British takeover.

During this period in European medicine, literal quicksilver was commonly administered as a therapeutic, and various antidotes to counter poison were thought to gain power by being mixed inside carved unicorn horns (though in the *General History of Drugs*, King Louis XIV's pharmacist Pierre Pomet opined that these purported horns were mostly counterfeit from narwhal tusks).[130] It's possible that the conceptual overlay of *likornia* was inspired in part by colonial medical practices like these or by conversations with European traders searching for unicorns during their scientific and trade expeditions in the Caribbean and Latin America. Because of the high price that unicorn horns could fetch on the medical market during this period, colonial traders and naturalists looked for them obsessively. Unexplored territories of the Americas became the place in which unicorns were most suspected to live. When artist Julius Goltzius sketched his vision of four continents, Europe was portrayed as a chariot pulled by horses, Africa as one pulled by lions, and Asia by a pair of camels, while America was represented by an Indigenous woman in a chariot pulled by unicorns.[131]

Somehow the notion of *likornia* took shape in close exchange with such colonialist fantasies and European commerce. As one Dutch explorer lamented of American unicorns thought to live in the interior: "Because of their fleetness and strength, they were seldom caught."[132] Maybe people on Saint Vincent heard of the creatures that kept eluding colonial harnesses and admired their powers of evasion and survival, or somehow came to link their qualities with the name for a potent antidote against death.

Licorne was also one therapy that Europeans could not steal through bioprospecting. Its essence still remains some part of Garifuna metaphysics today, at least according to the puzzles that language leaves behind. All I can say for certain is that by the time of my work, people said that quicksilver was a formidable method the old ones had of "fixing life" in a person. Garifuna scholar and priest Jerris Valentine has published on this "complex and controversial" substance in careful detail:

> *Likornia* . . . is a substance that the ancients put into the system of their grandchildren as a prevention from harm. It is administered orally or it is absorbed through the pores of the skin. This seems to be a very potent mixture that could kill if too much is administered. With the correct dose, however, nothing—obeah, ghost, gunshot, etc. and nobody—can harm whoever has it. *Likornia* has been explained as something like quicksilver because it "travels" all over the body. A person who has *Likornia* will find it difficult to die. For some it is impossible until *Likornia* itself dies.[133]

Loosening such a hold could require different things, people said: lime juice, prayers, sometimes a specialist. Arreini's quicksilver was somehow also part of her physiology. I only ever met a few old women who were said to have *likornia*, but for me the substance seemed forceful as a concept as well as a treatment. I used to picture diaspora as fragments—but over time came to think of it like quicksilver, traveling droplets that can become scattered yet keep regathering into new wholes. This fluidity is something not captured in the English sense of *mercurial*—which suggests unpredictability but misses how changeability can at times be a responsive form of staying power. Quicksilver shares with epigenetics an unfixed kind of fixing.

Yet "fixing" took many forms, which often entirely blurred the mundane and the supernatural. Two months before my time in Belize was over in 2010, Arreini began planning a trip to Chicago. Her Charcot ulcer still had not healed; the infection kept subsiding and reappearing again, despite an endless string of antibiotic pills and herbal treatments. The tissue had seemingly lost the ability to heal itself, and her doctor in Belize City had again suggested cutting her foot off (apparently as a precaution so that she wouldn't lose the whole leg or succumb to bacterial blood poisoning). She was going to the States to try to save her foot and also to visit with her family there. Several of her children lived in Detroit and Chicago, and one son had even taken out a U.S. health insurance policy for her. She said that her husband wanted her to "come back" and visit him there too, but she was unsure. "I buy this love for myself," Arreini said.

We were finishing our meal together on the wooden bench when the cordless phone started ringing from inside the bulging pockets of Arreini's apron. Her Garifuna grew loud and anxious, but I couldn't understand. She hung up the phone, her head bent down in silence. "She do complicated," she finally said out loud, more to the yard than to me. "Whole lot of complicated upon this world."

Finally looking back at me, Arreini shuffled around in her apron pockets and lit her pipe, stuffing it with fragrant leaves that sounded brittle in the darkness. She told me that Guillerma's dialysis portal was infected, her chest on one side swollen with the sickness. The surgeon was going to "bore another hole" in her chest the next day to open a second portal, on the opposite side of her heart this time. "It's rotting," Arreini said. "Now she has three things—the sugar, pressure, and the rotting, like a cancer [used colloquially for any decaying body part]. There is no remedy for that." Arreini was mad at Guillerma for sharing a dinner with her daughters of red *recado* and rice that night. "How's she going to pay when she needs the hospital? Not on my string."

She fell quiet, looking around at the yard she was about to leave behind. "Well, only Jesus knows," she said. Alongside all of Arreini's arts of *taking care* (which more often meant *giving care* to the person or situation in question), there were also points where holes were not always patchable. Arreini suddenly said out loud that as long as she was still alive, she would bury Guillerma in the village. "Here with me," she said, staring at the dirt road. Her voice sounded far away as she puffed on her pipe. Although she did not look back toward me once, I felt it was the most intense conversation we had ever had.

"I can't stop the deadness," she said.

Earlier that evening, Arreini had packed for her flight to Chicago (two suitcases and a vinyl *krokos* sack patterned with Disney princesses), so she could go to bed early and be ready for the dawn bus the next day. She asked for help as we stood up from the wooden bench and leaned heavily on me as she got to her feet, her stiffness surprising me, a jarring reminder that she was over eighty. As she moved her bamboo staff into place after tilting the bench in her usual nighttime routine, I wondered if I would really see her again.

"I will miss you, my husband. O!" she laughed at me, in a generous way that made you feel in on the joke whether you understood it or not. I still enjoyed being labeled with her kin terms of endearment, although I wondered by then if she called me by intimate terms in part because she forgot my actual name. For Arreini, the months of evenings we had spent together perhaps blurred into a long line of visitors. She proudly cultivated external interest in her life and was surprised only by how much the size of our interview recording machines had changed over time.

But for me it felt like a brush with a singular legend who turned out to be real, and in that moment we were walking together. The pressure of her weight on my elbow seemed at odds with her intimidating carriage, like edging arm-in-arm across the sand with a geriatric titan. I tried to memorize the scene: the spiced smell of her teas, the dozens of blackbirds that lived in the high tree above her kitchen. "You know who has all my important books," she reminded me, clenching her jaw when pressure fell on the tender foot as we moved toward the back house with slow steps. "Write the thing about what you learn from us here, and send it to me for Christmas."

Once, she had sat in the passenger seat of a truck I had borrowed, calling out greetings to everyone we passed through the open window and growing furiously animated ("Son of a Fock!") when we drove past a foreign real estate company's FOR SALE sign marking another plot of land her family had once owned.

SEQUENCING

Recognition or misrecognition of "biologies of history" materially shapes the future—in part because such accounts impact how science and technology get invested in and scaled up moving forward. People living with diabetes in villages around the world today are more likely to have had their genomes sequenced for risk than to have access to dialysis that might actually mitigate its consequences. As Stefan Helmreich writes: "The biology, as astonishing as it is, does not tell us *what it will mean*."[134]

In 2019, the company 23andMe announced that diabetes risk profiles would be an option on their ancestry testing. Although looking for a combination of genes rather than one alone, this procedure casts uneven distributions as something naturally inside people—and assumes that family patterns are due to DNA, not fluid bodily responses that point toward the need to focus on larger systems. "In a press release, the company noted that they have a partnership with . . . an artificial intelligence coaching platform that can guide users through, among other things, diabetes prevention programs—for $19.99 a month."[135] 23andMe also partnered with the pharmaceutical company Glaxo-

SmithKline to design new drugs from their database of DNA test results.

Some researchers have proposed that the best response to a disease like diabetes would be to create a "trauma pill" meant to work by wiping away epigenetic memories of a body's past molecular strains. But this presumes, among other things, that the traumas are over and their impacts solvable by consumers paying for a pill. Depictions of a "trauma pill" in sci-fi films like DuBois Ashong's *No Boni*, in contrast, portray nearly the opposite fantasy: imagining pharmaceuticals that do not make cells in bodies forget but make people in societies remember.

These instances stand as a reminder that diabetes research remains haunted by the phenomenon that Primo Levi's words hint at in this chapter's epigraph. In *Periodic Table*, Levi recalled being enrolled into bench science for a Swiss pharmaceutical company that was trying to make a new diabetes pill from flower petals. He realizes in this flash instant (when he sees himself being viewed as part of a "basically human race") that his own family risk for diabetes would make him a valuable human subject for pharmaceutical experimentation, for reasons quite related to the Nazi logics of scientific racism—the labeling of human difference by which he was soon afterward sent to the concentration camps of Auschwitz. The experimental science of diabetes therapeutics can be disturbingly coterminous with the types of patterned violence and histories of racialization that contribute to certain populations being at disproportionate risk for chronic disease in the first place.[136]

For this reason, research projects today eagerly collecting bodily samples from populations for epigenetic sequencing (often inner-cheek swabs to measure DNA methylation and unshampooed strands of hair one inch from the follicle tested for cortisol) raise their own deep quandaries. The legacy of collecting biological tissue from Indigenous and other minority populations also trails heavy colonial histories.[137] Under the guise of diabetes testing, Indigenous people's blood has long been collected for genome projects and a range of medical research. It is no wonder that many scholars today worry that epigenetic research based on human samples could reproduce similar ethical issues. The question of who benefits from collected biocapital accumulating in freezers around the world certainly remains salient, whether investigating theories of changing bodies or static ones.

Garinagu had an entire volume of the series *Current Developments in Anthropological Genetics* focused on them as scientific curiosity, a patchwork of studies carried out by researchers in the 1970s with an array of strange metrics: measuring the length of people's noses and their "trunk sizes"; employing a technique the researchers called "dermatoglyphics" to graph out the loops and whorls on fingerprints as a racial index; using light-reflecting meters to measure skin pigmentation from their armpits; and collecting blood samples for various analyses of genetic markers.[138] Garifuna biological samples were measured and employed to test mathematical equations of various "racial admixtures" that scientific researchers at the time were constructing—"constitutive elements [that each] operates within a loop of circular reasoning," as Kim TallBear writes in *Native American DNA*[139]—with some idea of a benefit to science writ large, but ultimately with little material benefit to the communities whose bodily tissue made up the researchers' physical samples.

In some ways, any kind of specimen collecting from racially categorized bodies can risk taking on echoes that recall Anderson's scientific search on Saint Vincent for Carib skulls to study and measure. The bodily specimens he categorized also became props in a political apparatus that was much larger than any particular scientific project or actor involved. By trying to identify and schematize inherent bodily differences linked to race, Anderson (like Linnaeus) played some supporting role in helping to produce and renew ideas of "natural" human difference. Yet these classifications *did* hold potential biological implications—coming to normalize violent reorderings of plants, places, and people—by constantly placing focus on narratives about the misbehavior or disordered biologies of populations, rather than the unequal harms alive in precisely that moment.

Any writer or researcher selects specific details that become part of the case being built; the setting of any narrative already establishes certain terms for its unfolding plot and will have much to do with what will count as its resolution. Perhaps this is as true for epigenetics as it is for anything. Start the story in a laboratory, and you will end the story seeking a solution in a laboratory. Start with a gene, and you will end up targeting a gene. But how to start the story somewhere else, such as with the interactive phenomena causing injuries in the first place?

Many conquest-era plant specimens from stolen islands such as Saint Vincent are now extinct in the wild. Some are alive only in British greenhouses, like the huge Victorian glass atriums at the Kew Royal Botanic Gardens. In their attached archives, a kindly curator led me through wheeled-open aisles. Their drawers contained thousands upon thousands of seeds and plant specimens gathered from across the colonial world, especially the former British Empire. Packed with jars and boxes of seeds surrounded by living gardens, many from plundered lands across the Caribbean and around the world, such collections are also part of the biologies that were rearranged by trans-plantation.

When I photographed the Kew archives' specimens from Saint Vincent, I thought they would start making sense later. Were some of these jars and boxes of foodstuffs and plant life actually among any of the seeds from Garinagu's lost ancestral foods and vegetables? Or just reminders that such seeds had once existed? I didn't know what meaning they might hold for people I knew in Belize, if any, but took notes to ask about them: a jar of seeds labeled "Black Mauritius Beans"; cardboard boxes of unshelled peanuts; a round gourd fashioned into a canteen with a woven sisal strap labeled "Black Caribs of St. Vincent"; herb seeds like *Ochroma pyramidale*, barks like *Combretaceae*; dried-up fruits from the *Couroupita guianensis* nut tree and gummed sap of *Dacryodes hexandra*; cassava in every form: boxes of chunks, flakes, ground in jars.[140]

One archivist told me about recent genetic sequencing of certain food plants like taro. By testing the colonial samples now at the British Museum of vegetables taken from their lands, and comparing these genomes to the remaining crop varieties grown today, some groups are now using genomic testing to learn what ancestral food crops their ancestors lost during colonial incursions. For a moment—standing amid the botanical volumes and specimens in an archive of empire—I imagined a mapping of DNA and diabetes risk that focused exclusively on the genetic sequencing of plants instead of humans, studying vegetable genes to tell better histories of which humans domesticated them and who gained or lost food options in the past five hundred years.

As of 2019, Garinagu in Belize are trying to receive official recognition from the state as "Indigenous" people. Their collectives are frequently excluded from internationally backed land advocacy projects, Joseph Palacio notes, because "the funders, who are mostly North American, have difficulty accepting black people as indigenous people."[141]

"Altho' originally Africans, from the mixture and connection with the American Indians they were what we may call a hybrid race from the two," Anderson had concluded on the last page of his report back in 1796. It did not seem like a coincidence, after his long efforts to foster doubt about whether Black Caribs were truly Indigenous, that he revised his assessment as soon as they were on board the ships deporting them from their homeland.

Anderson ended his life obsessively editing his old cursive manuscripts, especially his account of Garifuna exile. He drew *X*s over each
instance of the word "Island" and replaced it with "Rising Colony."
His papers at the Linnean Society are schizoid documents, with entire
pages crossed out, showing both a tug of conflicted conscience and a
compulsion to tell a revised story about why events could not have been
otherwise. Anderson lived to see the worsening environmental erosions
of the forestlands that became plantations. Before his death on Saint
Vincent in 1811, he wrote at least four versions of an unpublished novel
about apocalyptic climate change flooding, titled "The Delugia." He
climbed Mount Soufriere, once the ancient symbol of Carib sovereignty,
to study the signs of rising atmospheric temperatures and climate
change.[142] But Garifuna people, Anderson wrote around 1800, were
"now nearly extinct." In the last line of *Geography and History of Saint
Vincent*, he concluded his natural history with the prediction that it
"will soon be forgot that such a race ever existed."[143]

Each year, hundreds of Garifuna people living around the world travel
to Balliceaux to memorialize the April anniversary of their ancestors'
captivity there. The story of Garifuna insurrection was taken up widely:
in 1823, the first known script written by a Black playwright in the
United States was set in the lost Garifuna homeland. Named for the
Garifuna leader Satuye (Chatoyer), the play's title was translated as
King Shotaway. (Shortly after its performance in New York City, African Grove Theater was burned to the ground.) Today the Garifuna-run
museum in Dangriga is named for Gulisi, daughter of Satuye, who
helped keep memories of what happened alive in oral history. As one of
her descendants, Felicita Francisco, retold the story to Joseph Palacio:
"Having experienced the massacre of our people in St. Vincent and the
miraculous way how we survived the surrender, the diseases, the inhu-
man conditions. . . I wanted the little ones to know the very strong met-
tle of their forefathers and be proud of them."[144]

In some recent epigenetic research, the increased risk for diseases like diabetes gets described by certain researchers as "vulnerability" or "frailty."
The enfeebled sound of these terms amazed me the first time I saw them on
the pages of a medical journal. Whatever is happening to Arreini and her
family as the diabetes epidemic roils through their far-flung community—
with its many mysteries and mechanisms and injustices, molecular or
otherwise—I feel certain that *frailty* is not the right word.

The last time I saw Arreini was several months before her death. We were sitting in the dark under a night lit with summer stars, sipping Nescafé with clots of dried milk. I stared out toward the water and dimly recalled that there is a Garifuna word for this luminescent glow on the sea at night, *úhuyu*. Arreini began reciting her evening prayers. She required no statues or icons, only her plain-beaded rosary, beginning each day and ending each night with the words she called her *misas*. Most of the spiritual practitioners I had known in Dangriga focused on altars crowded with a ceramic pantheon of saints, such as Saint Christopher. Some say you could tell a lot about a person's prayer work based on whether their Christopher statue could be separated into two, since it was not the saint but his detachable baby who did the spiritual dirty work. Many others relied in particularly hard times on Anthony, the region's patron saint of shadow mischief and supernatural errands.

But in the end, she kept returning to Lucas. Her mind was growing confused, and it was one of those touchstones that kept coming back as a steadying point. Arreini spoke obliquely of the prayer's force: "With this, nobody can do anything to you. You can go anywhere and they cannot touch you." The sea was crashing maybe a hundred yards from us, more of a character than a landscape as we talked in the night. It was a constant setting for the ancient histories she cryptically evoked, for episodes of unspeakable violence and unfathomable tenacity "written in water" and leaving no traceable trails. Even documented histories were not safe from its ruin; once, in Belize City, the country's archives were put on a ship for safekeeping during a Spanish attack, but then the boat hit a reef, and all the country's written records sank into the sea. *Crónicas* of Garifuna history, because they were preserved orally by those who survived the journey to Belize and whose stories are still told in Dangriga today, ironically proved less fragile.

Lost but also present, how do you prove a history? When do its effects begin or end? What are the politics of reading bodies as an archive of what is missing? Were those even the right questions? As Arreini spoke, the ocean—like blood sugar—seemed a kind of liquid unconscious that contained something more than either of us, or the sciences swirling around us, could really say. Listening back now, I feel she is trying to tell me something I don't really understand: about the metaphysics of improbable love and raw struggle, their elusive forbearances and transmutations through the blood and pain of history, and other things that cannot really be written down into books. Not this one either.

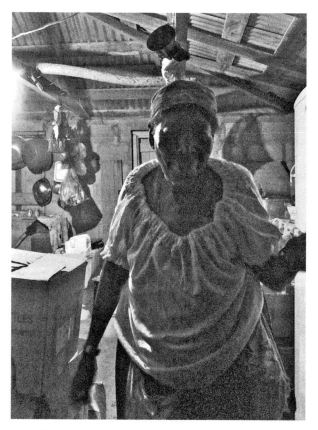

Arreini in her kitchen.

Prayer of Saint Lucas	*Oración de San Lucas*
Holy Spirit	*Espíritu Santo*
(three times, three crosses— watch how it's done)	*(tres veces, tres cruces—mira cómo)*
I love you through anything	*Te amo cualquier*
And anything is mine	*Y cualquier es mío*
[inaudible in wind] the sky	*[. . .] el cielo*
Come to us	*Vénganos*
Here we have the miracle.	*Aquí tenemos el milagro.*

Crónica Four: Repair Work

Maintenance Projects with Laura, Jose, and Growing Collectives

Everybody wants to build and nobody wants
to do maintenance.

—Kurt Vonnegut, *Hocus Pocus*

When Laura told me in 2010 that she hoped she wouldn't need dialysis, I thought back to the hospital garage. Being led through its padlocked door felt like stepping into an abandoned museum of medicine. The cavernous room, with a high tin roof set aloft by wooden rafters, was crowded with aging machines that were once used to restart American patients' hearts or wash their blood. Some of the devices were coated in sawdust and trailed electric cords and tubing, with piles of lumber and paintbrushes tucked around them. Others were wrapped in mummy-tight bundles, layers of cellophane revealing only the vague contours of an engineered anatomy underneath.

"People just keep bringing them down here. Mostly our American volunteers," a kindly hospital administrator named Ethan told me, explaining that most of the analog machines reached Belize in boxcar-sized containers carried by barge across the ocean. "I feel bad because they pay a lot for shipping," he added. "They really think we are going to be able to use them somehow, even the old dialysis machines with no cartridges and pieces missing." Ethan was quite sympathetic to the caring sentiments that motivated the volunteers' donations, if somewhat perplexed with his role of curating these fossils of good intentions. Yet he seemed unwilling to throw the broken machines away, searching fondly amid the hodgepodge to show me his favorite specimens with archaic buttons and retro dials.

We also encountered some recently opened cardboard boxes of building materials. Ethan explained that several years ago, an NGO had donated these tiles for a building project but had not included the specialized foreign laminate needed to actually install them. But a maintenance man at the hospital had figured out a method to soak the tiles in a bathtub to loosen the adhesive on their backs, which could then be scraped clean, one by one, and installed without the missing custom laminate. The workers subsequently began using these painstakingly modified tiles to help build what, as we spoke in the summer of 2010, everyone hoped would soon become the region's first public dialysis center.

The artifacts disintegrating in the garage seemed to demonstrate—or even caricature—the hidden sides of intervention practices focused on chronic conditions in Belize. It was hard not to be disconcerted by the gap between the volunteers' well-intended donations and the reality of what a hospital infrastructure needed. A colleague who once ran an NGO clinic in Sierra Leone pointed out to me that equipment donations mismatched with local needs were not always innocent—there could also be an unintended "dark side of bricolage."[1] It was often cheaper for U.S. hospitals to dispose of old or unwanted equipment as a donation (and tax write-off) rather than pay for safe local disposal. Overstretched clinics abroad might then be left to manage accumulating unusable equipment—a particularly complex issue because such machinery often leaks toxicants as it ages, adding to accumulating chemical exposures that could well contribute to chronic diseases of the future.

On the other hand, the jumble that Ethan showed me was also something more than a dumping ground. The retooled floor tiles had arrived in unusable condition but were now being made into the foundation for one of the most innovative ongoing clinic projects in the country. Their team was taking up the work of receiving, and *activating*, the parts that came their way to remake this flotsam and jetsam into usable goods. "To create a life," Kwame Anthony Appiah writes, "is to create a life out of the materials that history has given you."[2]

HALFWAY TECHNOLOGIES

Diabetes treatments often rely on medical objects that have been called "halfway technologies"—devices that address "symptoms or manifestations of disease, rather than the underlying pathogenesis." Such *halfway technology* "does not treat the underlying disease itself, but reflects the absolute failure of all efforts at medical and conservative therapy and is a last ditch, gerry-rigged lifesaving solution." And yet, the physician-author adds, "when a 'halfway' technology is also lifesaving, its value cannot be underestimated by the individual patient."[3]

A common answer to *How are you doing?* in Belize was "trying to maintain." When it comes to living with diabetes, organs, limbs, and senses will wear down without care. How does a body and its injuries interact with the infrastructures around it? According to the World Health Organization, around 80 percent of medical equipment in low- and middle-income countries is either donated or funded by foreign donors. Yet only a small fraction of this donated equipment—between 10–30 percent, depending on the country—ever gets working once it arrives. Another half of that breaks down in the first six months.[4] Technologies might allow health to be extended, but require that bodies and infrastructures be maintained together.

The importance of infrastructures often only "becomes visible upon breakdown," scholars of maintenance observe.[5] Working to counter this, recent projects by Steven Jackson and other writers focused on repair have generated fields of academic enthusiasm around "processes of breakdown, maintenance, and repair as central but neglected moments in our individual and collective relationships with technology."[6] This Science and Technology Studies lens follows objects' life cycles over horizons of time, linking up with insights that anthropologists of medicine offer about the "recursive cascades" of chronic conditions: tinkering is the kind of care work that will never be over, both for bodies and the technologies that might sustain them.[7] As Annemarie Mol puts it: "Try, adjust, try again. In dealing with a disease that is chronic, the care process is chronic, too. It only ends the day you die."[8]

Going further, Toni Morrison's use of the term "repair work"[9] several decades before Jackson's contains all this but also destabilizes it. In her account, bodily reckoning with the violence of colonial histories implies longer horizons of time, memory, and responsibility. Read against unjust colonial histories, all maintenance today takes place in the wake of racial capitalism's resource flows, legacies of five hundred years of material accumulations against which breaking even is not actually possible. In this context, risk and hurt are not evenly shared for venturing collaboration. Yet this fragility does not negate the force of people's slow work in the face of debility—it only deepens the stakes of what is meant by aspirations toward "the right to repair."[10] Whenever bodies and infrastructures of food and medicine are maintained together—or not—questions about the irreparable are present in the

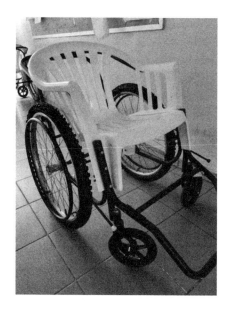

Hospital wheelchair in Belize City.

living histories in circulation. Yet these deeper contexts often get muted by the immediate minutia of surviving with chronic conditions in daily life. "Well, it is here," one community leader said to me matter-of-factly of diabetes. "So we must deal with it, true?"

Before it happened to her, Laura recalled that she didn't realize the acute danger because her leg had finally stopped hurting. It just felt like cement. She was the first to tell me another line that I would hear many times in Dangriga: "I was trying to heal [after the first amputation]. But then the infection was gone higher. The surgeon came back. He said, 'Let's go to the theater.'" Even the cells of her nerves struggled to fathom what happened next.

PHANTOM LIMBS

"The truth is, we all have phantom limbs superimposed on our real ones," Princeton psychology and neuroscience professor Michael Graziano notes, since our brains construct a "phantom map" of our bodies: "It contains no information about bones, tendons, or the biochemical basis of muscle contraction. The brain doesn't need to know those details in order to control movement. Instead, it generates a surreal description of magic segments connected by hinges. It's a phantom body." Scientists call such a map a *body schema,* and it helps explain the mystery by which an unused phantom map can remain in consciousness long after the limb it modeled is gone. Severed nerves' "trunks" also remain alive, akin to how a tree's roots at times stay alive in the ground even after the rest is cut down, still bearing signals.

Nearly all amputees report phantom sensation for at least a few days. For some, the sensation keeps returning in erratic flashes. A few feel them forever, Graziano reflected in "How Phantom Limbs Explain Consciousness"—as in the famous 1797 British case of Lord Nelson's arm, lost in war off the coast of the Canary Islands (also home to the colonial world's first sugar plantations): "For the rest of his life he could sense it, as though the appendage were extending invisibly from the stump. He supposedly claimed that he now knew there had to be an afterlife because if his arm could have a ghost, then so could he."[11]

Sometimes a phantom leg's locomotion is so distinct that someone still adjusting to an amputation can repeatedly collapse after standing without thinking about it. Strange ephemeral sensations also include tingling and itching, hot and cold, pressure or squeezing, wiggling toes, and the feeling of wearing shoes. Such perceptions offer clues about how our bodies perceive themselves in time and space more generally: *telescoping,* for example, refers to a phenomenon in which someone feels their ghost appendage getting closer to their stump as years pass—suggesting how phantom maps may be revised over time, but only partially.

Phantom limb pain is the more brutal aspect of this ghost sensorium, related to a nerve's memory of pain. Some amputees experience the feeling of being cut with knives or pulsing shocks in their missing limbs for the rest of their lives: "Severe post-amputation pains from phantom limbs have been recorded in survivors from World War II, some 50 years after loss of a limb."[12] Laura was among the people with diabetes I met in Belize who reported that blinding pains in her removed leg could be so overwhelming that on bad days she couldn't get out of bed during the day or sleep at night. But the lightning-flash pain that she described sounded less mysterious than many other aspects of phantom sensation—more like replaying a cut nerve's traumatic last memory of being electrically shocked and surgically severed.

Not long after we met in 2010 Laura had undergone the emergency procedure bluntly called a guillotine amputation. While the more common flap procedure gets closed with a seam of stitches, the harsher guillotine technique is occasionally necessary as an emergency measure to stop gangrene or sepsis from climbing further. This makes it harder to heal afterward since it leaves no healthy skin to suture. Laura had been through two such cuts (segments of the same leg) in one week. But the second amputation was better than the first, she noted, because there was anesthesia.

When she invited me to visit her at home a few weeks afterward, Laura wore a bright turquoise rosary. It was the only time before or since that I saw her in a wheelchair. Laura had to laugh at herself, she said, because she liked to cover her face with a pillow each time her cousin changed the bandage. She was praying hard to heal, and to be eligible for a skin graft surgery later that might make it possible to wear a new leg.

Delicate "nerve repair" surgeries are being pioneered in wealthier countries to manage postamputation pain. (Decades ago, back when painful sensations were assumed to be localized in cut nerve ends, some surgeons attempted to excise the ends with an additional amputation— but this tended to compound the problem into a phantom leg and a separate phantom stump, both in pain.) Today, by approaching nerves more like living electrical circuits, some surgeons are finding techniques for pain alleviation by wrapping the roots of cut nerves together with the nerve cords nearby. This type of rewiring goes a step further than more common pain relief procedures also relying on neuroplasticity, such as burying the nerve in muscle after an amputation. Nerve healing matters not only for chronic pain—it also affects how a stump can later join with a replacement limb, since "painful cut nerve endings often prevent effective fitting and use of even the most rudimentary prosthesis."[13]

From the outside, many amputations look more or less alike to a casual observer. But internally, very different neurological responses may be taking place. Pain can be caused by any number of typical things, including a bone spur (osteophyte) or a swollen ball of nerves (neuroma), especially painful if near the skin's surface or a bone. "There is a close association between the presence and severity of stump neuroma pain and phantom limb pain," as one pamphlet notes.[14]

At the level of nerve repair, pain's neurological networks become contiguous with other infrastructures of limb restoration. I have never heard of a surgical procedure done to reduce postamputation pain in Belize. The specialists pioneering these delicate procedures in wealthier contexts are largely plastic surgeons (a specialty very rarely practiced in Belize, as is the case in many small countries). Since statistics documenting how many people in the world get amputations due to diabetes are already elusive, it is doubly daunting to estimate what subset also experiences phantom pain. Percentages must vary sharply across different contexts, depending in part on factors such as access to anesthesia (and what kinds) during amputation and available remediation afterward. All of those I spoke with about losing limbs in Belize reported times of severe phantom pain, even those who otherwise felt only total numbness.

The article on "nerve repair" quoted above drew from research paid for (in part) by the U.S. Army. "'You hate to think that war is what drives technology, but it does,'" observed the vice president of prosthetics for Hanger, a major artificial-limb producer founded just after the U.S. Civil War.[15] One of the key centers for prostheses production today, Hanger is based in Manassas, Virginia, not far from where Confederate soldier James Edward Hanger got hit with a cannonball and became the first amputee of the Civil War. The legendary Hanger Limb leg was first whittled from barrel staves in 1861. Hanger's invention was legally patented under the Confederacy and, three decades later, also by the United States. This milestone in prosthesis innovation is indicative of a larger military legacy, including much of the literature on amputation as well as most funding for cutting-edge prosthetic design.

In Belize, I had encountered several elders who were veterans of World War II, Mr. P among them. England had enrolled soldiers from across its Caribbean colonies during the war, and each month Mr. P made a trip into town to pick up a small military stipend from the Crown. When Mr. P explained how he always went to pick up the money from England with another veteran who had lost a leg, I wondered if his companion had lost the limb in combat. "No. Sugar." At the time, I was already struck by how this different cause changed the *social* meanings attached to the injury. But it took me years to learn that losing a leg to diabetes also holds major implications for a person's *technical* options for prosthesis.

My previous imaginations of prosthetic limbs were informed by TV shows and movies: pro athletes running record-breaking sprints on carbon-fiber blades or advanced microcomputing robotics approaching the goal of what some designers call a "Luke arm" (so named for Luke Skywalker's prosthesis in the *Star Wars* movies, hardwired together with nerves to respond directly to brain signals). Although military priorities drive much of this development, at times so-called civilian spillover offers something relevant for other traumatic accidents.[16] Made to interface with lively nerves, however, these impressive advances in prosthetic limb technology are designed in a way that makes them hard or impossible to use following a diabetes-related amputation. The nerve and tissue damage that leads to diabetic amputation in the first place would require an even more sophisticated interface than those being developed for postcombat and traumatic accidents. For nerves worn numb by diabetes, such electric interfaces might not be achievable.

At the same time, nobody really knows what potential innovations go unimagined when diabetes-tailored research receives such little specialized funding. Very little money goes into design for diabetic limb loss, though "only about 15% of amputees are trauma victims or cancer survivors—the types of patients who most often make good candidates for high-tech prosthesis. About 80% of amputations are due to vascular diseases like diabetes," noted a piece titled "State-of-the-Art Prosthetics Are Incredible, but Not Always Useful."[17] This majority population tends to be much poorer and lower profile. Materializing what Lochlann Jain calls the "prosthetic imagination," many people and conditions are rarely imagined in design worlds where "certain bodies—raced, aged, gendered, classed—are often already dubbed as not fully whole."[18]

In some parts of the world, pamphlets that help prepare patients for amputation read something like this counsel from Johns Hopkins Medicine: "After surgery, you may have emotional concerns. You may have grief over the lost limb. . . . There are specialists who make and fit prosthetic devices. They will visit you soon after surgery and will instruct you how to use the prosthesis."[19]

Laura remembered what it felt like to lie in a hospital room in Dangriga afterward, trying to get used to the sight of where her leg used to be, without any expectation of a prosthetic limb or therapist arriving at her door. So when she heard the news that her roommate from the hospital would also be getting her foot removed due to diabetic injuries, she called her right away, hoping to improvise a kind of talk therapy.

"I told her that if you dwell in this depression, you can lose your whole body in it," Laura recalled. "We must survive. I want to see you again." Those talks had meant so much to each of them that now Laura tried to contact any of her neighbors going through their first amputation. "My love has a lot of meaning. It is not just family, or care. It is something I am creating—*the carefulness*. It is a bond."

Laura's legs and feet used to bear a constellation of small scars that looked like cigarette burns. In her telling, they mapped out constellations from decades of recoveries—she remembered each diabetic ulcer, when it had appeared, what she had used to heal it, and which nurses or friends had helped. She always used to call the leg they'd had to remove her "depend upon," because it was the side she always leaned her weight on.

The aftermath's mundane particulars made for a different kind of "uncanny ordinary," to borrow a phrase that Zoë Wool recalls from Stanley Cavell.[20] In older theories of "the uncanny," detached feet in motion symbolized Freud's concept of how traumatic separation created strange doubles and involuntary repetitions. But if there were any uncanny doubles that haunted the stories that Laura shared, it seemed to me that their most unsettling fantasy space was the prosthetic limbs everyone saw on TV and online but had no way to personally acquire.

On Belize's pirated cable, most any home could tune into shows like Smithsonian's *Incredible Bionic Man*, which featured a team of scientists cobbling a bionic robot entirely of prosthetic parts.[21] Globally, there have also been important advances around affordable limbs: some, like the famously versatile Jaipur Foot pioneered in India, date back to at least the 1960s.[22] Others, like teams using 3-D printers that promise to revolutionize affordable customized limbs, aspire toward a wide reach in future markets. But none of these were actually available to Laura in the time and place that she lived.

Somewhere, these phantom limbs meet each other: The synthetic limbs that she knew existed somewhere in the world. Specialized prosthetics for diabetic limb recovery that no one has ever invested (or likely will ever invest) millions into developing. And what she kept imagining; what her nerves kept imagining. The leg that she could still feel there sometimes.

Laura had, however, heard of one group in Belize who might be able to help.

SUGAR SHOES

Fede vaulted from the high blue pickup truck and spun his skateboard around on the street, reaching up to slam the driver's side door. Under his baseball cap, he had a quick smile and a salt-and-pepper mustache. He had offered to pick me up when a thunderstorm loomed on the afternoon of our planned meeting, arriving in a modified vehicle he drove with silver canes affixed to the gas and brake pedals.

As he jumped a curb from the rain-slick street up onto a walkway, I wondered whether Fede liked to show off his agility hard-won during the more than three decades since he was born without legs. Or maybe he just maneuvered so confidently that his routine methods of navigation appeared as acrobatic flourishes to a newcomer like me in Orange Walk Town—better known as "Sugar City" for its sprawling cane fields.

Propelling his skateboard toward the clinic's locked door, he fiddled with the key and waved me to follow inside. I jumped out of his truck's passenger seat and ran through the rain to catch up.

The workshop that Fede led me into looked the way I pictured a cobbler's workspace—only Fede did not make shoes. Their team made limbs. The room's shelves were stacked with feet in many styles, a selection of hinged legs and arms, and hundreds of appendages sorted in nooks labeled by features: heel height, shoe size, left or right. Some of the hands appeared to be holding each other. Other prosthetics around us sat in various stages of reconstruction, like one shoulder upside down near a toolbox laid close to a cabinet labeled "Extra Feet." One baby-sized foot rested on the floor next to a bag of cement and tubes of Epoxy.

I followed along as Fede gave me a tour of the adjoining rooms, wheeling alongside benches and explaining various workstations. One room had a wall of crutches and plastic orthotic braces. The smallest sizes were patterned with rainbows and Flintstones characters. Fede explained that the majority of their clients had diabetes, followed by people injured in traffic accidents. Still others suffered machete wounds or farm equipment injuries or were children born without legs. Saws, screwdrivers, and other tools hung from a pegged rack. Leaning on a low drill platform, Fede described the process of handcrafting each limb: casting, plastics and parts, shaping and reshaping. When they arrived, most of the prosthetic limbs were the color of beige Band-Aids designed for white skin. Fede described how he worked with new owners as part of their fitting to make the limb whatever color they chose, using a palette of custom-mixed colors. The adjacent laminating room held paintbrushes, bottles of pigment, and jars of resin in many shades of brown, yellow, red, and white.

Fede handed me the plaster cast of a knee as we spoke. Between waves of rain clattering on the tin roof above us, he described his first day of going to school as a child after his old prosthesis had broken, the day when the other children realized the extent of his disability for the first time. "It was devastating." He said that it had taken him many years of inner struggle to reach the place where he no longer felt concerned about wearing prosthetics for the sake of others' comfort around him. He now usually goes without them. But that childhood memory, Fede said, would always inform his work. "I will never operate something where only rich people can get legs. I think everybody deserves the right to walk."

The workshop we were standing in first began with a much more modest goal: a friend had fundraised to send Fede to Dallas back in

1995, in the hope that a professor of prosthetics she knew named Rob might be able to make Fede a new pair of legs. The three of them had formed a deep bond during the visit. Fede returned to Belize from Dallas able to walk with crutches and look people in the eye. Although he opted to return to his skateboard some years later, it was still greatly meaningful for him to have the choice to stand.

When their friend's NGO returned to Belize the next year, Rob asked to tag along, hoping to follow up with Fede and make sure his new prosthesis received maintenance. But he was "unaware that an announcement had been made on the TV and radio that the man who had made Fede's legs was coming to town and that if anyone needed a prosthesis, they should meet the team at The Diner." The resulting scene would be recounted later on their project's website: "Rob was astounded when the caravan pulled into the parking lot of The Diner and the patio was filled with amputees. . . . It was at this time that Rob learned that in the entire country of Belize, there were no prosthetic or orthotic services available to the citizens."[23]

That became the origin story of Rob and Fede's collaboration. Their first improvised evaluations began in the diner's parking lot that summer day in 1996. They were committed to doing the prosthetic fabrications there in Belize. Fede began on the path to an informal apprenticeship with Rob over the next four years, which grew into a partnership: Rob bringing supplies and students from U.S. universities several times a year and Fede providing coordination and day-to-day maintenance support in Belize. He also gradually learned certain technical aspects of prosthetics crafting through collaborations with Rob and his colleagues.

The makeshift team did their first fittings in Belize in 1997, working in a local high school's auto garage while the students were on break for the summer. They custom crafted limbs and taught people to use them. American Airlines pitched in, giving Rob's team waivers to transport start-up supplies. "It was before 9/11 then, so we could send these big boxes of supplies on the plane from Texas," Fede explained. Later, U.S. team members brought the specialized resins and prosthetics to Belize in their suitcases. "I asked them to teach me. I got to see all their tricks," Fede said. "So I make my own now." (Much later, I learned this was a very different take than Rob's intention of imparting skills to help with maintenance). Over the years, these partners had made prosthetic limbs for over four hundred Belizeans, Fede estimated. They had come to call their collaboration Project Hope Belize.

When Project Hope Belize had outlined policy recommendations, shoe safety was one of their most creative suggestions: "Proper footwear for diabetics is not available in Belize and importing shoes is likely to be cost prohibitive. The establishment of a diabetic shoe industry should be considered as a viable solution to poor foot wear options for diabetics in Belize in order to make low cost diabetic shoes, as well as create employment opportunities for diabetics."[24] Funding for this creative proposal never materialized. In fact, I was surprised to hear of the existence of shoes that help prevent diabetic amputations, since nobody I knew owned them. But a quick Google search yielded images of pairs fastened by Velcro, commonly called "sugar shoes." I thought uneasily of the growing need for artificial feet in relation to the lack of access to everyday measures like sugar shoes.

Constant fundraising went into keeping Fede and Rob's collaboration afloat. "The poorest patients might arrive here without a dime," Fede said. "They don't have money for a hotel or food while they are here. . . . all of that, even the bus fare to go back home, we take that all out of our pocket. So how can you turn something like this into business?" Fede said that before their workshop opened, some well-heeled Belizeans had purchased prostheses from Mexico. But the last he had heard, a leg in Chetumal cost around four thousand U.S. dollars.

"They just give the leg to you in a box with a little paper of instructions," he said. "How can you just hand someone the leg and say, go home and put this on? How will you know this person will not be in pain later? That is my job here. I listen to them, I teach them what I know. We adjust the thing together." Sometimes their team even refitted prosthetics that came from Chetumal, Fede said, "to make it fit the person for real." Their workshop in Orange Walk was located some forty-three miles south of the border town, along a highway surrounded by sugar plantations—some overgrown and abandoned, others active with trucks picking up bundled cane. In fact, Fede said, the cement building where we were talking that day had been built on land donated by a local sugar company. As a generous supporter of the country's only prosthetics clinic, the sugar industry in Belize helps to provide diabetes education and various social and medical assistance to amputees, in the tradition of company towns. Fede said that he had learned how to make prosthetic limbs strong enough that some of their workers had returned to work in the cane fields after losing a leg to diabetic sugar.

Diabetes limbs were the hardest, Fede said, because of the delicacy of putting pressure on the stump. "If the pressure points are designed in the wrong place, that could cause a blister. And then the person might need another amputation, even higher." Fede said he liked to meet the person they were making a limb for before beginning the work. That way he could get a better feel for their needs and help them to prepare. "Shrinker" socks were a crucial step in this, he said. They were made especially for prosthetics, to minimize swelling of the stump and improve blood flow. He showed me one. It looked like a tiny elastic white stocking. Shrinker socks were especially important when it came to diabetes, due to the related circulation and nerve damage.

Fede said the organization's waiting list was growing much faster than the pace at which they were able to make the prosthetics. Trying to imagine what it might mean to "scale up" such a personalized process, I asked Fede whether he envisioned becoming part of the national healthcare system in Belize one day. I was surprised when Fede said he worried that possibility could make their project vulnerable.

"Whoever is in power at the time, then the politicians will say you are supported by this party. Then the next party that comes in could squash you, especially how small we are. That would be the breaking point." Fede worried about sustainability—but, counterintuitively, he said that was the reason he had not kept pushing for incorporation into national structures. "It's hard, because then you don't have anyone else to help. But I just want to keep this all politically neutral. I want to do a good thing for the people of Belize."

Where, then, does one seek stability over time? That hovered as an open question. Fede said that he just focused on scheduling patients for the next of Rob's visits. Rob had last been there just the week before my arrival, Fede added, and had brought three students. "We fitted six legs and one arm." During these regular visits, amputees waiting across the country who had made arrangements with Fede would converge in Orange Walk for fittings. When he showed me the place where they set up handrails for people to try their first steps on a newly fitted limb, ready to make adjustments, I imagined Laura leaning on the metal bars. She was in touch with Fede by phone in 2010 and hoped to schedule a fitting sometime the following year. But it takes serious work to receive a prosthetic limb, even before an actual fitting. "Believe me, it is hard to wear a prosthesis. It takes a lot of strength. For someone who has been immobile, it is like learning to walk all over again," Fede said. "It will take work to learn to use it. You have to start step by step, little by little."

Some shelves were lined by more weathered limbs. On a wall by the door, I noticed one leg in particular that looked very heavy. Fede must have been following my eyes because he handed the artifact to me and noted the iron bar inside that the man had once used to walk, pointing out the stratigraphy of additions and repairs that he and its wearer had made together during repeat visits over the years: heavy resin, a plastic encasement, a bright yellow thigh strap to hold it in place. There was a string looped around the knee just below its hinge and a beige foot bolted onto the scratched plastic shin in mixed skin colors. When components finally arrived from Atlanta to craft its wearer a new prosthesis, the man autographed his old calf in marker for their collection: "Clay Crawford lived in this leg for 27 years."

"But it is better to keep on trying than not to try," Fede had told me as he turned off the workshop's last pull-string light bulb. I never imagined, back then in 2010, the tense situation that would unfold between Fede and his partners before the next time we talked. In fact, a painful falling-out would lead the organization to rebrand itself with a new name to signal a fresh start, Prosthetic Hope International, to which we will return later. But a snapshot of this place as it was then still captures a moment in time, and the complex social networks that both crafted limbs and people needing them in Belize have traveled through.

When her turn came to prepare for a prosthesis, Laura struggled with the shrinker sock. It squeezed her stump painfully, but she still wore it. "Darling," she said, "we must live on."

DIALYSIS: PRESSURE

I met one of Laura's brothers in Belize City, but her other brother I had seen only in photo albums. We sat together on her blue couch as Laura told me about his death from kidney failure. I suddenly realized why her younger brother sounded intense when I asked him an interview question about kidney disease. "Needing dialysis has been a death sentence here," he had said heavily. At the time when their older brother had needed dialysis, that was the harsh truth. As one Belizean news station described the situation back in 2003: "If you are acquainted with anyone who has suffered kidney failure, then you know that the unfortunate victim has two choices: go abroad for regular dialysis treatments or stay home and die."[25]

Diabetes is the most common cause of kidney failure, and kidney failure is one of diabetes's most predictable complications. Its temporary treatment, dialysis, is a classic example of generative tinkering. The first working dialysis machine was cobbled out of sausage casings, orange juice cans, and a clothes-washing machine during the wartime shortages of Nazi occupation in the Netherlands.[26] Dutch physician

Willem Kolff's tinkering produced the world's first prosthetic organ in 1941 and transformed the history of medicine. Early models featured a rotating wood drum and a jug to hold drained blood. Kolff never patented the invention, in the hope that keeping the design open would make future machines widely accessible to others.

That physician-inventor's dream of affordable dialysis—like insulin's original one-dollar patent—did not last long into the twentieth century and its many privatizations. Today a new, high-quality dialysis machine the size of a small refrigerator costs around fifty or a hundred thousand U.S. dollars.[27] It took more than half a century for such dialysis devices to first reach Belize. In 2003, kidney specialist Dr. Miguel Rosado opened the first dialysis unit at a private hospital in Belize City. But Dr. Rosado died tragically three years later, after a car accident in Belize left him in a lethal coma at the age of thirty-nine. The hemodialysis unit he had founded remained open, but the country had lost its only kidney specialist and biggest advocate.[28]

After Rosado's death, there was no nephrologist or endocrinologist practicing in Belize and no public dialysis unit in the country. By the time I visited the unit at the private hospital, dialysis sessions were available for a fee of around $680 a week, costly far beyond the reach of all but the wealthiest. This is not an unusual situation in the world, according to the U.S. National Kidney Foundation: "Of the 2 million people who receive treatment for kidney failure, the majority are treated in only five countries"—the United States, Germany, Italy, Japan, and Brazil—"yet this number may only represent 10% of people who actually need treatment to live."[29]

For those trying to enter this slim margin, that 10 percent implies other numbers that are harder to turn into statistics. One of them is miles. As I write this from my childhood home in the United States, for example, there is a DaVita dialysis center about a three minutes' drive away. In contrast, the first person I met receiving dialysis in Dangriga, a man in his fifties named Max, traveled by bus for eleven hours (each way) to Mexico three times a week. To make the trip to Mexico was his choice to try to maintain, he said. Max suddenly peeled back a patch of medical tape and showed me the bright blue valve and clear plastic tube sprouting out of his wrist. Max's wife, Elena, then showed me the balled-up plastic bags in her purse. (One of dialysis's common side effects is nausea.) She made the long bus trip with him every Monday, Wednesday, and Friday to Mexico.

In 2009, I started hearing about something unusual happening in Belize City. There were national news headlines about dialysis access and photographs of patients protesting in the streets. It was the first group protest of any kind I had heard about in relation to affordable health care in Belize (much in contrast to surrounding countries like Mexico and Guatemala, which have robust populist traditions of health protests). Late in 2010, I traveled to Belize City to learn more.

Before the Chateau Caribbean Hotel later burned down in 2016, the old colonial wooden building had long, narrow rooms and strange keyhole-shaped doorways—partitions left from when the hotel was still a private hospital and each room a ward built for eight or so beds. After checking in, I headed to the newer private hospital across town where, at the time, Belize's only dialysis unit was located. Unlike my hotel's aesthetic of a hospital ward, the private hospital's colorful furniture made its rooms look like welcoming hotel suites.

"We have a list of people waiting," Nurse A told me when I arrived at the dialysis unit. "Here, you will only meet the lucky ones."

Most of the people close to death I had met up until that point were spread out, but in the dialysis center they filled chair after chair. I recognized some of their faces and names from news stories about the recent protests, including a Kriol woman who waved me over. She introduced herself as Carmela and asked me to use her real name, as the national papers had; she was strategically trying to turn herself into a public figure. With changes on the horizon in partial response to their media work, the room's group of patients were learning to leverage the stories of their plights in new ways. "Share the story when you go home. Diabetes," Carmela said. If it wasn't for the dialysis, she added, "I would have died already." I had the sense of stepping straight into the news cycle stories that had brought me to that room in the first place:

> Carmela . . . told our newspaper that February 2009 will mark one year since she has been taking dialysis treatments. She, too, is concerned about the lack of a doctor at the dialysis unit.
> "I know that it's hard, because we don't have a doctor. When our pressure goes up, God is the doctor. When my pressure goes up high I pray God please help me and I beg him because I don't have any money for any doctor," [she] shared.[30]

"I didn't know how I was going to get here today," Carmela told me, repeating the worry she often emphasized when being interviewed by the national news stations. She wanted people to know about the dialysis situation in general, but also had a specific goal in telling her story:

Carmela was always trying to raise bus fare. The bus from Belmopan to Belize City cost three U.S. dollars for a ride of one hour and required a taxi (five U.S. dollars roundtrip) to reach the clinic from the bus station. She needed to make this trip three times a week. Every Saturday, Tuesday, and Thursday, Carmela spent most of her day telling her story to other Belizeans in the hope of raising sixteen dollars for the round trip so that every Monday, Wednesday, and Friday she could reach the dialysis sessions the government had begun unevenly subsidizing that year. Having media confirmation of the reality she was describing became a useful tool in this endless work. Carmela felt she had been very lucky to get on the list, reciting the others with diabetes in her family: a sister and brother both already "dead off of sugar," but also another sister trained in nursing who had managed to get a kidney transplant in Cuba. As we spoke, a loud Spanish love ballad floated over the clinic din from the next room. "That's my cousin." Carmela shook her head, smiling. "He likes to sing on the machine."

It felt intense to enter such an instrumental space of stories being performatively told and lived. Patients shifted restlessly in their chairs during the hours-long treatment, calling me over with things they wanted to say into someone's tape recorder: whether or not they were on dialysis "scholarships"; the ways they obtained money to take the bus here; whatever they knew about the person whose death opened a spot for them in this room.

On a Monday morning, after visiting the week before, I heard the news alongside the room of patients that one of the country's twenty-one dialysis patients had died over the weekend. Someone waiting would be bumped up the list kept on a paper taped to the desk near the phone. A new regular would be sitting in his chair by Wednesday. "I was just talking with him on Friday," reflected one man getting dialysis. "You can be walking today and by tomorrow morning you are . . . *not here*." The unit's patients on once-weekly treatment were dying so quickly that it created a palpable sense that everyone was sitting in someone else's former place, and that someone new would occupy their blue chair once they were gone.

I felt myself being immediately enrolled into some much more fortunate transient rotation, one in a long line of past and future storyteller-witnesses visiting that room. At times I stopped writing in my notebook because I was listening so intently that I knew each word would be imprinted on my mind later that night anyway. Other times I would stop writing for the opposite reason, because bodily I just could not take in anymore. Both limits left me feeling dizzy and spilling over. It was at times a physical relief to have a tape recorder rolling on those days, and to think it would be possible to one day process whatever could not be absorbed in real time. But later I found the tapes almost unbearable to listen to—piercing machines, background televisions, and bits of hardship coming from all sides that I found no way to process and share on a relevant interval. Many of the patients who were sitting in one of those chairs that day died many years before this book was finished.

But others have lived on and on. One young woman just a few years older than me, Katherine, covered 250 miles each week for the sessions. She wore her long dark hair straight down her shoulders. In her late twenties, Katherine said the diabetes and kidney troubles had developed during pregnancy. Her son, who was five by the time we met, lived far south with her parents in Toledo; Katherine didn't want him to move to Belize City because so many children had been caught in the violence. He loved Spider-Man, she smiled. I thought how his superpowers are also made possible by moving between infrastructures. Katherine's strategy was to arrive with her suitcase packed at every Friday session, ready to undergo the trip to her parents' village to see him for the day on Saturday before making the return trip on Sunday to be back in Belize City for Monday dialysis.

As Katherine told me this, intricate feats of fluid mechanics were occurring in tubes inside the machines around us. Blood flowed in one direction and clear dialysate fluid (technically, "a buffered electrolyte solution") in the other. The liquids were being brought together inside an encased plastic cylinder about a foot long, which is the dialyzer cartridge that actually serves as the "artificial kidney," dwarfed and fed by the larger mechanical apparatus. The cartridge simulates the work of a glomerulus (Latin meaning "little ball of yarn")—the knotted balls of vessels and fibers that make up the kidney's semipermeable membrane for filtering toxins. Today most semipermeable membrane simulations use a new mechanism, a far cry from the original sausage casings model. Blood is channeled inside tiny hollow fibers, each only about the width of three human hairs, capillaries submerged in a bath of dialysis solution inside the cartridge's inner chamber. Very small pores in the fibers' walls keep larger blood cells and proteins, which need to be returned to the body for survival, inside the filtering membrane. But smaller molecules of accumulating toxins, including excess potassium, sodium, and bicarbonate that can rise to dangerous levels in the blood without a kidney, diffuse through the membrane's tiny pores and dissolve into the chamber's fluid. Invisibly laden with waste, salt, and extra water from the blood, the used dialysis solution, going half a liter a minute, drains discretely behind the machine.

Meanwhile the filtered blood flows back into the patient's veins, preferably through a fistula in their arm. Natural looking once healed, a fistula is made by surgically joining a vein and an artery, which makes a bigger blood vessel but needs careful upkeep. Needlestick options alone include the ladder technique to allow for healing between climbs up the vein, or the buttonhole approach akin to a pierced ear. Either requires vigilant monitoring for infection along the length of the limb. Just that single entry point can reorient senses of bodily motion in many domains of life—for instance, patients need to avoid sleeping on their arm with the fistula. One dialysis center website cautions patients to listen to their fistula access for the sound of flowing blood—called the bruit—usually loud enough to hear even without a stethoscope. "If the sound gains in pitch and sounds like a whistle, your blood vessels could be tightening (called stenosis)," caution these instructions. The "vibration of blood going through your arm is called the 'thrill.' You should check this several times a day. If the 'thrill' changes or stops a blood clot may have formed."[31]

If a fistula surgery cannot be performed for a dialysis patient, then more obtrusive hardware might need to be installed, like a catheter or graft (plastic tubes used to surgically connect veins and arteries, which bulge under the skin). In Belize, the dialysis unit's walls had also been fitted with plastic tubing as part of specialized filtration hardware to supply ultrapurified water as the base for the dialysate fluid. I imagined these infrastructures of plastic tubing reaching between the building and its patients.

Yet not just dialyzing technology itself but also the very idea of a right to it was a front for tinkering. The expectations I heard in Belize were very different from, for example, what Sherine Hamdy has described in her work with dialysis and transplant patients in Egypt. In that case, patients asserted an idea that both their state and their kidneys had failed—charges and protests that also animated future demands in Egypt, and spoke of a responsibility (if a largely unfulfilled and highly contested one) that the state was widely understood to have toward its citizens in the first place.[32]

In Belize, I struggled to understand why I never heard anything like this. With so many people who had diabetes dying preventable deaths and sustaining other losses all around me, patients still seemed to implicate themselves and take the limits of the state system in stride. Some people called the opportunity to get one subsidized dialysis session a week a "scholarship" (although they needed three to survive). People in crisis largely focused on getting anywhere they *could* receive the sessions—trying to find some route to Mexico, Guatemala, or the United States, for instance—rather than agitating for change within their state. Economist Albert O. Hirschman famously described the channels through which people respond to social injustices: voice, loyalty, and exit.[33] It would be fair to say that most Belizeans facing trouble (health or otherwise) were in the habit of trying to exit their tiny country when survival became strained. Belizeans have never had a constitutional right to health, nor a patient activist group that had come together to leverage a particular demand from the state.

This was the backdrop against which I met Jose Cruz in Belize City in 2010. Cruz and the group of patients coalescing around his spokesmanship had reached a certain level of celebrity in the country, after initiating what was apparently the first rights-based patient activism movement in the history of Belizean medicine. Together with other dying patients and their families from the Kidney Association of Belize, they organized civic protests and generated collective momentum that eventually pushed the government into greater action.

"I didn't even know what the word *dialysis* meant when I heard he needed it," Jose Cruz's wife, Mileni, later told me. The costly sessions drained their life savings in a matter of weeks. After that, the generosity of a cousin carried Cruz through a few more months of sessions. But the others around them dying without dialysis were a constant reminder of this dumb luck.

"One day, a man from Dangriga came into the unit," Mileni would recall later. The man, Mr. Z, pleaded with the nurse to hook him up to the machine. He had managed the seven-hour journey through the Maya Mountains to get there, but just didn't have any more money. "I'm so sorry," the nurse told him, her hands tied by strict hospital policy. Cruz and five other patients hooked up to machines in the room that day looked on. They recognized how badly Mr. Z needed dialysis from the signs they'd each experienced when things got rough. And they knew how much those signs not only signaled danger but hurt—face so puffy the crescents under the eyes bubbled out, feet bloated to the point they no longer fit in shoes and looked about to burst the skin—the outward signs of kidneys no longer able to regulate fluid levels in the body.

Mileni remembered getting the phone call that morning. "Babe, how much money do we have?" Jose asked her, describing the scene in front of him while Mileni counted what she could get that day. It was a Monday morning. Mileni had the money already waiting for her husband's Wednesday dialysis session, two days later. Jose and Mileni agreed it was the right thing to do. She returned to the hospital and made a beeline for the cashier.

Mileni showed Nurse A the receipt. Surprised and relieved, Nurse A hooked Mr. Z up to the machine right away. As the three hours passed, Mr. Z's swollen face and feet melted back to their true size. He looked ten years younger, like a different person, by the time he shook Jose's hand.

Several weeks later, the same scene played out again: Mr. Z arrived in acute need of dialysis, his body looking so swollen after the long journey from Dangriga. Only in the repeat version, it was Friday. Jose called Mileni and asked the same question again. But that time, the couple had already used their cousin's weekly deposit to pay for Jose's three sessions that week and didn't have any cash that day to share with Mr. Z.

Absorbing the news, Mr. Z died right there in a wheelchair in front of them.

Jose couldn't sleep all week. "We need to find a way," Mileni remembers him saying.

"WE DON'T WANT TO DIE"

Ready to try anything, Cruz began a makeshift media campaign. He called in to Love FM, Belize's popular radio station, and described the situation. "People are dying, all the time." He was invited for an interview on air and told the story of his own experience and of the many people he was watching die around him. "The people of Belize need to know about this."

Not long after, a group of dialysis patients—including Cruz, his cousin Carmela, and Mileni—protested in front of the hospital, surrounded by news cameras they had invited to the event from the full range of Belize's media outlets. Their small movement had gained a powerful immediate goal when the group learned about a letter from a U.S.-based organization that had offered to supply dialysis machines and train personnel if the Belizean government agreed to refurbish two unit locations and commit to certain care criteria over time. Cruz called the U.S. organization himself when he learned that the letter had gone unanswered. The first time, the NGO office hung up, because they were not familiar with the sound of a Belizean accent.

Cruz called back. "Listen, don't hang up. I am a patient," he said, recalling the memory to me later. "Tell me what we need to do."

Together with the leaders of the Belize Kidney Association and a close-knit team, Cruz began assembling documentation that he hoped would be a step toward the government signing on to the agreement with the U.S. organization. He also continued going to the media and appearing on TV and radio, asking people in Belize to talk with each other about dialysis and the conditions that were making so many patients need it. His words hit home for many people dealing with kidney failure in their own families. Belizeans began calling in to the Ministry of Health from across the country, asking what they were going to do.

"When one media started, then all the media were interested," Mileni recalled. After Cruz caught the media spotlight, he worked to leverage the attention. Once the government began providing dialysis three times a week for him, he started agitating for the others who received just one session instead of three—and for those like Mr. Z still dying without any sessions at all. For a time, Cruz even boycotted his own dialysis until the government took steps to offer the same to others on the waiting list. As he told one news station:

> I need to see something happen. I am willing to stop doing my dialysis. I am willing to die for it.
> This is nonsense. People are dying for God's sake. . . . We have people dying, literally dying and nobody's paying attention. So I am making a stand today.[34]

His makeshift tactics kept changing as his body did. At one point, when Cruz was told he needed to go to Guatemala City to avoid losing his leg, he took that story to the media too. "It's going to be a toeless Christmas" ran a caption over a picture of his decaying foot.[35] Generosity poured in from across Belize, helping to fund the trip to a specialist in Guatemala. Later, Mileni would fondly recall the way the kidney specialist there spent a whole hour with her and her husband. "He said, 'Don't be afraid. People can live with this. This is what you need to do.'" The specialist patiently explained to them what each test meant, what Jose could eat with kidney failure, and what groceries to buy at the supermarket. The experience of repeatedly traveling to Guatemala City on the

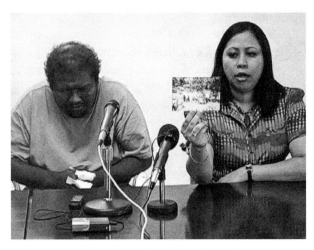

Jose Cruz convening a press release about his pending
amputations.

verge of death and returning feeling revived was heartening but eye-
opening. Seeing what was possible in Guatemala, Mileni remembered
the first time Jose said out loud: "Why doesn't Belize have this?"

Trying to bring attention to a system unable to support patients like
him, Cruz started convening amputation "press releases" for national
media outlets each time a part of his body was about to be cut off.

João Biehl describes two ways that patient-citizens in Brazil are
learning, in their words, "to enter justice" around their state's constitutional right to health: one can "enter through the court" (by filing a
lawsuit for access to medications) or "enter through the press" (by getting media coverage about missing rights that puts public pressure on
the state for upholding them).[36] But in a country like Belize without a
right to health written into its constitution or law, what do such tactics
become when they rely on the press alone? What bodies are stories like
this meant to put pressure on?[37]

"It is open for us to affect human history," Cruz had told me on the
morning we first met. By that time, in September 2010, he had already
gone blind and was missing one leg and several fingers. "I'm a young
man trapped in an old man's body," Cruz said with a laugh. A self-
declared "difficult patient," he preferred to arrive shirtless for his sessions and then be covered with a sheet. He was also known for his
overdone singing during the awkward first part of treatment getting
connected to the machine—mostly romantic Spanish ballads learned

from his grandfathers, one born in Guatemala and the other in Mexico. "It kills the time a little faster."

Cruz was diagnosed with diabetes when he was twenty-eight years old. "The problem with diabetes it that it has different effects," he said slowly. "For example, because they did not diagnose the problem in time, I suffer retinopathy in both eyes. . . . my vision went in a span of about two years." It turned out that Cruz had lived for many years with the diagnosis of diabetes before finally learning that his high blood sugar was actually rooted in a deeper pathology: polycystic kidney disease. This genetic disorder causes little cysts on the kidneys to grow and burst, triggering infection as well as Cruz's blood sugar spikes. "Over 500," he said of his glucose during times of infection. "When that happens, it makes dialysis . . . complicated."

For about four hours a day, three times a week, a dialysis machine removed and spun the entire volume of Cruz's blood outside his body every fifteen minutes, filtered it clean, and returned it to his veins. Unsurprisingly, this can cause blood levels of all kinds to tick up or down in ways that sometimes have an impact on the chemistry of treatment. Although rising blood pressure and blood sugar are concerning while "on the machine," the most immediate danger is crashing. Nowadays, glucose also gets added to dialysis fluid to prevent it from lowering the blood's sugar level while the fluids mingled during osmosis. But even with precautions, the unit was seeing more than its fair share of patients who suddenly stopped breathing.

In a country with no nephrologist, Nurse A—as the only nephrology-certified nurse in Belize at the time—fell under tremendous pressure. Participating patients each had to sign a waiver before getting hooked up to the machine, acknowledging that they accepted the risks of getting dialysis even though there was usually no doctor present. Whenever a patient went into crisis, Nurse A immediately phoned for the doctor on call to come. But there were many times when no doctor was available at that exact moment.

"She brought me back to life," Cruz told me. "Most of us in the room." A Maya woman whom Dr. Rosado had sponsored for a nephrology course before his accident, Nurse A had for decades been managing her own diabetes. She resuscitated many of the unit's patients over time, tense moments with the whole room watching. Several patients spoke of this as a profoundly personal connection, to know and trust the person who kept them alive through heart failure. Her role in their advocacy grew out of this intense context.

"She stood up for her patients," Mileni would recall later. At one point, Nurse A even resigned for a short time, leveraging her position as the only nephrology-certified nurse in the country at the time as her contribution to advocacy. She and the patients asked that a physician—any kind—be available on-site in case one of the patients went into heart failure or other crisis. Her patients protested in front of the hospital to demand she be hired back. In news photos of the protest, Jose Cruz held a message printed on yellow poster board that read WE DON'T WANT TO DIE.

In this context of normalized deaths, what gets branded as fatalism? Realism about the actual proximity of death could easily blur into what could be read as a certain resignation to it. It therefore became a major feat of advocacy just to counter the assumptions about diabetes and dialysis patients that were so often repeated.

On one hand, it was true that the extreme time and travel commitment required of patients needing dialysis meant some people did not consider the benefits worth the costs in their particular case, a deeply personal choice that each patient uneasily faced. On the other hand, the difficult decision made by some to forgo spottily accessible dialysis (given these numerous obstacles of various kinds) certainly did not apply to everybody in Belize—an inaccurate assumption I sometimes heard repeated to normalize gaps in dialysis availability for those people who *did* want and urgently need it to survive. Against this backdrop, Cruz and the other patients in their group made signs illustrated with skulls and crossbones, calling attention to the thin line between realism and fatalism. Many of them were indeed doing inner work to prepare for death—but that was the reality they were there to protest.

"I was told it couldn't be done," Cruz told me, flashing a mischievous grin. "But you can see the doctors are circling up already. That is what I'm doing. Despite the fact that I'm always fighting with them. That is part of it, fighting all the time, or it is never going to happen." At some point, fellow patients and their families began calling him "Dr. Cruz," a striking nickname to emerge from a context where patients were getting dialysis without a physician. Cruz became both patient in and doctor of the system.

Cruz's use of press coverage enabled a way to talk about the need for end-of-the-line treatments like dialysis—but he hoped that this might only be the first step in expanding chronic care more broadly. He worried aloud that many have come to accept the fragility of their systems— "they are used to it," in his words—and often ask for nothing more. "Because they determine . . . we're in a third-world country. That's the reason I am so much an advocate of critical dialysis," Cruz told me. "We deserve to have good healthcare in this country. For the individual . . . in the population, no? As part of the population."

On the day I left the dialysis center in 2010, Cruz was belting out "I'm Singing in the Rain" in a comedic opera voice, the patients around him laughing with a shake of their heads. He waved goodbye with a three-fingered hand, trailing tubes and singing like a showboat. I did not know at the time that he and his inner circle had begun receiving death threats for their advocacy work. But even then, the sense that his routine performances were a serious joke remained larger than life in my memory. And so did the first image I had seen of him on the news back in 2009. Cruz had both legs then, marching in the midst of a protest in Belize City. One of his hands still had all its fingers. But he held the sign in the other, the missing few fingers read as part of his poster's message: A PROMISE IS CONSOLATION TO A FOOL.

"This is the first time in [Belizean] history we have a group of actual patients suffering from an ailment come together and demanding what they want," Cruz told one Belizean news station. "I hope that the Belizean people are taking notice."[38]

FOOD INFRASTRUCTURES

As Laura fought to recover in 2010, she hoped to grow a few vegetables around the ramp that her husband built for her on the back of the house. A local hardware store kept a rack of seed packets near the cash register for aspiring gardeners in Dangriga, packaged by a U.S. seed company based in Philadelphia. For lack of alternatives, this was where the local Belize Diabetes Association pointed people with diabetes if they wanted to buy vegetable seeds. Garden projects like this were markers of how infrastructures of food and of medicine are connected—reminders that dialysis machines and prosthetic devices were intimately related to another set of missing tools and apparatuses, namely, around land and agriculture.

In another vegetable initiative, members of the Dangriga BDA discussed the possibility of a "field trip," traveling together by local bus to a nearby Mennonite village to buy vegetables. It was heartening to hear neighbors come together in trying to figure out ways to reach the healthy foods they could not affordably purchase in their own town's market. But their proposed weekend plan also struck me for the problem being underlined yet again: even for people living in a district capital, actualizing the option of a large supply of affordable vegetables would require a trip that took hours. And not only that—getting outside food desert conditions meant a trip to its whitest villages. How was it that agriculture had been so incentivized for Belize's recently arrived Mennonites, when farming was systemically discouraged for so many others attempting similar projects in the country's history?

Mennonites came up in other conversations about diabetes care as well. I once met a woman named Lucy who had worked for decades with Honduran laborers in the southern banana villages of Stann Creek. She and her daughter both had diabetes and helped each other with insulin shots. They sat side by side on a threadbare red couch adjoining their kitchen, surrounded by posters emphasizing the family's East Indian heritage. Lucy removed a sandal to fully display her foot, missing two toes. She credited a Mennonite hospital with the fact that she was able to keep the rest. "They saved it," she said, even after being told in the hospital that the entire foot would need to be amputated. Lucy described the treatments that the Mennonites had used to restore the imperiled tissue: homemade herbal poultices applied to the wound, periodic massage, a strict diet of raw vegetables fresh from their gardens, and a cryptic process that she described as "removing stones." It was one of several Mennonite medical rescues I had heard about from people living with diabetes around the country, several of whom reported "miracle" cures, such as salvaging dying limbs that hospital experts said would certainly need amputation and restoring eyesight that no one had expected to return.

One day in August 2010, I set out to find the place that Lucy had described to me as a "vegetable hospital." The road stretching north was unpaved but freshly graded, grayish and chalky in comparison to the orange-red soil of Stann Creek. It passed through a village where the aboveground cemetery looked at first glance like a city of miniature cathedrals. A little later, the sugarcane plantations turned into cornfields, and the tractors rolled on metal claw wheels instead of tires. We were in Mennonite country.

"Their vehicles can have an engine or rubber tires, but not both," one traveler named Saul explained, since the compressed air to fill tires is considered a restricted technology. He said of one Mennonite town: "We call these ones Mechanites, because they like these machines. But some of the stricter kinds won't use any machines at all. Some of them won't even use paint. And the ones who do cocaine crossings and drug stuff we call Moneyites, because of how much money they have now." We passed a small lake. The farmhouses were spread far apart, set back from the road on a hill. Besides the bearded driver of a horse and buggy, the only people we saw outside were three young children with white-blonde hair in front of a farm. They ran away barefoot into the house, dressed in the suspenders and modest dresses of tiny adults. "They are so pretty, but they always hide," Saul laughed of the shy Mennonite children before returning to a story about his own life passion, caring for wounded alligators.

It took me a while to find the clinic, a sturdy cement building reinforced inside with rebar. Disappointed that the clinic appeared closed for the weekend, I copied the handwritten text of the sign on its door:

Open Monday
Tuesday + Wednesday
Offen fuer Deutche
Freitag u Sonnabend

I don't speak any German, but a colleague in Belize once described this Plattdeutsch language to me as "like coarse Prussian from the 1830s."[39] The Mennonites have been political exiles for centuries. Originating from an Anabaptist group in which many of the founding leaders were killed for their subversive teachings, this violent history is recounted in the 1660s book *Martyr's Mirror*.[40] Survivors scattered across Europe and later the world, developing distinct sects. Today, Mennonites live in at least fifty-one countries across the globe, a range of diasporic histories cataloged in the *Mennonite Historical Atlas*.[41] During the 2010 census, there were over ten thousand Mennonites in Belize.[42] Mennonites are known for large-scale agriculture of their land and itinerant autonomy. By last national count, 6 percent of Mennonites in Belize had diabetes, the second-lowest rate for any ethnic group besides "White."[43] (For context, it is worth noting that Mennonite in Belize would code as appearing of distinctly European descent—in contrast to other sects in countries like Guatemala, where converting local residents has been more central to Mennonite presence.)

A Mennonite woman approached me as I was copying the sign into my notebook. She said that she and her husband together owned the clinic and asked why I had come. Her bright blue eyes matched her plain dress, though her gaze cast to the grass as we spoke. Her head was wrapped in a black scarf held in place by a single bobby pin, and her black apron partially covered the subtle pattern of tiny purple flowers on her dress. When I explained my project, she visibly relaxed and introduced herself as Elizabeth. Opening the clinic door, Elizabeth quietly explained that she was descended from apple farmers in Canada. I would later read that the Mennonite population there originated from a group sent to the gulags of Siberia and Kazakhstan after becoming embroiled in World War II, when Germans invaded the area of the Russian steppes they had been farming. Many of the Mennonites who made their way to Canada had escaped from Western Siberia by dogsled.[44]

Inside, the clinic opened into a small wooden room. It strongly resembled my imagination of a nineteenth-century apothecary shop. Behind its narrow counter, there were shelves crowded with herbal medicine bottles: bee pollen granules, evening primrose oil, horsetail and black cherry concentrate, capsules of manganese and chelated zinc. Intermixed with the Puritan's Pride–brand selenium and dolomite bottles, there were also a few more decorated boxes, like one of Korean ginseng tea and Nin Jiom Pei Pa Koa from Hong Kong. Next to a grandfather clock with a gold pendulum, a 1988 *Physician's Desk Reference* leaned against an antique brown book with a battered leather cover embossed with a gold filigree O. Elizabeth's husband, Isaac, shyly explained to me that the book was over 140 years old and showed me the second crumbling page that was signed "Cincinnati 27 November 1863." Those were the only words I could understand, save a handwritten recipe tucked between the pages; the rest was written in German. Isaac told me that the book was about herbs, and he returned it to its prominent place next to bags of psyllium husks and licorice root.

Elizabeth brought me into a back room to explain her collection of essential oils for massage therapy, which she kept in a row inside a handmade cabinet. She opened one vial at a time and had me guess the smells: lavender and lemon, peppermint and thieves. "These oils can get so deep," she told me, explaining they are a key treatment for the limbs of patients who are facing possible amputation. In the room, she had a massage table alongside a regular bed. As we walked down the hallway, I saw other tiled rooms as well, where patients could stay overnight if they wished. There were two beds with simple frames and pristine white sheets, the rooms' only decoration a clock and one seashell.

We sat in handmade mahogany chairs as I told her more about my research. "Diabetes is the most complex disease," Elizabeth said. "It is difficult to be released." She did have several patients who no longer needed their hospital medicines though, she said, and even some who no longer needed herbs. "But when the symptoms come, blindness or wounds and nerve issues and so, these are the last signs," she explained.

"We try to get to the root, to understand why the body is suffering with these signs." She showed me acupuncture charts of the bottoms of two feet and a diagram of the organs associated with various nerves along the spinal column. There were also diagrams of two eyes sectioned into slivers, which they studied when people came to the clinic with symptoms of diabetic retinopathy. When I mentioned how the woman I met spoke of "stones" removed from her, Elizabeth went to a stack of pictures and pulled out two, explaining their scale: "These are a little larger than life. Here, this one is of the real size." The pictures showed brown egg-shaped lumps, glistening an iridescent greenish color with purple around the edges. "These are gallbladder stones," she explained. "It usually takes one day and one night to pass these." Kidney stones, on the other hand, had to be treated for a longer period prior to passing, to wear down their razor-sharp edges. "With that, it comes out more like a dust. Sometimes I tell people to let a glass of their urine sit for half a day, and then you can see it on the bottom."

Elizabeth next produced a series of photos documenting patients' excrement, highlighting specimens with distinct patterns: bulging and swirled, narrow and ribbed. These forms each meant something different, she explained. Not all patients chose to share this, but it helped with diagnosis. Elizabeth handed me another of her favorite herb books, describing wild carrots and chokecherries, dandelion, cattails, and acorns. "These books have taught me a lot," she said. "But something of experience teaches you too."

Elizabeth's husband was a soft-spoken farmer who kept his thumbs tucked in his suspenders. The six languages he spoke (including fluent Spanish and several registers of German) encoded his family's layered histories and the Mennonites' seemingly paradoxical entwined values of nomadic staidness: after his family left Mexico, Isaac said, he had lived in Spanish Honduras for a number of years before finally settling down in British Honduras in 1961.

"Probably about 60 percent of our patients have diabetes," Isaac estimated. He described one woman who came on the bus all the way from Nicaragua, her knees swollen because of excess uric acid. "She felt good when she left here," he said. Then he picked up a photo they had on the shelf of a woman with gangrene. In the picture, her foot was black and its toes white. She had spilled boiling water on her foot, Isaac said, but because of her diabetes she had not been able to feel the injury. By the time she reached their clinic, the woman had already been told the foot would have to be amputated. Isaac and Elizabeth had worked with her closely during her stay, supplying fresh vegetables to eat in addition to her other treatments. In another photo, a Kriol woman wearing an orange American flag T-shirt looked amused, staring down at the dead foot as Elizabeth tended it. "Her flesh came back, and it could feel again," Isaac said. "The feeling came back. Her sugar was 500 when she came, and it was below 200 when she left. It was working." He looked sad as he described the hope the woman had left with, but she had trouble affording vegetables every day at home. They heard that not long after, her foot suffered a relapse and had to be cut off a few months later.

While we spoke, Elizabeth was bustling around blending the powders from foil bags. She knew how to mix custom-made powdered ingredients for each patient. Once the various green, brown, and earth-colored dusts were ready, Isaac's role in their partnership was to mix the powders together in a bag and hand make each pill by pinching the mixture into clear gelatin capsules that twisted close. "I can do about two hundred in an hour," he explained. In the room where Elizabeth made her mixtures, she had over three hundred ingredients tucked in tiny wooden drawers. There was a scale for measuring powder on a silver plate. It rested next to a hemoglobin meter and an unlit oil lamp, its glass lantern patterned with Spanish dancers. Elizabeth showed me olive leaf powder and spikenard root dust. "It's what Mary used to wash the feet of Jesus, in his Holy Scripture," she added. Whenever she handed me a bottle or fresh sprig, she always said the same thing of each herb: "It is so precious."

Before I left, Elizabeth took me to her garden, where we stepped between seedling orange and lime trees. She pointed out a new tree she was trying to grow under a wooden crate. Its leaves were yellow next to a cracked eggshell. Back past the water tank, wild spinach grew among the sorosi. Next she showed me the leaves of yucca and sweet potato, which can be eaten like lettuce. We picked some for lunch, and she gathered sprigs of spinach and greens for me to take back to Dangriga, their stems wrapped in wet napkins so they could be replanted.

I put the spinach in a water bottle until my next visit to Laura's house, for her new garden. For a while, the greens grew near the ramp to her kitchen, eventually producing a single salad. Trying to understand the space between Laura's dream of a garden and the actual difficulty of starting one up is the reason analysts talk not only about garden projects but also about *food infrastructures*.[45] That term emphasizes that even for those who want to grow some vegetables or try a kitchen garden, there are many bigger issues at play that make the dream easy or difficult. What growth gets capacitated by institutions?

What gets discouraged? Land titles, start-up capital for machinery, state-guaranteed markets or support, tax incentives, trade deals, legal protections for small collectives, and easy access to meaningful seed supplies all come together in how Elizabeth and Laura were part of different food infrastructures.

The historical idiosyncrasies of the Mennonites' situation are illuminating to think with but impossible to replicate. No other ethnic group sits outside national tax structures (the Mennonites pay no agricultural taxes due to religious exemption). This is a major part of what allows their community to be actually self-governing and independent from global food trade policies. I heard that certain Mennonite sects elsewhere focus on social justice outreach such as access to repairable technologies, like machines to grind peanuts. But the only people I met in Belize who had acquired farm machinery from the Mennonites purchased it at their John Deere store, in an agro-industrial community where (many other Belizeans were quick to note) the well-paved road ended immediately at the town's edge.

Actually, a machine for processing peanuts had been the dream of one local Garifuna farmers' cooperative. The group had been looking to market a nutritious protein cereal—Cerebuitu, they named it, Good Cereal—as a grassroots business, hoping to supply nearby school breakfast programs. The cereal they envisioned could be made not only from organic rice but also from banana, yam, and breadfruit. To start out, they had perfected a recipe with a base of organic peanuts and rice, flavored with ground ginger and nutmeg. When I sampled the bag they shared with me, it tasted nourishing and subtle, reminding me of something from a high-end health-food store. But the collective needed a particular machine from Guatemala City in order to process a market volume of peanuts. The group's leaders had met with government officials and NGOs, typed up an itemized budget, and even visited Guatemala City to price and photograph the necessary machine. It cost six thousand dollars. By the time they showed me its picture, they had been looking for a funder for many years.

Three farmers from the collective brought me to a building full of drying sesame. By that time, their collective was contemplating turning the space into a tilapia farm to finance equipment for the cereal initiative. As we walked through waist-high grasses, a farmer with loose silver dreadlocks told me how their collective had grown a huge quantity of peanuts that first year, hoping to launch the cereal project. They had

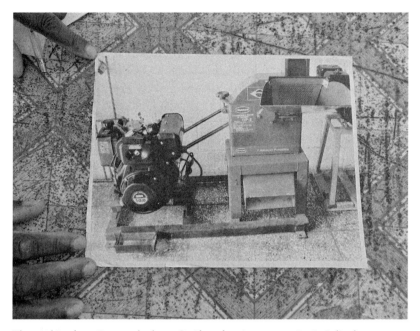

The machine from Guatemala that a Garifuna farming cooperative in Belize hopes to buy for their healthy cereal project.

a hand-crank grinder meant for family supply and had printed some labels for packaging. But the group had not been able to track down any governmental or other support to scale up equipment or distribution. I was surprised to hear about the difficulty because foreign peanut supplements like Plumpy-Nut have become well funded among donors concerned with childhood nutrition. But after sharing, selling, shelling, and grinding all the peanuts humanly possible without an industrial machine, the farmers eventually had to agree there remained a large quantity of peanuts beginning to rot. Maybe the next year, they hoped, things would work out with the machinery. Before the remaining crop became a nightmare to haul, they returned it to the village ecosystem— micronutrients for crabs and fish, fertilizing the land and water system they would grow from again next season.

Or at least, that was the most optimistic way to think of seventy-two thousand pounds of organic peanuts, grown with dreams of starting a healthy Garifuna food program for children, that had to be dumped into a swamp.

Another major Garifuna food sovereignty project underway in Honduras is spearheaded by Miriam Miranda, president of the Black

Fraternal Organization of Honduras, whose work has helped capacitate a generation of thriving Garifuna farmers along the Honduran coast. Recently, a Canadian investor announced plans to build a series of "charter cities" as part of a tourist megaproject on their land. The collective is now also battling this planned foreign construction across the land of twenty-four Garifuna communities.[46]

This especially tense case in Garifuna Honduras amplifies certain contradictions of food infrastructures. But in more subtle forms, they are actually quite common. People with diabetes are frequently made to feel like it is their responsibility alone if they develop chronic health conditions. But it takes rather extraordinary and personally risky measures to try reforming the agricultural *systems* that make such conditions likely for many. When Miriam Miranda won a food sovereignty prize in 2015, her traveling companion to the United States, Lenca Indigenous activist Berta Cáceres, was assassinated at home shortly after the two returned. Miranda has continued her work even after multiple death threats and a kidnapping.

Collaborating between the Garifuna communities of Belize and Honduras, collectives at work on food justice issues have continued despite rising violence toward environmental activists in Honduras. In November 2015, two Garifuna activists there were run off the road. The next month, the president of the Garifuna Land Defense Committee was shot in his driveway in Honduras, after speaking out against a land grab by Canadian tourism developers; he survived the three bullets, one in his lungs.[47] Several other Garinagu were killed by police in Honduras amid strange circumstances in 2016, 2017, and 2018 (events linked with a growing U.S. military presence, according to activism and solidarity statements by the Belize National Garifuna Council). But you won't find any of that on the clinic educational pamphlets suggesting that patients with diabetes reduce their stress and eat more vegetables.

BETWEEN HURRICANES

Chronic weather was what Laura used to help explain her diabetes: she said it felt like watching a hurricane approach. Good cooking had always been very important to her because it was a way she could live with "open hands," sharing with her family and giving to neighbors even though there wasn't extra money. "You can't eat the money!" she would laugh. It was an upsetting dilemma for her to realize that the food she had always cooked with love—with ingredients that could be stretched widely enough to have extra to freely share—was part of how she ended up losing a leg. Speaking with tenderness of both past and future generations, Laura merged collective memories of hurricanes like Hattie with her views on how foodways have changed to explain to me how it felt to watch an emergency approaching so slowly.

Her metaphor began with a memory of storms. "We used to have a big house, but not cement. A wooden house on the beach," she described. "And right there, you could stand up inside and see when the water was coming [when the sea levels rise during a hurricane]. We were just little kids, but we weren't scared. . . . family members and neighbors would come. This house was full of people. But how many people would die in that house because we didn't move from out the sea?"

That was what diabetes felt like to her, Laura said—a hurricane coming. It was part of a system much bigger than any individual, but there were certain measures that people knew to take nowadays to protect themselves and their families, she explained. But back then, it was different: "We didn't know," she recalled of the way her family used to stay in their wooden house during hurricanes. With what they know now, "even if I have a big house, if a certain category of hurricane comes, I wouldn't stay there. Because it's coming! It's going to come at me." Laura evoked a sense of food climates and weather systems together reaching their tipping points. Her sense of chronic risks and the long-term patterns that precede a crisis made me recall how diabetes is biologically characterized by overheating on the cellular level, both kinds of warming gradual in accumulations and then suddenly erupting into crisis.[48] Laura stayed with these overlaid images, returning to Hattie: "God saved our lives again. . . . My mother was just fighting her way through. My mother didn't even know to move from there." In contrast, Laura said, "What I wouldn't do now! I wouldn't stay here, with my grandbaby. So it's funny, the eating . . ."

As Laura spoke, we both kept looking out at the sea in front of her sister's house. During my time in Belize in 2010, already Hurricanes Alex *and* Karl had hit, and Hurricane Richard struck weeks afterward. In that moment, her analogy about food climates and hurricanes felt like more than a metaphor. What happens when not only houses and bodies but shorelines and atmospheres are in need of repair?

There is something in diabetic foot care known as *demarcation*—slating a body part to amputate itself at a particular line and choosing not to intervene with an active procedure. It seemed to me that demarcation was increasingly being applied to the changing landscape: Certain sections of the Mesoamerican reef closest to tourist markets in

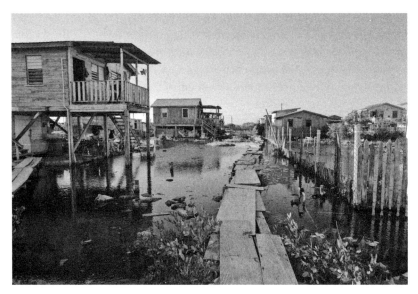

"London Bridges" in Belize.

Cancun had received health insurance policies for emergency care in cases of a hurricane. ("If you cut any place of your body, and you get attention very quickly, you have more possibility for getting healthy. It's the same with the reef," explained the backing insurance company.)[49] Some Belizean groups like Fragments of Hope work to replant nursery corals on metal rods, like little prostheses for dying sections of the reef, trying to shore up against the warming ocean. But other places were not considered salvageable. "The problem of the twenty-first century is the problem of the water line," Stefan Helmreich observes, as global warming interfaces with the long-standing color lines that W.E.B. DuBois famously described.[50] "The entire Belize City will be submerged by an encroaching sea in under 7 decades," the Belize Ministry of Health replied when asked about one eroding coast.[51]

In Belize, this problem feels both old and new: about 1 percent of the population already lives in "London Bridge" communities over water. As one official in Belize explained to anthropologist Herbert Gayle, "That is the only place where I see such unity among the poor. They come together and extend the bridge to each other's shack."[52] Cobbled from improvised scraps, London Bridge homes often emerge in flood zones, where the state has little presence with infrastructure or roads. Their architecture is named for the nursery rhyme: *London Bridge is falling down. . . . Build it up with wood and clay. . . . Wood and clay will wash away. . . . Build it up with bricks and mortar. . . . Bricks and mortar will not stay. . . . Build it up with iron and steel. . . .*

Even in some of the bleakest areas, an unlikely infrastructure of collaborative maintenance sometimes emerges. "What people call [a] nice place now was morass and people dump it [in the] same way. We put the plan in place afterwards. . . . Belize City sits on a delta. The people of old have been doing this, so we're learning the technique and we're creating another space," explained one resident.[53] Such chance bits sometimes come together in rearrangements more meaningful than any of their single pieces—structures that contain shards of painful history but sustain new possibilities, with the force of jagged affinities and unauthorized tinkering.[54] Yet there are places where it is nearly impossible to travel with crutches or a wheelchair.

PROSTHETIC HOPE INTERNATIONAL

When Laura received a prosthetic leg from Fede, her granddaughter called it their household "robot foot." But the leg hurt, Laura said. On the day I visited to see it, she was stretched out in a hammock and the leg was in a corner, a folded napkin in the socket.

Diabetic stumps in particular often swell and contract, even in the course of a day. It is not uncommon for a prosthetic socket that fit when made to later need modification, because stumps' shapes often change over time. So Laura's concerns did not strike me then as out of the ordinary. In my mind back in 2010, Laura's work getting a leg from Fede was one of few stories that seemed to have a sort of resolution: cobbling across the odds, Belizeans in partnership working hard to help other Belizeans recover. But looking back, I realize that I had trouble hearing her that day. She tried to tell me that the limb was not free of charge, after all. (I had figured this must be a misunderstanding.) And more than that, she told me that the socket was not fitting right. She said that she'd had trouble sorting out an adjustment with its cobbler and could barely even use it just to wear in church.

Setbacks are integral to the realities of maintenance stories, so it wouldn't feel right to leave this next part out: Laura wasn't the only one who ended up in this kind of situation. I was surprised to learn years later that Fede had been let go from the organization, in tensely fraught circumstances. Several people told me that Fede had started charging patients "under the table" for limbs made by the organization—in some cases exorbitant prices, even for patients with few means or for poor-quality legs. By the time I followed up on our earlier interviews, Fede was no longer working for what was once called Project Hope Belize. In the aftershocks of their schism, the organization had shut down for several years to rebrand and rebuild. Fede and Rob both offered to share a retrospective comment about what happened.

Fede and I met up at a Chinese restaurant, his flashy pickup truck long gone by then. He arrived on a hand-pedaled bicycle. Charismatic as ever, he focused his narrative on the more philosophical aspects, which were easier to talk about: What was a good enough foot and for whom? Fede said he worried that prosthetic students passing through from other countries made limbs for Belizeans *as if* they were going to get maintenance. He said that his constructions were considered rough and overly heavy by those working in other contexts; but that he'd seen people's legs snap, even top-of-the-line models, because their parts weren't engineered for tropical environs like Belize. Some clients worked in heavy labor in agricultural fields, or lived on the beach and needed a leg to walk on sand, or otherwise asked him to make something that would last five or ten years. By the time we spoke, Fede explained he was down to the dregs of his supplies. But he said there were people who came to him because they didn't want to wait many years in hopes of a better leg. That was his side of the story.

Yet something is not always better than nothing, Rob said with worry when I caught up with him later in Atlanta. A poor-quality prosthesis can be dangerous. "She had a right amputation, he offered her a left leg," one of these stories began. I told Rob how I was struggling to write about what had happened, and felt uneasy now writing about the way things had appeared back in 2010. He felt uneasy too, and told me that I wasn't alone in wishing there was a way to rewrite the past few years. Rob spoke passionately about the work ahead but honestly about the pressure. "You want to go down to Belize and make legs for people, there's all this other stuff you gotta do to keep the machinery running." He realized that many Belizeans were waiting for his team in order to get a limb and wished he could be in two places at once. Rob said it was a strange feeling to keep going without Fede, some twenty years into their collaboration. He sounded just as sad about the lost relationship as Fede had. "You know, we were in our twenties when we met. He was one of my best friends."

After lunch, Rob waved me into the shade of an enormous warehouse. Recycled objects were stuffed in a maze of cardboard boxes on red shelves stacked four high, with lumber piled on the highest tier near the tin roof. Many boxes held retired Delta Airlines uniforms, but Rob's section had very specific labels, like "left foot shells" or "6 ply socks." Rob pulled down a crate of right feet to show me some of the supplies for their next trip to Belize, coming up in a few months. Rob and his partners renamed the organization to signal a fresh start: Prosthetic Hope International. The group has started working more closely with the Belize Assembly for Persons with Diverse Abilities (BAPDA). They estimated that around two hundred people are currently on the waiting list for either new prosthetic limbs or old ones needing repair. One of them was Laura.

Last I heard, Fede was contemplating moving to Guatemala, which would leave no one I know currently living in Belize who makes or repairs prosthetics. Rob remained committed to going to Belize several times a year, and is working to collaborate more closely with the Belizean government now that the issue is more central on their radar. He hoped to secure a grant to team up with a Belizean craftsperson for on-the-ground daily repairs and expand care.

If the whole situation was a parable, it might be about how each collaborator could use a figure like the other: balancing global resource flows with consistent presence and local knowledge, bringing distinct kinds of expertise together.

This is not a parable though, just another tough reality faced by many countries. One thing is sure: the demand for prosthetics is not going anywhere. The last thing Fede told me was that he feels worried about his kids since the whole family now lives on his wife's grocery clerk salary of one dollar a day, which means that most days they can only afford meals of plain noodles. While Fede was born without legs, he said his mother recently lost both of her legs as well, to diabetes.

HOLDING MEASURES

Mileni told me she dreamed of one day continuing the dialysis and advocacy work that she and her husband, Jose, began. Most people who pass Mileni in her unassuming cleaning uniform don't realize the kind of life she has lived since childhood, which warrants a book of its own. But that is a story for another time, Mileni added with a laugh. For now, she wanted to tell me how her fight at Jose's side had ended.

All the couple's possessions had been stolen from their home shortly before his death. Mileni recalled how someone broke in and took their mattress, couch, and furniture. They even took the little plastic egg that Jose had bought as a surprise for her birthday one year, a funny gift that she missed more than the wedding ring it used to hold. But they didn't take the box of her husband's papers about the advocacy movement, so Mileni had been saving them for many years. The box held the bureaucratic traces of their fight: Jose's back-and-forth with the U.S. dialysis organization and Belizean officials. Shuffled in with the rest were also news clippings, love poetry, medical records, and eleven cassette tapes on which Cruz recorded his own narration of his advocacy projects and life chapters, bearing sticky labels in his handwriting with titles like "Fudge: His Life."

In retrospect, Mileni thought Jose somehow knew clearly when it was coming. She remembered her husband's urgency on the day before he went into heart failure, when he suddenly wanted a burrito from his favorite restaurant, owned by a close friend. Later, she said, the proprietor had told her that Jose said goodbye that day. It gave her peace to be able to give thanks for how it happened: "My husband died of natural causes." Her favorite way to remember him was singing karaoke—like at her friend's wedding, when he had surprised her by getting up in front of everyone. Already blind and missing a leg by then, he sang the Bryan Adams classic "Heaven," a Belizean favorite, dedicating the song to Mileni. Jose had a pitch-perfect voice after singing in so many dialysis sessions. Whenever the song came on the radio, Mileni said, she felt him near.

Later, I wasn't sure how to read that year's protest events: Was the dialysis patient activism I had seen in 2009–10 a citizen consciousness that might continue growing around other aspects of healthcare or an evanescent moment that coalesced around a few charismatic individuals? I don't know if it might be a story still unfolding. But since Cruz's work to create an idea of rights took place largely through the news stories written about him, I am trying to take seriously the different work of narrating these stories myself. As always, the center of gravity shifts depending on where you stop or start the story.[55] Being in dialysis units made me think of people I'd met who couldn't access them—how there was nothing to say when twenty-year-old Jordan showed me his bloated feet and said that he was not even on the waiting list. Apparently his kidneys were so bad that he was considered a poor candidate for the costly treatment. I remembered, too, how when Cresencia's legs filled with fluid, she could find relief only in ancestral interventions.

But I could also tell a more heartening story about what I saw when I returned to Belize years later, to the same location where, almost five years earlier, Ethan had shown me the space being prepared for the newly arriving dialyzers they hoped to install. Ethan was gone by then, having moved on to work elsewhere. Jose Cruz died on a December morning, three months after I interviewed him in 2010. But there it was on the hill, landscaped with dirt from recently dug oil wells in a Mennonite town nearby: a low building and a small sign directing patients into the Jose Cruz Memorial Dialysis Unit.

It took me a minute to compose myself enough to take a picture of the open clinic, thinking of the past lives its sign marked and the ongoing ones it might now extend. But I suppose you can't freeze-frame a happy ending any more than a tragic one. Inside the unit, two visiting dialysis nurses bustled around. Later, a government official worried aloud to me that the U.S. donor who had originally funded the center had now drawn back after three years of training and support, as had been planned, leaving the machines to the state for maintenance. A large percentage of the Ministry of Health's entire operating budget was being spent to keep dialysis centers running, although there were still shortages around more basic technologies—such as glucometers and strips for home testing (too expensive to be provided by the state) and insulin (provided by the government in three of the country's six districts)—which will mean more Belizeans needing dialysis in the years ahead. After hard work by the policy planning office, some 25 percent of patients who needed dialysis in the country were now receiving it, up from what was initially 10 percent. But the other 75 percent were still waiting. Government officials were looking for investors to help them maintain the units, hoping to find a potential partner abroad.

But also there in the clinic, getting dialysis in the room that morning, was my old friend Guillerma. It was striking to see her in that room after our earlier conversations in such a very different context all those years ago, when her mother, Arreini, had hosted an ancestral meal for protection, at a time when Guillerma was understood to be dying from diabetes complications and could not get dialysis at all. The last time I had seen Guillerma was in a Belize City hospital at the end of 2010, when she had just started getting one of the three dialysis sessions she needed each week, due in large part to Jose Cruz's advocacy. It was a fraction of the care she needed but had still opened some precarious margin of survival.

Sitting there in the Jose Cruz dialysis unit, where Guillerma was now getting all three weekly sessions, these histories meant something different to both of us already. But they were also part of the "repair work" that had sustained her until now. I showed Guillerma the picture I had taken during my last visit, when she had been sitting in the same chair in Belize City where Jose Cruz once received treatment—though the two had never met, she told me. "Let them know, I am still right here fighting it," Guillerma said, four years later then. Three mornings every week, she woke up at 4:00 A.M. and took a taxi and then a public school bus three hours in each direction to receive her hard-won 8:00 A.M. session. "I look *good*. People don't believe I am on dialysis until I show them my fistula."

We watched from the window as people walked down the big hill. It was so hot that with the steep climb, many patients who had just gotten off the machine had fainted at least once while walking down it. ("They boxed me up," Guillerma once laughed while we waited for the bus, recalling the last time she was slapped back to consciousness by her favorite nurse.) I thought of the evening when Arreini had first told me about her daughter's "dialys" and the place in her village she had planned to bury her. Instead, all these years later, Guillerma wanted to share pictures of the beautiful deep-red dress she had bought to walk her own daughter down the aisle.

The dialysis machine whirred and beeped next to us the entire time we spoke, like a shrill but persistent third voice in our conversation, as it removed accreted toxins from Guillerma's blood. In many parts of the world, dialysis is considered a "holding measure"[56] until renal transplant becomes possible. But in Belize, where no renal transplant has yet been performed in the country's history, dialysis was instead a "holding measure" against death.

I remember how mechanical those exact machines had looked back in 2010, still stiffly wrapped in factory plastic, when I had photographed them in their storage room with the air-conditioning blasting to preserve their delicate parts. It was somehow comforting that the medical tubes now carrying her blood into one of those very machines looked more pliable than I expected: less the electrical circuitry of a cyborg, more like an umbilical cord. Guillerma followed my eyes. "Still alive," she smiled. The electrodes and wires threaded the air between us, awkward and alive, into its tenuous machinery. Together we watched the centrifuge wheel her blood backward like a broken clock, trying to turn back enough time for the week ahead.

THE GRADUAL INSTANT

Public health and medical sciences read very differently when juxtaposed against the lived histories of people actually navigating care for chronic conditions. Their arts of survival and repair often ricochet against any assumptions that take for granted what diabetes looks like and where it comes from—bringing attention to what James Baldwin once called "the questions hidden by the answers."[57] At the same time, this account has tried to do something more than note diabetic sugar's many complicated questions, by also following along with those trying to put pieces slowly together into habitable stories. Guided by people "still fighting it" (as they say in Belize) and trying to work up to their insights and craft, this book has attempted to assemble pieces together in ways that more closely reflect how they were lived: as material fragments searchingly rearranged into whole worlds that often astonished me with the force of their improvisation and pain, but also with their persistence and love.

"How's our miracle?" Laura's surgeon liked to ask, which always made her laugh.

"I'm doing good, doctor."

Whenever Laura recalled again her story of getting those amputations of the same leg only days apart, the awfulness of the procedure was not the part that made her emotional. "It was funny," she said. "It was quite funny." Laura kept replaying that scene in her mind. She could never talk about it now without crying, she explained when her voice started to break a little, because that day in the hospital, she had seen her whole family unexpectedly gathered together.

Laura saw her brother pacing in the hallway, scratching his head (an anxious habit of his that she remembered from childhood). She saw the expression on each of her children's faces as they realized they might lose her, and she heard the way her husband called out to her, "*Tone, gial,*" like back in the days when they had first fallen in love, after the hospital staff told them it might be the last time they saw her. Laura wanted to tell them all, "I will be okay, either way," but she could not talk. Laura said that she would never forget the image she had seen in that moment when the nurse wheeled her through the door of the operating theater: her entire family watching, each one of their faces. "How much they love me."

That, for her, was the day's gradual instant. Listening, I realized that my first impulse had been to describe the events with an emphasis on what led to hardship, the accumulations that necessitated the cut. But in Laura's telling, she focused on the slow care that got her through it. "I wish everyone with this sickness would know, please try to take care.

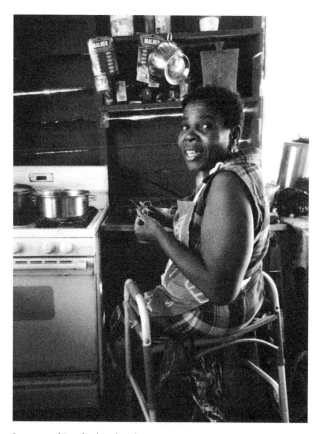

Laura cooking for her family.

Because it's not just you," she said. "It is your whole family that goes through it with you."

By the end of 2010, Laura had invented a way to turn her walker into a makeshift seat, affixing a blue strap borrowed from another appliance and weaving it through the handlebars. Using this makeshift chair of suitable height to sit by her stove, Laura could begin cooking again, which had once been her profession. Her favorite dish to make had always been *darasa*, a Garifuna word meaning "slow." Laura laughed about this and the slow work she was trying to do for her family—to keep herself healthy enough to avoid the dialysis her doctor said she might need otherwise; to make her mother's and grandmother's family recipes while tinkering with their ingredients; to take the time to shred carrots and prepare vegetables in special ways to bridge tastes. "Look at my grandbabies," she smiled to herself, and called out to a four-year-old playing near us. "K, come here love. Do you like broccoli?"

"It's delicious!" said K, running behind the couch and peeking warily at me over a pillow.

"It's delicious," Laura repeated with an amused grin. Her granddaughter was learning to like vegetables for the taste, with no idea yet of the cost of broccoli; or that generations before her had not eaten this recipe; or what her grandmother was trying to protect her from, in the daily labor of making special recipes and shredding carrots into a more tender dish of peels.

"Nothing is sudden," Anne Michaels writes. "Not an explosion—planned, timed, wired carefully—not the burst door. Just as the earth invisibly prepares its cataclysms, so history is the gradual instant."[58] If slow violence is characterized as difficult to discern, slow care might be even harder to see: meal by meal, gesture by gesture. Its culmination is not the moment when something dramatic happens. Its culmination is every day that it doesn't.

"I will never ask God why," Laura had said and nodded toward her remaining leg, which she used to consider her worst side because of its two amputated toes. She laughed when she told me of her daily prayer: "Just please leave this one for me. So I can still hop around the house."

It was such a profoundly humble petition that, eight years later, my stomach knotted when Laura told me over the phone that she had lost the second leg too. It brought to mind the pains she often described and what difficulty she'd already gone through adjusting to the first prosthetic leg that Fede had made her. I wondered what she was going to do, now that the country's only prosthetic workshop was in transition and unstaffed by a repair person on a day-to-day basis.

Yet when I arrived the next day, trying to hide my dread that I might find Laura disheartened after also losing her "hop around the house" leg she had prayed to keep, the scene was the exact opposite of the tragic immobilization I had imagined. Actually, it was the most nimble and confident I had ever seen Laura. Even when she had both legs, their pain and numbness had meant she walked slowly. Rather than dreaming of a second prosthetic leg this time, Laura said, now she suspected that she no longer needed any prosthesis at all. She was wearing a tight green tank top that showed off her arm muscles. "My son said it looks like I'm going to do yoga," she laughed of the athletically styled shirt.

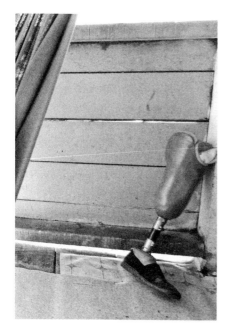

The prosthetic leg that Fede made for Laura, now no longer needed.

Her husband made us popcorn, which he had begun selling in plastic bags from his cart some days instead of ice cream.

Laura and I sat on the porch floorboards and listened back to our interview from 2010, as she helped me pick the best parts to highlight here. "You know, it's amazing for me to hear my own voice," Laura said when the recording ended. She joked about the old tape recorder we had been listening to play back her words: "I never knew this gadget would be here for me!" I asked if she had anything she wanted to add, these years later.

"This is for any friends or public," Laura started a bit formally, as she tried to imagine you who might read her words one day and what your reasons were for picking up this book. "It is good to learn from each other, from inside the life of one living it. What is reality? What you can't change. I'm not hiding away from that. You just have to take care, as much as you can. Right? We must set our minds to what we can do."

In Laura's case, what she could do included a combination of strength and balance exercises that began slowly rebuilding her muscles and dexterity, until the day when she was sure she would be able to visit her relative's house again—even though it had high, steep stairs. But Laura wanted to surprise her family with the ability she had been honing. She turned down her son's invitation to carry her up into the house. Step by step, Laura did not look down at them watching on the road below, moving up each rise of the wooden stairs by balancing the weight on her palms—steps as slow as the years it takes most anything to change; as difficult, local, and specific as the stairs at home for someone walking on their hands.

When Laura got to the top, she didn't want her daughters to make a fuss if she looked back, so she just called out a little joke to them over her shoulder. Whenever I try to imagine the scene now, her words feel like an open question for all of us:

"Well, are you people coming?"

Epilogue

Out of the strong came forth sweetness.

—Biblical riddle used as a corporate slogan to market
   Caribbean sugar, as seen on a deserted factory in London

I used to think that diabetic sugar was too elusive to be captured in a single, stand-alone picture. But right before this went to press, I encountered one photo that changed my mind. Nurse Norma sent it to me in 2018. The picture showed a candlelight vigil that Norma's collective had organized in Dangriga for World Diabetes Day on November 14. Gathered at a park near the water, a few dozen people had arranged themselves into the shape of a circle, matching blue balloons in hands, candles lit, and heads bent. A number of participants in the circle held photographs of their lost loved ones who died with diabetic sugar. The sturdy picture frames looked borrowed from tabletops and living room walls. I knew some of the faces, but most were unfamiliar.

I sat with the picture of these photos for a long time. It reminded me of seeing Mr. P's album ten years before and the sense of watching a loved one slowly disappear from a family archive. I recalled the matter-of-factness of his voice as he turned each page of his album and repeated the word *sugar*.

Different versions of that tenderness and disappearance have been playing out in family photos across the country, long outpacing my short time there. But the vigil brought together versions of those shared stories over and over again, across time, in one place. The collective repetition began to seem like a time lapse of something else—not receding but expanding. Instead of individuals sealed tightly into frames of loss, the mosaic of images opened up the broader realities of dying and living with sugar.

The care reflected in their composite image of the vigil was a pointed reminder to me, too. It has been jarring to see the ordinary gravity of slow vanishing happen in such patterned ways across my own photos. Although those pictures are different in so many ways than a family album, when people ask what I've been writing about, I never know where to start. Most times I just answer with a line borrowed from Mr. P. "Sugar".

Over the past decade, a great deal has changed in global policy stories about diabetes. The topic now feels everywhere across media headlines and in health debates, changing the public arenas that these chapters' stories might enter. I tried to write with the ethics of a "slow pen,"[1] checking back with people as they helped me revise. Yet pictures I wanted to give back to project contributors in the form of this book weren't always the same pictures I thought might allow outside readers to think about expanded care. The tension between those versions has made it hard to let go of these images.

Some of the pictures that didn't fit in this book found a place in other homes. When I handed Tobias the picture of his sister Sarah that I had left out of this book, he smiled to himself. He told me about his new garden of organic beans and repeated again the story of his journey to receive treatment from Dr. W in New York. I thought of the hyperbaric chamber that simulated the act of plunging him under sixty-six feet of seawater day after day until the oxygen was enough for his body to heal itself. In the photo of Sarah I handed Tobias, she was holding the device she called a sugar machine. "That's a good one. Do you know she could flip the mattress over all by herself?" He asked me if there was any way to make a bigger copy for their wall. "Just a little memory," he said.

When I visit Belize now, my old pink local flip phone is filled with dead people's numbers. It feels wrong to delete them, but there is always a split second when I'm scrolling with my mind elsewhere and it feels like I could give any one of them a call. Sometimes moments like that send me back to old recordings that I can't bear listening to, or can't stop listening to, depending—either one suspended in closed loops of unfixed errata. Sugar can make time feel sticky; at times I got attached to feeling stuck.

Sometimes I tried to get out of it. Once in 2018 I traveled to England, thinking that I might find clues by walking the global circuit of sugar's commodity chains. On the wharves of east London, the cold wind smelled like burnt sugar. Boats of sugarcane from Belize still arrive regularly along the river's shores. I wondered why I had really come there.

Maybe I was looking for something like a nemesis. But that wasn't what I found. Today nearly all of Silvertown's other factories have been abandoned, but not the sugar refinery. KEEPING SWEET, its signs read. TASTE THE SUNSHINE.

It was a far cry from the "Sugar Mile" famously depicted by Sidney Mintz.[2] Long gone are the days when business was so good that the Tate & Lyle Company could market a line of sugar cubes exclusively for circus bears. Most labor-level jobs have long since been taken over by machines; someone said the few remaining human positions in the factory mainly belonged to engineer types with PhDs who monitored chemistry or programmed computers. But there is still a building called the "Royal Sugar Shed" for the queen's personal supply (today owned by a U.S. conglomerate), with piles of white sugar as high as sand dunes.

I took pictures as I walked through the parking lot of one of the nineteenth-century jam factories from *Sweetness and Power*. Someone had left a single shoe in the watchman's booth. The walls were marked with graffiti from long-lost union strikes against bankrupt or offshored companies. The abandoned factories reminded me of a biography called *Sugar Girls* that I had noticed in the London airport.[3] The book profiled the British women who worked at the sugar factories of Tate and Lyle Company, to which Caribbean cane had long traveled for refining. The book's subtitle—*Tales of Hardship, Love, and Happiness*—could also fittingly describe the Belizean women who gave themselves the nickname "sugar girls": Antonia, Dee, and Cresencia. Groups of friends on both sides of the Atlantic had jokingly arrived at the same term of insider distinction and endearment for each other. But all four of the "sugar girls" in England were still alive and in their eighties.

Bent parallels: the sugar that the British nickname referenced was former factory labor groups, while the Belizean nickname referenced rising sugar inside consuming bodies. Mintz's imagined production-consumption dyad not only seemed to have inverted poles, but dissipated and permeated its unequal climates and atmospheric textures. "It is not the specifics of any one . . . set of events that are endlessly repeatable and repeated, but the totality of the environments in which we struggle," Christina Sharpe writes of such uneven embodiments, "the machines in which we live; what I am calling the weather."[4]

I stood at the water's edge and looked through the fog at the abandoned industrial mills and distant cranes putting up glass condos, rumored to be mostly owned by investors from China and Dubai. Locals said that digging releases smells from the earth of whichever factory used to sit above: creosote, telegraph rubber, perfume chemicals. "In understanding the relationship between commodity and person, we unearth anew the history of ourselves," Mintz wrote as his book's last line.[5] Watching the cranes, I wasn't sure what was being unearthed in this history of ourselves, except that commodities' potent afterlives lingered in bodies of all kinds.

Maybe I traveled there searching for some kind of acknowledged interrelation. But the closest thing to that I found was the warped slogan "Out of the Strong Came Forth Sweetness" flaking off the derelict Lyle sugar factory's giant golden molasses tin, dominating the landscape with its eerie image of bees emerging from a dead lion. Not the parable I was looking for, just another unresolvable riddle. I was trying to locate a sign of responsibility for linked histories but found only empty houses all around the sugar factory, some bearing little notes on their doors: POSTMAN—NOBODY LIVES HERE.

The day before, I had traveled up to the highest point in the city, the Coca-Cola London Eye. From inside its wheeling glass pods,[6] I looked out from this latest sugar machine toward the museum exhibit on sugar and slavery that I had visited inside an old Docklands sugarhouse. Its narratives recounted how ships from the Caribbean routinely arrived there to be unloaded in "Blood Alley"—named not for the humans carried in the same holds during another leg of those vessel's triangle trade routes, but because the cones of crystalized sugar had sharp edges that cut the British laborers carrying them. More severe injuries elsewhere were present mostly in cryptic traces: the museum displayed a drinking ladle from the slain Garifuna leader Satuye, which had been mounted like a trophy and traded to England by former French allies once Garinagu ancestral lands were turned into sugar plantations.

Staring through the corporate soda logos emblazoned on the glass pods' windows, I could see Buckingham Palace and the Parliament buildings where historian Hilary Beckles and other leaders from CARICOM[7] countries like Belize gathered to present their policy proposal, including healthcare investments for diabetes as a form of repair and apology for colonial injustices. I had told myself the U.K. trip made sense, in part, to better reckon with my own position in sugar's connected histories. Perhaps that had been another displacement, I realized, looking out onto London's skyline through a U.S. corporate emblem. In fact, the sugar machine near Sarah's house in Belize that used oil for distilling molasses was installed by a slave owner born in Pennsylvania, minutes from where I grew up—histories not as distant as I wanted to think.

But the sugar machine was also unfixed in time, and maybe the machine that mattered most to the story of sugar's future was whatever transformations the earth and atmosphere had undergone through these long centuries of slow violence. Considering one postcolony from the sky above its former metropole, the sugar machine made me think of the engines of the war machine: "It could do anything but stop."[8]

The sturdy brick around east London's sugar factory had been designed to double as a seawall, someone said, in case the area flooded. Its protection reminded me of how the land where I did my first interview in Belize is already underwater. The place along the southern coast where I spoke with a gardener back in 2008 was part of the shoreline now under the ocean in his southern Kriol village, along with the soccer field, more than twenty houses, and parts of the village cemetery. I watched on YouTube as residents piled sandbags around loved ones' tombs to try to prevent them from opening in the sea. Families are not sure how or where to rebury their dead.

The time-lapse quality of disappearances from photo albums is now happening not only to people, but also to shorelines and other places gradually disappearing piece by piece. These scales of chronic global consumption—of carbohydrates and hydrocarbons, the fuel of people and machines—have been materially linked for centuries. "Oil and sugar would seem to have little in common," Vincent Brown adds of evolving forms of hydrocarbons, yet "we are reminded of how the consumption of fossil fuel has been closely associated with the machinery of death."[9] Those stories are there in the coal- and oil-powered factories once populated by the British laborers consuming sugar, and in the ways Caribbean sugar requires coal or other fossil fuels for heat to refine.[10] They are there in the petrochemicals that contribute to diabetes entering bodies, and in the calories of fuel spent on transporting calories of food,[11] as overheating climates remake center and peripheries. Like wild cane growing ragged along roads in Belize, the English sugar refineries puffing on without working-class labor appeared both evacuated and alive, continuing to unleash forces in the world.

Many scientific models of the coming century suggest grim forecasts about these material afterlives: that sugar will do harm in an increasing number of bodies, and that carbon's atmospheric effects will harm many living things' chances to survive. One could imagine, from London, a future where the fixes of "halfway technologies" like geo-engineering are enough for a while: carbon capture filtering the atmosphere something like the washings of dialysis machines; solar engineering projects injecting particles into the stratosphere as routinely as people inject insulin. One could imagine that these stories about struggles for access to technologies in the face of chronic wear may grow to an atmospheric scale; that unequal infrastructures for repair work could produce unevenly normalized death for planetary bodies, in addition to human ones.

But set against those ominous thoughts of looming global histories in Silvertown, I also heard there was an improvised museum of sugar factory artifacts inside the old Tate Social Institute, assembled by its migrant squatters who recycle and repair computers. I was glad to find that tiny crack of ethnographic surprise amid bleak thoughts of models. The cracks in models are filled with people, and people are doing things that posit a future.

The day before their vigil in 2018, the Dangriga branch of the Belize Diabetes Association arranged a group walk through town. Nurse Norma and the other branch leaders had gone door to door to gather support for these community activities and series of memorial events. Their new banner showed a clasped fist and a magnifying glass. "KNOW diabetes, FIGHT diabetes," it read. Two young people up front held the banner's corners as their crowd walked down the main street. For Norma and for many in their group, the route for the march was also their daily exercise loop through town: the bridge across the south creek, the park near the beach, a road where the river meets the sea.

Laura wore diva sunglasses and a checkered cap that day, her daughter pushing her chair in the middle of a crowd. I recalled the routine domestic vigils that I used to notice in Laura's kitchen: a white candle burning next to a glass of water on the table while she cooked. When we were both ten years younger, I had asked her about it once, remembering that thirst is a symptom of diabetes. She smiled gently at my awkward question. Laura explained how it was her way of praying to her mother, who had lived and died with diabetes before I knew her family. Lighting a candle for someone helps their spirit find you; the glass of water because the dead arrive thirsty from their long travels.

Last time I saw her, Antonia said she saw Cresencia's spirit moving across the room between us. She said that I should feed her something sweet and ask for help with writing this.

The group in Dangriga had designed T-shirts that said "FAMILY & DIABETES," and many participants wore them to the vigil. The hurtful aspects of diabetic sugar were plainly visible among those like Laura who were working to recover, and evident across time through the gathered names and family photos; but those tributes and losses were being marked by the slow care of loved ones coming together to honor their fighting grace and to continue on. It was "wake work" in the full sense that Christina Sharpe describes, as their group came together to keep watch for the dead and remake life in the present. "We're all positioned by the wake, but positioned differently," she adds.[12]

Looking at Norma's picture, I felt that difference as I saw how their group had created a living, beautiful thing much greater than whatever accounting I had been trying to grasp toward with this book. The image that mattered for the future was their circle, one of many gathering each November in places across the world. Their small collective stood still with candles near the sea as if outlining time and space between misaligned statistics and many thousands gone, a place where no one had lost count. Holding little kids' hands and careworn photos, they said each name in the dark.

In loving memory of the contributors who made this project possible:

Mr. P and Mrs. P

Sulma

Elisa

Ára

Sarah

Theo

Grace

Nel

Cresencia

Francisco

Jordan

Sadie

Nancy

Juanita

Sammy

Toribio

Alexandrina

Leanna

Angel

Calvin

Mr. R

Arreini

Jose Cruz

All author proceeds from this book will go toward supporting food justice projects and chronic disease care and recovery groups led by people in Belize.

Learn more about these groups' work at www.travelingwithsugar.com.

Acknowledgments

I am so grateful to have known the people to whom this book is dedicated. Yet to speak of the dead, in many Belizean languages, already also implies "those who will carry on." These individuals' families and loved ones also remade my understanding of so many things beyond diabetes, and I hope they know what their trust meant to me.

Love and admiration to those "still fighting it" in Belize and beyond, especially Nurse Norma, Dr. W, Mileni, Laura, Antonia, Tobias, June, Nurse A, Carmela, Katherine, Guillerma, and Lorel, as well as the many branches of the Belize Diabetes Association and the Diabetes Foot Care Group. I am grateful for the leading lights of Phyllis and E. Roy Cayetano, and for the teacher who asked to be called here Igemeri, to whom I owe a true debt. Joseph Palacio's inspiring work and early messages were heartening to me. Warm thanks also to the leaders and members of HelpAge, to Rob Kistenberg and Prosthetic Hope International, Nurse Obi and the Dangriga Cancer Center, and to Peter Ciego and the teachers at the Gulisi School and Museum for generative conversations together.

Dr. Phillip Castillo has been a steadfast mentor and source of inspiration in Belize. Drs. Marvin Manzanero and Ethan Gough at the Belize Ministry of Health were also instrumental in getting this project off the ground and improving it since. At the National Institute for Culture and History in Belize, Drs. John Morris and Jaime Awe helped with the paperwork to launch this project a decade ago, and Rolando Cocom and Nigel Encalada, Phylicia Pelayo, and Selene Solis at the Belize Institute for Social and Cultural Research helped me to explore its second phase and more widely share its findings. Dr. Espat, Nurse Lee, Dionne Anne, Lynn, Jo, Terese, the amazing Nuñez family, and Nurse Suzanne and her family were always so kind, as were my landlords and many more not named here (who are thanked by pseudonyms or appreciated between the lines). In Belize City, Lorraine Thompson, Dr. Beer, Dr. Bulwer, Dr. Hidalgo, and Dr. Arriaga kindly took time to speak with me.

I owe gratitude to Michael Polonio, Ernest Castro, and the National Garifuna Council for their support in launching this project and to Sandra Miranda for finding time to continue the conversation. Thanks to Ivan Duran and Stonetree Records for possibilities ahead. Artists Pen Cayetano (from Dangriga, Belize) and James Young (from Shreveport, Louisiana) each shared their talents to create illustrations for this project, and I am deeply grateful for their beautiful contributions. At Cayetano Studios, I also owe thanks to Ingrid Cayetano for her help behind the scenes. Sherine Hamdy encouraged me to pursue the artistic possibilities of ethnographic engagements.

The Department of Anthropology at Princeton was a wonderful place to learn as a graduate student. I especially thank João Biehl for his insistence on attending to the lives of real people, and for being such a humane thinker to continue learning from. Carol Greenhouse, Carolyn Rouse, and Jim Boon extended a generosity of time and thought that pushed this further. I also owe thanks to Abdellah Hammoudi, Rena Lederman, John Borneman, Isabelle Clarke-Decès, Alan Mann, Elizabeth Davis, and Lawrence Rosen, as well as to Carol Zanca and Mo Lin Yee. This project benefited from conversations during graduate school with Michael Stone, Joseph Amon, Claire Nicholas, Nikos Michailidis, Gwen Gordon, Peter Locke, Ramah McKay, Peter Kurie, Mark Robinson, Sam Williams, Bridget Purcell, and Saul Schwartz, Serena Stein, Jessica Cooper, and so many others. Richard Sha and Roberta Rubenstein propelled this work in its very earliest stages; Betty Bennett told me it was possible to get a PhD. She is missed.

For the time I was a postdoctoral fellow at the Department of Anthropology at Brown, I owe special thanks to Daniel Jordan Smith, Bhrigupati Singh, Paja Faudree, Jessaca Leinaweaver, Rebecca Louise Carter, Elizabeth Hoover, Stephen Houston, Kate Mason, and Ellen Block for engaging with this project, and to Brown's Cogut Institute for the Humanities, Center for Population Studies, and Program for Science and Technology Studies for research support. The Rachel Carson Center for Environment and Society offered a writing fellowship where

I was fortunate to meet Christof Mauch, Ursula Münster, Helmuth Trischler, and an inspiring community of scholars.

Over the past four years, I have had the very good luck to complete this book as a faculty member in the MIT Anthropology program. I am truly grateful for the inspiration and conviviality of my colleagues Stefan Helmreich, Heather Paxson, Chris Walley, Manduhai Buyandelger, Susan Silbey, Graham Jones, Jean Jackson, Michael M.J. Fischer, Bettina Stoetzer, Amah Edoh, and Héctor Beltrán, as well as the sage advice of Erica James. This manuscript became much better through the insightful comments and caring encouragement they provided in response to an earlier draft of this work, especially at a book workshop in 2016. Joining us there, Elizabeth Roberts pushed me to define the para-communicable, Lesley Sharp offered incisive comments and helped me realize how much this project was about mobility, Michael Montoya urged me to pull fewer punches, and David Jones pushed me to sharpen the critical medical science.

With true kindness, Irene Hartford, Amberly Steward, and Barbara Keller in MIT Anthropology have helped to coordinate more details than I could count and made things feel like home. Elsewhere at MIT, I am grateful for conversations with Jose Gomez-Marquez, Anna Young, Dwai Banerjee, and Robin Scheffler, as well as with HASTS graduate students, including Elena Sobrino, Beth Semel, Tim Loh and Luísa Reis Castro. I am fortunate to be part of ongoing conversations with Mary-Jo and Byron Good and the Harvard Friday Morning Seminar community. The undergraduate students in my classes at MIT and Brown also nourished this project and helped to improve its storytelling.

Fact-checker Ben Phelan helped to verify technical aspects of many rabbit holes I wandered down, at times far outside my areas of expertise. Ari Samsky came through with brilliant and caring final edits. Laurence Ralph offered sharp comments that greatly improved several chapters. Readings by Colleen Lanier-Christensen, Esther Lee, Kimberlee Manora, and Stephanie Kim were enlightening. Over the years, this work has gotten better through conversations with Adriana Petryna, Cornel West, Hannah Landecker, Vanessa Fabien, Kim and Mike Fortun, Alice Street, Harris Solomon, Alex Blanchette, Tatiana Chudakova, Nick Shapiro, Emily Yates-Doerr, Nadine Levin, Chris Cokinos, Michele Friedner, Ieva Jusionyte, and Susan Ellison.

Archivists Tom Rosenbaum and Mary Ann Quinn at the Rockefeller Archive Center in New York provided help tracking diabetes in policy histories. In London, warm thanks to the Linnean Society of London and the guidance of Isabelle Charmantier, who took time to bring me into the vault of Linnaeus's original papers; Paul Talling for a walk through the Sugar Mile; Fred Rumsey at the British Museum of Natural History; and Sara Edwards, Frances Cook, Mark Nesbitt, Sue Zmartzy, and Craig Brough for hosting such a useful week at the Kew Herbarium and Archives.

At University of California Press, Reed Malcolm acquired this book, and Kate Hoffman was an astute production editor. Archna Patel coordinated many details, and Tom Sullivan deserves warm thanks. I am especially grateful to Anne Taylor and Wendy Lawrence for their caring dedication with copyedits, and to Nicholle Robertson and her team at BookComp, Inc., for their excellence in the home stretch. Peter Redfield and an anonymous reviewer for the press provided feedback that proved transformative in reframing this work. Portions of chapters appeared as articles in *New England Journal of Medicine, Cultural Anthropology, Global Public Health,* and *Limn*; thanks to each for the permission to reprint.

This project took clearer form through the help and grace of writers I trust. Erin Kane has been reading and thinking with me since first grade and commented on key portions of this text; I am so glad to be in the world with her. Ongoing conversations with Adia Benton reshaped many concepts on these pages. David Bond provided generous insights in pivotal moments. Just when it mattered most, Lucas Bessire's rogue wisdom and soul friendship helped me take the hard road, and kept me trying to live up to his writing partnership and existential company.

This research and writing were made possible by the Wenner-Gren Foundation, the American Philosophical Society, the Rockefeller Archive Center, the Mellon-American Council of Learned Societies, a U.S. Department of Education FLAS Grant, the Princeton Program in Latin American Studies, the Woodrow Wilson Society of Scholars, the Princeton Institute for Interregional Studies, Princeton Health Grand Challenges, the MIT School of Humanities, Arts, and Social Sciences Dean's Fund, and the Alfred Henry and Jean Morrison Hayes Career Development Professorship. I am very grateful for their support.

Immeasurable thanks go to my mother, my first and best editor, who taught me how to listen and burned the midnight oil with me through many revisions. I am profoundly appreciative for her steadfast love; and for the care and support of Karen, Nora, Evie, Rick, and Gary, who all helped in their own ways. Deep thanks also go to Bill, Annette, and Keith and to many across the extended Moran, Thomas, and Rossi families—especially Nereo and Lola, for their true example of love and for the extraordinary man they raised. Franco Rossi and I have been growing up together since I was eleven and he was twelve. On the wildest day of this ten-year project, when he told me to count the things in the room that were real, I counted him first.

I hope that those thanked here feel it from the heart—even though, as Stuart Hall once put it, "A book is not a consensus." This work offers my own interpretations that others surely have their own perspectives about. I look forward to dialogues ahead, but no one except me bears responsibility for this book's remaining errata.

About Translations

The people whose stories appear in this book speak not only English (Belize's national language) but also Belizean Kriol, Garifuna, Spanish, Mandarin Chinese, Low German, and Mopan, Yucatac, and Kekchi Maya. It is due to these contributors' expertise across languages, rather than mine, that we could easily talk in a language they spoke fluently. Although moving across these many vernaculars might help capture a sense of social fabrics, the limits of this approach are important to note.

The translations I struggled with most of all in writing this book were those conversations that unfolded using different versions of English. The majority of the dialogues recorded here took place with me speaking my version of English and Belizeans speaking either their version of English or Belizean Kriol. There is a large gray area between these registers, and the orthography of Belizean Kriol is just starting to be standardized. Although it is the most widely spoken language in Belize, accents, inventions, and mixtures between English and Kriol grammar vary widely from speaker to speaker. On the one hand, it felt odd to transcribe recorded interviews as if with a correcting pen, changing people's shifting grammar into "standard" U.S. English. On the other hand, using notations commonly accepted within Belize (transcribing with orthographies that might change from speaker to speaker and even sentence to sentence, as Belizean national newspapers at times do to reflect each individual speaker's actual words) felt charged with a troubled racial history when writing from a U.S. university for English speakers who have different associations with such spellings.

In the end, I am a white foreigner and writing from a country where the orthography of English dialects is a tangled thicket of stereotypes. Ngugi wa Thiong'o has noted of nation languages: "Their orthographic representation is problematic, and they are often written as if they were misspelled English or French words."[1] Without a background in linguistics, I felt underequipped to render Kriol words as they were spoken without these knotted issues obscuring the content of what was actually being said. Ultimately, it is *because* I believe it is crucial to treat pidgins and creoles seriously as languages that I chose to translate Belizean Kriol expressions and terms into standardized English (just as I did with words from Spanish, Maya, or Garifuna).

In the end, I hope these caveats are actually invitations. Some expressed interest in possible critical annotation and potential translation efforts for portions of this text into Garifuna and other Belizean languages, or perhaps public radio, collaborations that I hope might be realized to improve and extend this project. Until then—as Adrienne Rich once put it—"this is the oppressor's language, yet I need it to talk to you."[2]

Image Credits

Left: Enslaved man who has had his leg cut off for running away. *Right:* The invention of a French man in Martinique to prevent slaves from escaping. After a sketch in *Relation d'un Voyage fait en 1695, 1696, & 1697*, by Francois Froger. UIG/Getty Images / 36

A sugar machine at Indian Church, Belize. Photo by James Meierhoff / 52

Dr. W at work with a Doppler machine, Dangriga. Photo by author / 55

Nurse Norma doing foot care: "Eyes on Diabetes." Photo by author / 67

Stock photo of a hyperbaric chamber in a dive shop. BSIP/Getty Images / 84

Diabetes "Limb Salvage Form," Dangriga. Photo by author / 92

Casa de la Crónica, Chetumal. Photo by Carol Ailles / 95

Plastic washed up from the ocean tide, Stann Creek District, Belize. Photo by author / 104

Aerosol FISH chemicals for sale in Stann Creek District, Belize. Photo by author / 106

Retina angiograph showing the risk of glaucoma linked to diabetes. BSIP/Getty Images / 114

Cresencia in 2010: "Take it before I start to smile." Photo by author / 138

Five Decades. Rosary made of insulin syringe and diabetic medications. Photo by author / 146

An acrostic from Sadie's book, which she titled "Don't Feel It to Know It." Photo by author / 158

"Testing Strips for a Variety of Glucometer Models." Amy Moran-Thomas, "Breakthroughs for Whom? Global Diabetes Care and Equitable Design," *New England Journal of Medicine* 375:2317–19. Copyright © 2016 Massachusetts Medical Society. Reprinted with permission. Photos by author, arranged by *NEJM* graphics / 170

Portrait of Jordan as a Teenager, in Broken Glucometer Parts. Collage by James Young / 184

"Hi." Photo by Barb Wagstaff, www.diabetesadvocacy.com / 188

Sugarcane mounted and classified by Carl Linnaeus as the species *Saccharum spontaneum*. Used with permission of the Linnean Society of London. Photo by author / *194*

House on Saint Vincent plantation, circa 1898. Jean Blackwell Hutson Research and Reference Division; Manuscripts, Archives, and Rare Books, Schomburg Center for Research in Black Culture, New York Public Library. Ref. No. Sc Rare 917.29-H, Robert Thomas Hill, 1899 / *207*

Hurricane Hattie Belize, by Pen Delvin Cayetano, 1996. 104 × 75 cm. Oil on Canvas. © 2018 Artists Rights Society (ARS), New York/ VG Bild-Kunst, Bonn / *218*

Portrait of Arreini in her kitchen. Photo by author / *239*

Hospital wheelchair in Belize City. Photo by author / *243*

Jose Cruz convening a press release about his pending amputations, 2010. Photo courtesy of Channel 5 Belize News / *262*

The machine from Guatemala that a Garifuna farming cooperative in Belize hopes to buy for their healthy cereal project. Photo by author / *272*

Homes in a "London Bridge" area of Belize. UIG/Getty Images / *275*

Laura cooking for her family in Dangriga, 2010. Photo by author / *283*

Prosthetic leg that Fede made for Laura, now no longer needed. Photo by author / *285*

Notes

APPROACH: EMERGENCY IN SLOW MOTION

1. See Subramanian (2009).

2. IDF (2010, 7); see de-Graft Aikins, Agyei-Mensah, and Agyemang (2014); Bukhman et al. (2015); Beran and Yudkin (2006); Hall et al. (2011); Mbanya et al. (2010); Reynolds Whyte (2014b).

3. H. T. (2013).

4. Belize Ministry of Health (2017).

5. Castro (2005).

6. IDF (2017).

7. Ahlqvist et al. (2018).

8. IDF (2017).

9. Anderson-Fye (2004; 2010); Awe, Gonzalez, and Ken (2007); Baines 2015; Balboni, Palacio, and Awe (2007); M. Johnson (2018); Kane (1998); MacPherson (2007); McClaurin (1996); Moberg (1997); Moss, Stone, and Smith (1992); Palacio (2005a; 2005b); and Wilk (2006a, 2006b).

10. World Bank (2018).

11. Some 24 percent of adults in Stann Creek and 31.6 percent of women had type 2 alone (Gough et al. 2008).

12. For perspectives on the negotiation of these transnational formations, see "How Did the Garifuna Become an Indigenous People?" (Palacio 2007) and *Black and Indigenous* (Anderson 2009).

13. Palacio (2005a).

14. Excerpted from the "Health" section of "The Garifuna Agenda" by the National Garifuna Council of Belize ([1998] 2015). This is a striking contrast to the U.S. context, where many minority groups instead feel they have been historically over-researched rather than neglected when it comes to diabetes issues. This was distinctly not the case in Belize; in fact, diabetes is the only

topic I've ever researched in which many patients and caregivers have reached out to ask to be interviewed.

15. See Kincaid (1988).

16. In the age of Facebook and social media, "public figure" has become a less obvious designation; as these pages describe, some people were trying to reach out in crafting a public advocacy persona for themselves.

17. Crosbie (2005, 78). Thanks to Melissa Johnson for a very helpful conversation about this term.

18. Gonzalez (1988, 78).

19. Palacio (2005c, 54).

20. Garifuna Women's Project (2009), with vocals by Chella Torres.

21. More elaborated notes and further sources, trimmed for space here, are available on the project website.

22. Whipps (2008).

23. Pringle (2010).

24. Since colonial records referred to this population as "Black Caribs" throughout the time they inhabited Saint Vincent, some historians use this name as well when describing that specific time period, uncertain exactly when this population began to call themselves *Karifuna* or *Garifuna*. As an anthropologist, I often use the names *Garifuna* and *Garinagu* even in cases where a historian might find this anachronistic because it was the way people I was speaking with talked about their ancestors, including in deeper time.

25. Beckles (2013).

26. Bailey (2004).

27. Sweeney (2007, 34); Adams (2002).

28. For a persuasive critical history of *epidemiological transition* and the historical changes that such teleological terms can normalize, see Vaughan (2018).

29. These explorations have been guided by thinkers such as Beckles (2013); Hatch (2016); Whitmarsh (2011, 2013b); and Agard-Jones (2015).

30. See Ferreira and Lang (2006); McMullin (2010); Smith-Morris (2006); Rock (2003); Wiedman and Lang (2005).

31. Mintz (1985).

32. Mintz (1974); cf. Behar (2003); Biehl (2005); Jackson (2011); Kleinman (1997); Rosaldo (2004).

33. The term *racial capitalism* signals long ongoing conversations about the ways capitalism as we know it is in fact built on the history of slavery and Indigenous dispossession (Robinson 1983). Mintz's discussion of this in relation to global sugar is but one instantiation of a lens that might be taken on most any capitalist commodity (cf. Beckert 2014). Walter Johnson provides a useful definition of *racial capitalism*: "That is, as a history of the relationship of Europe, Africa, and the Americas. The Americas, in particular, represented a new era in the history of the world: the era of both the dawn of capitalism and the emergence of categories of racial differentiation as primary organizing categories for thinking about exploitation, solidarity, and entitlement." See W. Johnson (2018) and a range of responses in the "Slavery, Racial Capitalism, and Justice" issue of *Boston Review*, which is also where Mintz's earliest iteration of *Sweetness and Power* first appeared.

34. Biehl and Petryna (2013, 11).

35. Biehl (2016); see Biehl and Locke (2017).

36. See discussion of this term by Good, Good, and Grayman (2010), developed as part of their work on "postcolonial disorders" (Good et al. 2008) that inform these thoughts on metabolic disorders.

37. Lauren Berlant's concept of "troubled knowledge" (2008, 7), in dialogue with her discussion of weight and "slow death" (2007), inflects the way "slow violence" is approached in this book.

38. Jung (1989); Dalí ([1952] 1998, 34).

39. See also Das and Han (2015).

40. Garcia (2010); Jain (2013).

41. Cayetano (2009, 224).

42. Or, at least, that is one way of interpreting my jarred field notes from that time. *March 23 2010: Tonight I had a dream that I was at the Shell gas station in Dangriga. In the middle of a conversation with some nurses my wrist starts spurting blood, so dark and thick it's almost the color of motor oil. I scream and feel an urge to run but people gather around, watching; there is an unbearable pain in my right hand. When I look again, my right finger has a faint but distinct black line all the way around it; leaning in close, you can tell the line is actually a series of small but messy stitches, as if my finger had been cut off and half reattached. In fact my whole hand looks patched together like Frankenstein's creature, with mismatched fingers of different sizes and colors. I feel a wave of dread that whatever has just overtaken my hand will consume my whole body. When I look down again, it is clear that each severed part of the hand belongs to a dead person I have known here: the worn Garifuna palm is Mrs. C's, a young man's finger mottled with the underlying pallor of anemia belongs to Jordan. But I am most disturbed by the tiny, mismatched thumb with the tiny blue crescent nail of a baby. I try to move the hand, not sure if it is still mine, but the fingers wriggle easily, their sutures twitching like worms. The last thing I remember before waking up is calling out frantically for someone to bring me Neosporin and holy water. Now it's four AM and I can't go back to sleep, although the dream didn't really surprise me; on some level, I have felt for awhile emptied of myself and filled with other injuries, as if becoming someone else's zombie. Maybe these are just the raw sutures of an anthropology without enough distance. Or maybe when working closely with people, we all take pieces of them with us; probably we all lose parts of ourselves along the way in this kind of research, although it is hard to say what is gone or where it was lost. But I'm not sure how to closely engage sick people's lives alone here without also carrying their deaths. I don't know how to absorb people's own understandings about what is happening to them without also absorbing something of their pain and its violence, even when I feel it overtaking both my conceptual frames and the person I used to be. But one thing I do know, is that I've been kidding myself to think that these fieldnotes about dying friends and strangers are anything so elegantly tragic as death masks. They are more like the stitched-together monster made from bits of people whose lives and deaths now feel grafted to my own.*

43. Strangely, some historians have interpreted John Canoe and other colonial satires in the West Indies "primarily as the products of a surge of blood sugar" during plantation holidays (Schuler 1989, 248).

44. Two of the people included in the dedications list died of causes other than diabetes, Leanna and her grandson. His mother, Gia, asked me to include her baby next to her mom's name and suggested the name Angel for him.

45. "Cancer, diabetes, heart diseases are no longer the diseases of the wealthy. Today, they hamper the people and the economies of the poorest populations even more than infectious diseases. This represents a public health emergency in slow motion" (Ki-moon 2009).

46. IDF (2017).

47. Bourgois (2009).

48. Nixon (2011).

49. Berlant (2007).

50. Puar (2017).

51. Anishinaabe theorist Gerald Vizenor offered the term *survivance* as a way to speak of historically patterned oppression against Indigenous peoples while at the same time keeping focus on the survival, endurance, and vitality of those most affected by these ongoing injustices. In Vizenor's (1999, vii) now-famous definition: "Survivance is an active sense of presence, the continuance of native stories, not a mere reaction, or a survivable name. Native survivance stories are renunciations of dominance, tragedy, and victimtry." This book attempts to relate its stories of diabetes's injustices in this register, in which even those individuals whose deaths are here acknowledged are part of the much larger story of Garifuna persistence and survivance (see Cayetano and Cayetano 2005; Ávila 2009; M. Palacio 2011; J. Palacio 2005a; 2005b).

52. Mintz (1985, 7).

53. Bessire (2014, 222).

PAST IS PROLOGUE: SUGAR MACHINE

1. *Sugar* is also a common name for diabetes on both sides of the Atlantic: see, for example, *Sugar Disease, Bitter Medicine: Living with Diabetes in Ghana* (de-Graft Aikins forthcoming) and *Sugar and Tension: Diabetes and Gender in Modern India* (Weaver 2019).

2. Crosbie et al. (2005).

3. Type 2 diabetes prevalence among adults in Stann Creek was 24 percent, nearly double Belize's national average of 13 percent. The prevalence of type 2 diabetes among women in Stann Creek was even higher, 31.6 percent. More than half of known people with diabetes reported either not being able to afford their medications or only being able to with much difficulty (Gough et al. 2008, 62, 64).

4. PAHO (2002).

5. Hussein (2017).

6. Simmons (2001).

7. The name *Belize* was in use even before the country became the colony of British Honduras, and so I use it anachronistically to refer also to this period of history. In an interesting contrast to typical struggles for colonial territories, the British administration actually tried to evict all British settlers from Belize in 1682 "on the grounds that the country was Spanish and the trade valueless" (Burdon 1931, 42). But the British Crown troops in charge of evicting these

English settlers in Belize mutinied en route, deciding to become pirates themselves, thus marking the first in a long string of failed attempts at colonial intervention in "the Bay of Honduras." In all, Belize spent over two centuries as a squatter community of uncertain status—settled by unauthorized British rogues on Spanish-owned land yet under the consolidated control of neither England nor Spain and largely inventing their own laws—before the settlement finally became recognized as British land in 1850. This means that Belize did not even *become* a European colony until the countries surrounding it (Mexico, Guatemala, and Honduras) had already won their independence from Spain and became sovereign nations. Belize thus spent much more time in this liminal phase of its existence (230 years) than it did as an officially recognized British territory (21 years), as a Crown colony actually governed by England (110 years), or as an independent nation ruled by a constitutional monarchy (with an elected Belizean prime minister and the official head of state remaining the Queen of England) from 1981 until the present. Yet even early in its origins, the people who lived in Belize wrote of "their country" and used the name Belize, although the place was part of no nation's empire. When Clifford Geertz spoke of the "central interpretative issues" raised by the "uncenteredness of modern times," he thus hit on a question that Belize has wrestled with continuously from its early history: "What is a country if it is not a nation?" (Geertz 2000, 228).

8. Trouillot ([1995] 2015, 14).

9. Mintz (1985) borrowed this formulation from Eric Williams (1944).

10. Toomer ([1923] 2019, 14).

11. Scheper-Hughes (1993); see Dunn (1972) and Brandes (1997).

12. Johnson (2007, 184).

13. Scott (2018, 2).

14. Taylor (2012, 124).

15. Shoman (1994); Bolland (1977).

16. Bolland (2003); Bolland and Shoman (1977).

17. Meyers (2012); Sweitz (2012).

18. Gann (1918, 18).

19. de las Casas ([1474–1566] 1906, 342).

20. Barrett (1970).

21. Ibid., 3.

22. See Singerman (2015).

23. Barrett (1970, 58–61).

24. These associations also traveled full circle back to Europe. In "Blood Sugar," Timothy Morton (2000, 194–97) examines a colonial trope he calls a "blood sugar topos," "a powerful and ambiguous metaphor in which sugar stands for the blood of slaves." Abolitionist drawings showed workers falling into vats and rooms with severed limbs lost to machinery nailed to the wall. "Perhaps there had been joy for them in finding that sugar could be made from blood," one of Edwidge Danticat's (2004, 175) enslaved characters muses. This "anxious play" intertwining violence and sugar even resurrected a poetic form called *gluochotes*, traceable through the antislavery writings of English poets such as Samuel Taylor Coleridge and intended to raise abolitionist consciousness.

25. Barrett (1970).

26. Brown (2008, 118); Brown (2010, 142).
27. Taylor (2012, 80).
28. Voltaire ([1759] 1918, 90).
29. James ([1938] 1989, 12).
30. Beckles (2014).
31. Beckles (2013, 36).
32. Benítez-Rojo (2001, 131–32); Walker (2014).
33. The kind of petroleum now being drilled in Belize is "sweet crude," which literally has a sweet smell (and taste, according to old prospectors) due to its low sulfur content—linked to higher market value because it can be processed into gasoline. At the time of my work, oil and sugar were tied as Belize's number one national export.
34. Song (2004).
35. Herbert (2009).
36. Darcel (1954, 3).
37. PETA (2019).
38. Fanon (1963, 64, 71).
39. Moore (2000, 426).
40. Kaiser (2011).
41. Belize Ministry of Health (2014, 32).
42. Alegria, Carvalho-Knighton, and Alegria (2009).
43. Mesnage et al. (2017).
44. Agard-Jones (2015).
45. See Abramiuk et al. (2011); Graham (1994).
46. Clegern (1967, 66).
47. Ibid.
48. Wilk (2006a, 63).
49. Dawdy (2008).
50. As James Boon writes, "It is important *generally* to undo pat sequences of 'isms,' which do not happen the same way the world over" (1999, xix).
51. Gálvez (2018).
52. Ibañez and Katsikis (2014).
53. Marx (1964).
54. The metabolic "absorption" (Solomon 2016) hinted at here is discussed more fully in "Coral Gardens and Their Metabolism."
55. Trapp (2011).
56. United Nations (2014); Gayle et al. (2010).
57. Gayle (2019).
58. Rodriguez (2007, 221).
59. Deborah Thomas describes *simultaneous time* as a texture "where the future, past, and present are mutually constitutive" (2016, 183; see 2011).
60. de la Monte and Wands (2008).
61. Mol (2002).
62. Taylor (2012, 16).
63. Describing Mol (2002).
64. Sebald (1998, 194).
65. Stapleton et al. (2018).

66. Crist (2018).
67. Hatch (2016).
68. Laymon (2018, 8).
69. Sharpe (2016).
70. Simpson (2014, 6).
71. Diaz (2012, 16).
72. Since people in Belize come from many backgrounds, including the Garifuna's identification as both Black and Indigenous, these ideas draw from a range of concept work in various arenas of critical race theories, settler colonial studies (which have specific resonances in Central America), and decolonial debates—trying to think across these conversations with the *"transversal politics"* that Patricia Hill Collins (2017) has proposed, while staying attentive to different textures of racialization and their distinct articulations for each contributor.
73. On the contemporary worlds of sugar byproducts, see Ulrich (2017).
74. McCutchon, Samuel papers, 1832–1874, in "Records of Ante-Bellum Southern Plantations from the Revolution through the Civil War, Part I." See Stoler (2013).
75. CABI (2018).
76. Deane (2019).
77. Sutherland (1998); see Gordillo (2014).
78. Manjapra (2018); see Beckert and Desan (2018).
79. Sen and Sarin (1980, 695).
80. Jain (2013, 12).
81. Whitmarsh (2013a).
82. Biswas et al. (2010).
83. Taussig (1989, 14), reflecting on missing ethnographic grit in *Sweetness and Power.*
84. Puar (2017, xvi).
85. Ibid., xviii.
86. *Damages* is an English word that came up frequently in the language of those I spoke with, yet it had a specific texture in Belize. I am grateful to the scholars whose work helped me rethink the ways my earlier uptake of this term could hold a more uneasy meaning and to those who taught me alternative terms. Sarah's formulation of the hurtful here resonates with the work of influential scholars such as Eve Tuck (2009) to turn away from damage-based research that frames pathology within people and instead more rigorously chart the violence of systems. This narrative unfolds along these troubled edges of engagement.
87. See, for instance, the economist's policy recommendation on page 187.
88. Hartman (2007, 31).
89. Contrast with Tsing (2015).

WHAT IS COMMUNICABLE?
CAREGIVERS IN AN ILLEGIBLE EPIDEMIC

1. Nerlich et al. (2000).
2. Pecoraro, Reiber, and Burgess (1990).

3. Klonoff (2015).

4. Linguists trace this to Garifuna exchanges with French colonists on Saint Vincent, from the old Latin root *chirurgia*. It also resembles the contemporary Spanish term *cirujana/o* for surgeon.

5. Herr ([1977] 1991, 18).

6. Ralph (2012, 2014).

7. Kistenberg (2005, 38–39).

8. Ibid., 41.

9. Armstrong et al. (2017).

10. Elgyzri et al. (2013). This figure specifically tracks ischemic ulcers, the most common type of diabetic foot ulcer.

11. Armstrong et al. (2013).

12. Armstrong, Wrobel, and Robbins (2007).

13. Armstrong et al. (1997).

14. Neil (2015).

15. Yaghi et al. (2012).

16. Armstrong et al. (2013).

17. Haagsma et al. (2016, annex).

18. Among a U.S. audience, a leg "getting cut" is assumed to mean a scratch, laceration, or incision. In Belize, that same phrase is used to mean an amputation. I occasionally add cut *off* to clarify, although this phrasing sounds harsh in Belize, where learning to speak gently of common injuries helps others cope with their omnipresence.

19. Benton (2015, 56).

20. *Curtis v. DOJ*, 2009 U.S. App. LEXIS 17200 (Federal Circuit, August 2009).

21. Browne (2015).

22. Nelson (2016).

23. Kistenberg (2005, 16).

24. Wright (2017, 25–26).

25. Ibid., 26.

26. Livingston (2012).

27. I am grateful to Ahmed Ragab for the suggestion to sharpen these notions of diabetes surveillance as something beyond biopolitical framings. The phrasing of "para-sighted" surveillance (Sweeny 2005) for anthropologists also brings to mind methods of juxtaposing para-sited fieldwork (Marcus and Fischer 1996).

28. Sontag (1988, 57).

29. See also Lakoff and Johnson (1980).

30. These are all Dr. W's words, distilled from a much longer conversation; several words were rearranged from the exact sequence in which they were spoken.

31. Geary (2011, 100).

32. Briggs and Mantini-Briggs (2016); Briggs (2017).

33. Belize Ministry of Health (2017); cf. Gough et al. (2008).

34. Brandt (1997, 56).

35. Rosenberg (1992).

36. Caduff (2015); Fassin (2011); Lakoff (2017); Packard (2016).
37. Redfield (2013, 72).
38. Wald (2008, 3).
39. Anderson (2006, vii).
40. Dodu (1967, 474).
41. Litvak (1975, 317).
42. Neel and Sargis (2011).
43. Bertazzi et al. (2001); see Fortun (2001).
44. Bowe et al. (2018).
45. Plumer (2018).
46. Selin and Kwon (2018).
47. Velmurugan et al. (2017).
48. Colburn, Dumanoski, and Myers (1997).
49. Parreñas (2018, 185); see Paxson (2013).
50. Fischer (2013); Scheffler (2019).
51. Solomon (2016).
52. Lamoreaux (2016); Roberts (2017).
53. Landecker (2015).
54. Niewöhner and Lock (2018).
55. Martin (1990); Landecker (2013a).
56. Glover, Rayner, and Rayner (2015).
57. Hoover (2017).
58. Landecker (2013b, 2018); Blanchette (2018).
59. Krieger (2012).
60. Lilienfeld (2000).
61. Benton, personal communication.
62. Fischer (2013).
63. Mendenhall et al. (2017); Seeberg and Meinert (2015); Moran-Thomas (2010b).
64. Mueller (2019); Livingston (2012); Walley (2013).
65. Fortun and Fortun (2005); Kenner (2013); Whitmarsh (2013a).
66. Nash (2007).
67. Bullard and Johnson (2000); Shapiro (2015); Murphy (2017).
68. Langston (2011).
69. Oreskes and Conway (2011).
70. Nestle (2015).
71. Mendenhall and Singer (2019).
72. Roberts (2015).
73. This phrasing is indebted to Elizabeth Roberts and the members of our 2018 American Anthropological Association panel "Communicability in Crisis," and to Lawrence Cohen for his insightful comments as a discussant.
74. Quammen (2018, 245–46).
75. Jain and Barman (2017, 692).
76. Saguy and Almeling (2005).
77. Farmer (1999, 226–27).
78. IDF (2017).
79. Farmer (1999, 255; italics in original).

80. Yates-Doerr (2015).

81. Vas, Edmonds, and Papanas (2017).

82. Porter and Teisberg (2006).

83. Mendenhall and Norris (2015).

84. Gutierrez-Sumner (2019).

85. @nutriliciouscorner

86. Fausto-Sterling (2016).

87. Montoya (2014).

88. Mauss (1966, 76–78).

89. Wirtz (2019); see Weisz and Vignola-Gagné (2015).

90. See Edwards (2010); Lucas (1967).

91. In the United States and other parts of the world, blood plasma is sold by the poor as a source of emergency funding (Desmond 2016). Because it may decapitate the donor's own ability to heal, people with diabetes are supposed to be discouraged from blood plasma donation, but in certain markets there is little regulation of this restriction.

92. Wilkinson, Chapman, and Heilbronn (2012).

93. Mobile Equine Hyperbaric Oxygen Therapy (2019).

94. Barbados Defense Force Hyperbaric Chamber (2011).

95. Dr. W described using 3 Atmospheres for very serious ulcers, for example, those verging on necrosis; but more routine hyperbaric treatment for a diabetic ulcer would be 2 or 2.5 Atmospheres.

96. Armstrong et al. (2013).

97. Wald (2008, 14–15).

98. Durkheim ([1912] 1995, 619).

99. Benn Torres and Torres-Colon (2018).

100. Simmons (2017).

101. Stevens et al. (2014).

102. Baldwin (1998, 83).

103. Compare WHO (2016) and IDF (2016).

104. Cole (2017, 180).

105. This quote from Dr. W, like the passage earlier, is distilled from our longer conversation.

CRÓNICA ONE: THRESHOLDS

1. Canguilhem (1991, 78).

2. Ibid., 190.

3. Ibid., 197.

4. Bond (2013).

5. Richardson (2009, 33).

6. Haraway (2015, 159).

7. Singh (2015, 402).

8. Petryna (2018, 573).

9. Canguilhem (1991, 236).

10. Canguilhem (1991); Murphy (2017).

11. Hardin (2018).

12. Whitmarsh and Roberts (2016).

13. Turner (1967). Some scholars today actually prefer not to use the word *ritual*—but in this context it was an ethnographic recursion, since past anthropological theories were already in circulation and shaping people's ideas of practice. The National Garifuna Council proudly has a "Ritual" tab on its website, and Garifuna travelers to Saint Vincent occasionally append slides of their trip photos with bibliographies that cite Turner and other anthropologists.

14. Jackson (2005, 332).

15. Garcia (2010, 149).

16. Kleinman (1997, 3–4).

17. Jusionyte (2018, 24).

18. Turner (1974, 33).

19. Green Reef (2010).

20. Malinowski (1935, 219).

21. Beliso-De Jesús (2014, 503).

22. Solomon (2016, 5).

23. Kolbert (2014, 142).

24. Innis (2016); see Braverman (2018).

25. McCollum (2019).

26. In Foster (2000, 155–56).

27. As measured in metric tons of carbon dioxide equivalent (a unit constructed to compare global warming potential of emissions), Belize's was only 0.6—compared, for example, to the United States at 5270 MtCO2. See http://www.globalcarbonatlas.org/en/CO2-emissions.

28. U.S. Environmental Protection Agency (2008).

29. Vogel (2009).

30. Well-heeled Belizeans could still buy fish, but at twice the price. Many families and businesses on tighter budgets gradually started serving more chicken because it only cost half as much (despite widespread rumors about chemicals the Mennonites were said to use in raising chickens). Families who were really struggling to make ends meet increasingly ate white rice or flour tortillas without any meat or chose lower-grade cuts (see Gewertz and Errington 2010).

31. My guess is that this odd term for insecticides has origins in a 1920s-era Rockefeller health campaign, which sought to decrease malaria by mandating the placement of live fish into barrels of household drinking water.

32. Pepper et al. (2004); see Todd (2017).

33. Hayes and Raz (2016).

34. See TallBear (2011).

35. Horton et al. (2014).

36. Masco (2010); Hecht (2019).

37. Weston (2017).

38. Foucault (2007, 22).

39. Sharpe (2016, 40–41).

40. Perhaps this was a form of naiveté, too—at that time, I hadn't yet read how aging appliances can leak toxic chemicals.

41. Cayetano (2009, 222–35).

42. Feudtner (2003, 146–47).

43. Ibid.

44. Balsells et al. (2009, 4290).

45. Kerns (1983).

46. Nading (2016).

47. Belize Ministry of Health (1996, 15).

48. Murphy (2013, 1–2).

49. A biomedical doctor might term this Charles Bonnett syndrome—but that is only one among many interpretive thresholds for such visions, and attributions also transform and shape experience.

50. Borges (1995, 345).

51. Residents may be interested in further examining the loss of locally owned land in relation to diabetic injuries, with a version of the methods Joseph Palacio, Carlson Tuttle, and Judith Lumb (2011) have exemplified elsewhere.

52. Young (2008, 22).

53. Flomenhoft, Cayetano, and Young (2007).

54. See Vaughn (2017).

55. Das (2015, 23).

56. Rhodes-Pitts (2013, 238).

57. Ibid., 12.

58. Sweeney (2007).

59. In Bolland (1977, 132).

60. In Gonzalez (1988, 109–10).

61. Bolland (1977, 133).

62. Ibid., 134; see also Stone (1994).

63. Bolland (1977, 144–45).

64. Wilk (2006b, 75).

65. *Great Britain* (1965, 51).

66. Palacio (1982; 1983, 153).

67. Gonzalez (1988, 103).

68. Trethewey (2010, 43).

69. National Garifuna Council of Belize ([1998] 2015).

70. Cayetano (1993, 69).

71. Aciman (2016).

72. Rabinow (1995).

73. Peterson (2014).

74. Patient Safety Authority (2010, 9).

75. Batalis and Prahlow (2004); Russell, Stevens, and Stern (2009).

76. Asking who should or shouldn't get insulin due to these real safety questions again raises the problematic "good patient" question that plagues so much chronic disease care, as Carolyn Rouse's work (2009) has shown.

77. "You will be a good friend, but you will pay for your passage."

78. In Wilk (2006b).

79. Ibid., 135.

80. Ibid., 130.

81. Ibid., 131.

82. Vannier (2011, 6–7).

83. Ibid., 2.
84. Ibid., 6.
85. See Holmes (2013).
86. Guthman (2011); Patel (2012).
87. James (2010).
88. As James Baldwin ([1964] 2011, 81) once borrowed this line from Henry James.
89. Palacio (2005a).
90. Foster (2005, 167).
91. Ibid.
92. Ibid., 169.
93. Taylor (1951, 141).
94. Ibid., 100.
95. Interview in Castro (2005).
96. From Greek *diabē-*, to stride or stand with legs apart, cross over, straddle.
97. Staiano (1986, 142).
98. Jain (2007, 2013); Garcia (2010).

CRÓNICA TWO: INSULA

1. Banting and Best were building on many predecessors' work in this finding—including English physiologist Sir Edward Sharpey-Schafer, a close observer of the pancreas who is credited with first deriving the name *insulin* for the islet's secretions some years earlier in 1910.
2. In Bliss (1982, 191).
3. O'Rourke (2014).
4. Arnqvist et al. (1993).
5. Rock (2005a).
6. Wendland (2010, 27).
7. Beard (2006).
8. Johnson (2016).
9. Oldenziel (2011, 13).
10. Wilson (1990).
11. Walcott (1992).
12. Morrison (2008).
13. Bliss (1982, 161).
14. Blakeslee (2007).
15. IDF (2015).
16. Moran-Thomas (2010a).
17. Ibid.
18. Belize is being heavily pressured by market institutions such as the International Monetary Fund and Greylock (which renegotiated Greece's national debt) to again "restructure," a watchword of neoliberal policies related to structural adjustment through which funding to state services (including health care) can be curtailed due to external pressures to reduce government spending. See Pfeiffer and Chapman (2010).
19. Hacking (1986).

20. Leinonen et al. (2001, 1501).
21. Trujillo (2007, 94); Bell et al. (2012).
22. Durnwald and Landon (2011); Torlone et al. (2009).
23. Leinonen et al. (2001, 1501); see Persson, Norman, and Hanson (2009).
24. Ringholm et al. (2012, 565).
25. Leinonen et al. (2001, 1502).
26. Sovik and Thordarson (1999).
27. Nguyen (2010, 90).
28. van Crevel, van de Vijver, and Moore (2017).
29. Cavell (1986, 92).
30. Bliss (1982, 136).
31. Ibid., 171–72.
32. Wendt (2013).
33. Bliss (1982, 186).
34. Ibid., 182–84.
35. Gebel (2013).
36. Ibid.
37. Wardian (2018).
38. Greene and Riggs (2015).
39. Idlebrook (2014).
40. Beran, Ewen, and Laing (2016).
41. Kelley (2013).
42. Gomez-Marquez (2016).
43. Ofra (2019).
44. Schaffer (2019).
45. Beran, Ewen, and Laing (2016, 278–79).
46. *People v. Latham* (2012).
47. Shobhana et al. (2002).
48. Mendosa (2000, 1–6).
49. Clarke and Foster (2012).
50. See Moran-Thomas (2016).
51. Grondahl (2012).
52. Moran-Thomas (2017).
53. *HLN News Now,* CNN International Television, June 7, 2012.
54. Redfield (2012).
55. Turkle (2007).
56. Alcorn (2019).
57. Mendosa (2000).
58. Stewart (2013).
59. Rettig (2011).
60. IDF (2005).

61. Technically, *muerto* means a dead person while *muerte* means death, but this translation from Spanish is more complicated than it might seem because of linguistic overlay in Belize. It was used in a place where people often speak "kitchen Spanish" as a third or fourth language, in very loosely improvised and Kriolized forms. Because of this, even though Jordan's nickname was literally Muerte, I heard it to mean something more like Dead than Death. This is why I offer two possible translations.

62. See the discussion of mangos and diabetes in Solomon (2016).

63. Fullwiley (2010, xviii–xiii).

64. Ibid., 67.

65. Mintz (1985).

66. Zhao et al. (2008).

67. Biehl (2005, 22).

68. See Scheper-Hughes (1995; 1993) and her discussion of Buber (1952).

69. Evans-Pritchard (1937).

70. Berg, Tymoczko, and Stryer (2002). This detail was striking to me, but aspects of this biochemistry are still debated even by experts; see project website for details.

71. Geissler's reflections on health projects and clinical contexts as "archipelagos" describe an African setting but have resonance for describing uneven constellations of access across the world. See Geissler (2013).

72. Feudtner (2003, 211).

73. Moran-Thomas (2017).

74. Fidler (2008).

75. Benjamin (2015).

76. See Collier et al. (2017).

77. Akrich (1992, 211–12).

78. Street (2017).

79. Akrich (1992, 222). A range of glucose measurement devices are now being envisioned as projects of "equitable design," though none yet implemented to a scale that reaches Belize.

80. See Sangaramoorthy and Benton (2012); Adams (2016); Biruk (2018); Nelson (2015); and Street (2014).

CRÓNICA THREE: GENERATIONS

1. El-Haj (2007).

2. Montoya (2011); see also Bliss (2012); Duster (1990); Finkler (2001, 2003); Fullwiley (2011); Rapp (1999); Rabinow (1999); Whitmarsh (2008, 2013b); Whitmarsh and Jones (2010).

3. Paradies, Montoya, and Fullerton (2007, 203).

4. Benyshek and Watson (2006); Poudrier (2008); Rock (2005b); Whaley (2003).

5. Fee (2006).

6. Hatch (2016, xii).

7. McDermott (1998).

8. Wailoo, Nelson, and Lee (2012).

9. "The notion of *generation* invites us to inquire into the distinctive consciousness that characterizes those who experience fateful historical events," write Susan Reynolds Whyte and colleagues (2014a, 13).

10. Marks (2007, 28); see Gould (1996).

11. Linnaeus's codification of scientific racism reflects colonial common sense of his time, which drew on geo-humoral theories from ancient Greece, but with added twists. For example, his taxonomy's suggestion that Black women were believed to produce "too much" breast milk served to rationalize violent

plantation norms such as forced wet nursing of white children—casting this practice as a medical cure for enslaved women's dysfunctional biologies, instead of violent deprivation of nutrition for their own infants.

12. Roberts (2012).
13. Ibid.
14. Landecker (2015).
15. Stevenson (2014).
16. Roberts (2016).
17. Anderson ([ca. 1798] 1983, 42).
18. Kim (2014, 226).
19. Ibid.
20. Anderson ([ca. 1798] 1983, 43).
21. Buyandelger (2013).
22. Han (2012, 31).
23. Jax (2010).
24. Landecker (2013a, 501; 2013b).
25. Hurley (2013, 53).
26. Walvin (2018).
27. Royal Botanic Gardens, Kew (1893, 233, 292).
28. Osseo-Asare (2008, 271).
29. Reynolds (1911).
30. Kew (1892, 92).
31. Howard (1996, 12).
32. Kew (1892).
33. In Handler (1969, 47).
34. Kim (2014, 229).
35. Gonzalez (1988, 32).
36. See Palacio (2005c).
37. Taylor (2012, 138).
38. Ibid., 141.
39. Ibid., 139.
40. Sweeney (2007).
41. Taylor (2012, 143).
42. Ibid., 151.
43. Reid et al. (2018, 16). List that follows is also from this source.
44. Grove (1995, 294–97).
45. Ibid., 285–86, original emphasis.
46. Gonzalez (1988).
47. Adams (2002, 58).
48. Palacio (2005a); Sweeney (2007).
49. Taylor (2012, fn192).
50. Ibid., 147.
51. Beckles (2013, 36).
52. Taylor (2012, 142).
53. Anderson ([ca. 1798] 1983, 95).
54. Hugh-Jones (1955).
55. Zuidema (1955).

56. Kinnear, Grillo, and Elliot (1964).

57. Shaper (1964).

58. Dodu (1967); Gill et al. (2011); Mohan et al. (1985); Morrison and Ragoobirsingh (1992); Rao (1988); Tripathy and Samal (1993).

59. Abdulkadir et al. (1990); Belcher (1970).

60. Alruhaili (2010); Wang et al. (2003).

61. Alberti (1998); Tripathy and Samal (1997).

62. Alemu et al. (2009); Nwokolo (1986).

63. Abu-Bakare et al. (1986, 1135).

64. Samal, Kanungo, and Sanjeevi (2002).

65. Mbanya et al. (2010); Mauvais-Jarvis et al. (2004).

66. Gill et al. (2009).

67. Grove (2018).

68. Gardner (1999).

69. Tulloch and MacIntosh (1961).

70. Niewöhner and Lock (2018); see Lock (1993).

71. Neel (1962, 2011).

72. Diamond (2003).

73. Benyshek and Watson (2006).

74. *Chicago Tribune*, July 1900; see Smith-Morris (2006).

75. Lim et al. (2011).

76. Fasting as a diabetes cure is also the premise of recent trends such as that in the *Diabetes Code* (Fung 2018).

77. Barker (2003); Barker et al. (1993); Gluckman and Hanson (2006); Hales and Barker (2001); Wells (2007).

78. Benyshek, Martin, and Johnston (2001); Begum et al. (2012); Buckley, Jaquiery, and Harding (2005); Godfrey and Barker (2000); Martin et al. (2000); Nolan, Damm, and Prentki (2011); Phillips et al. (1994); Stocker, Arch, and Cawthorne (2005); Yajnik (2004).

79. Yates-Doerr (2017); Hanson and Gluckman (2011); Hales and Barker (1992).

80. Konig and Shuldiner (2012).

81. Osgood, Dyck, and Grassmann (2011).

82. Schulz (2010); Hopkins (2011).

83. Heijmans et al. (2008); Rodriguez (2015); Sepa, Frodi, and Ludvigsson (2005).

84. Godfrey et al. (2011).

85. Handy, Castro, and Loscalzo (2011).

86. Corruccini, Handler, and Jacobi (1985, 114).

87. Corruccini and Handler (1983, 72).

88. Ibid., 72–73.

89. Ibid., 73.

90. Ibid.

91. Wolfe (2006); Kauanui (2016).

92. Brown (1959, 277).

93. Pollin (2011).

94. Fassin (2007, 32); see Kuzawa and Sweet (2009); Lock (2013).

95. Sweeney (2007).
96. McMillan and Geevarghese (1979).
97. Mathangi et al. (2000).
98. Schnell, Carvajal, and Anchustegui (1993).
99. In Chakrabarti (2010, 23).
100. Cain (1933).
101. Bolland (2003, 167).
102. Edgell (1982).
103. Avocados are called pears in Belize.
104. Gonzalez (1988).
105. Ibid., 21.
106. Ibid., fn35.
107. James (2010, 164).
108. Gayle et al. (2010, 296).
109. Ibid.
110. Ibid., 300–302.
111. Ibid., 301.
112. Ibid., 122.
113. Ibid., 313.
114. See Ralph (2014); Bourgois (1995).
115. Gayle et al. (2010, 50).
116. Bulwer (2010, 2).
117. Ciego (2012).
118. 7 News Belize (2012).
119. Kim (2011).
120. *Amandala* (2010).
121. Bodden (2010).
122. *Belize Times* (2010).
123. Ali (2011).
124. Vasquez (2011).
125. Cayetano (2011).
126. Bullard (1973).
127. Blass and Shide (1994).
128. Elmore (2016).
129. This Garifuna version of the novena was adapted from Roman Catholic custom of nine days of mourning prayers leading up to the *beluria* celebration on the ninth night. See Valentine (2002, 13–15).
130. Pomet ([1694] 1712).
131. Metropolitan Museum of Art (2013).
132. van der Donck (1655).
133. Valentine (2002, 4).
134. Helmreich (2014, 59).
135. Wetsman (2019, 1).
136. See Tuchman (2011).
137. Radin (2017).
138. Crawford (1984).
139. TallBear (2013, 6).

140. It would take further research to know which species were imported later into British plantations created on Garifuna territory, and which descended from plants growing on that land before the 1796 dispossession.

141. Llewellyn (2013).

142. Grove (1995, 297–308).

143. Anderson ([ca. 1798] 1983, 98).

144. Palacio (2005c, 159).

CRÓNICA FOUR: REPAIR WORK

1. Mika (2015).

2. Appiah (2005, 231).

3. Brown (1996).

4. Jones (2013); see Strebel, Bovet, and Sormani (2019).

5. Star (1999, 382).

6. Jackson (2014); Russell and Vinsel (2018).

7. Manderson and Warren (2016); see Manderson and Smith-Morris (2010); Kleinman and Hall-Clifford (2010).

8. Mol (2008, 20; 2009).

9. Morrison (1987).

10. The movement for "The Right to Repair" (https://repair.org/stand-up) holds implications for technologies treating health conditions linked to historical repair (CARICOM Reparations Commission 2013; Coates 2014).

11. Graziano (2016); Rugnetta (2018).

12. Neil (2015, 107).

13. Anderson (2014).

14. Neil (2015, 108).

15. Hanger (2015).

16. Geil (2017).

17. Eveleth (2014).

18. Jain (1999).

19. Johns Hopkins Medicine (2018).

20. Wool (2015); Cavell (1986).

21. The show's subtitle, "Million Dollar Man," played on both the military-restoration sci-fi movie *Six Million Dollar Man* and the approximate cost of the prosthetic parts used in the show.

22. Jaipur Foot, Rajasthan, India, jaipurfoot.org.

23. Prosthetic Hope International (2011).

24. Kistenberg (2005, 50–51).

25. Woods (2003).

26. Blakeslee (2009, 1).

27. This estimate is for U.S. hospital-quality models (but lower-quality used machines can be found for much less).

28. All the dialysis described here is hemodialysis.

29. U.S. National Kidney Foundation (2018).

30. 7 News Belize (2009); Ramos (2009).

31. Davita Kidney Care (2018).

32. Hamdy (2008, 2012); see Sharp (2013).

33. Hirschman (1970).

34. This quote by Cruz comes from a television interview with channel 7 News Belize on December 30, 2009.

35. Ramos (2009).

36. Biehl (2016).

37. Nikhil Anand (2017) explores situations where infrastructures reveal the ways different kinds of "pressure" are made by people. People in Belize spoke constantly of rising pressure, which commonly went hand-in-hand with high sugar. In the common phrasing "I have *pressure*," it was often literally impossible to tell if someone meant blood pressure or social pressure.

38. Channel 5 News Belize (2010); Ramos (2010); 7 News Belize (2010a; 2010b; 2011).

39. I realized later that this sign doesn't seem to be a bilingual translation after all; the English gives one set of hours, while the Plattdeutsch adds "Open for Mennonites on Friday and Saturday."

40. Published in Dutch by Thieleman J. van Bragt around 1660, this book is a catalog of Christian martyrs that begins from the first century and prominently includes Anabaptist persecutions in the sixteenth century. Along with the Bible, it became a major document for many Mennonite sects.

41. Schroeder and Huebert (1996).

42. Statistical Institute of Belize (2011).

43. Gough et al. (2008, 51).

44. Schroeder and Huebert (1996).

45. Frohlich et al. (2014).

46. Bartlett (2015); Nobel Women's Initiative (2015).

47. Cuffe (2015).

48. Hayden et al. (2005).

49. Flavelle (2017).

50. Helmreich (2016, xxi).

51. Ramos (2017).

52. Gayle et al. (2010, 134).

53. Ibid.

54. Although Claude Lévi-Strauss (1966) famously envisioned the bricoleur (a figure of constant tinkering) and the engineer (a scientist who lays out design plans ahead of time) in contrast to each other, London Bridges serve as a reminder that such practices and ecologies are not always in easy opposition after all. Sometimes the bricoleur defines the contours of where the engineer will one day work; their practices can be intertwined and cumulative.

55. See Han (2012); McKay (2018).

56. Mitaishvili (2010).

57. I first encountered this quote in Claudia Rankine's *Citizen* (2014). She noted in a recent interview (Schwartz 2016): "I thought I was writing a book about why things like diabetes and high blood pressure disproportionately affect black communities. I was thinking: What are the stresses that bring these things on? For me, these stresses were connected to the negotiation of racism."

58. Michaels (1998, 77).

EPILOGUE

1. Tsing (1993, 7).

2. Mintz (1985).

3. Barrett and Calvi (2012).

4. Sharpe (2016, 102–34) developed her conceptualization of weather from Morrison's closing lines of *Beloved:* "By and by all trace is gone, and what is forgotten is not only the footprints but the water too and what is down there. The rest is weather . . . Just weather" (1987, 322). For a resonant public health perspective on unequal bodily "weathering," see Geronimus et al. (2006).

5. Mintz (1985, 214).

6. Its structures reminded me of the "glass cages" of the panopticon that once served Foucault and others as an iconic figure of infectious disease control (2007), but emblematic of a new era of chronic health conditions. The Coca-Cola London Eye's carnival ride–like pleasures and distractions seemed a fitting icon of displaced surveillance—not designed to keep watch on those below in order to interrupt para-communicable transmission, but rather primarily to collect data on those inside for purposes of future advertising.

7. The regional alliance of CARICOM (the Caribbean Community and Common Market) includes not only island nations but also mainland countries such as Belize, Guyana, and Suriname.

8. Herr ([1977] 1991, 230).

9. Brown (2008, 124).

10. In *Carbon Democracy,* Timothy Mitchell describes a British history of coal that interlocks with the economies of sugar noted by Mintz: "Coal made available thermal and mechanical energy in unprecedented quantity and concentration, but this energy was of no benefit unless there were ways to put it to work. . . . In acquiring lands for sugar and cotton production in the New World, Europeans had relied on the total dispossession of the local population and the importing of slave or indentured workforces. . . . These colonial arrangements secured the extensive, solar-based production used to supply agricultural goods in quantities that allowed the development of intensive, coal-based mass production in the towns and cities of Europe" (2011, 16–17).

11. Wilk (2007).

12. Sharpe (2017; 2016, 21).

ABOUT TRANSLATIONS

1. Thiong'o (2009, 44).

2. Rich ([1971] 2016, 304).

Bibliography

7 News Belize. 2009. "Dialysis Patients Protest." December 30. http://7newsbelize.com/sstory.php?nid=15872.
———. 2010a. "Jose Cruz Needs $15,000 to Save His Fingers." January 15. www.7newsbelize.com/sstory.php?nid=15995.
———. 2010b. "Jose Cruz Refuses Dialysis in Protest." Accessed August 12. www.7newsbelize.com/sstory.php?nid=14397.
———. 2011. "Dialysis, Finally a Public Health Reality." February 4, 2011.
———. 2012. "Doctors Protest Colleague's Murder: Go-Slow & March." June 19.
Abdulkadir, J., B. Mengesha, and Z. Welde Gabriel et al. 1990. "The Clinical and Hormonal (C-Peptide and Glucagon) Profile and Liability to Ketoacidosis during Nutritional Rehabilitation in Ethiopian Patients with Malnutrition-Related Diabetes Mellitus." *Diabetologia* 33 (4): 222–27.
Abramiuk, Marc, Peter Dunham, Linda Scott Cummings, Chad Yost, and Todd Pesek. 2011. "Linking Past and Present: A Preliminary Paleoethno-botanical Study of Maya Nutritional and Medicinal Plant Use and Sustainable Cultivation in the South Maya Mountains, Belize." *Ethnobotany Research and Application* 9:257–73.
Abu-Bakare, A., R. Taylor, G. V. Gill, and K. G. Alberti. 1986. "Tropical or Malnutrition-Related Diabetes: A Real Syndrome." *Lancet* 1 (8490): 1135–38.
Aciman, André. 2016. "The Life Unlived: On W. G. Sebald and the Uncertainties of Time." *American Scholar*, December 5. https://theamericanscholar.org/the-life-unlived/#.XHyTZZNKjfY.
Adams, Edgar. 2002. *People on the Move: The Effects of Some Important Historical Events on the People of St. Vincent and the Grenadines.* Kingstown: R & M Adams Books.
Adams, Vincanne. 2016. *Metrics: What Counts in Global Health.* Durham, NC: Duke University Press.

Agard-Jones, Vanessa. 2015. "Chlordécone." Manufacturing of Rights: Beirut, May 14. https://www.youtube.com/watch?v=yvqVkR4Iuqs.

Ahlqvist, Emma, et al. 2018. "Novel Subgroups of Adult-Onset Diabetes and Their Association with Outcomes: A Data-Driven Cluster Analysis of Six Variables." *Lancet Diabetes Endocrinol* 6 (5): 361–69. doi: 10.1016/S2213 -8587(18)30051-2.

Akrich, Madeleine. 1992. "The De-Scription of Technical Objects." In *Shaping Technology/Building Society: Studies in Sociotechnical Change,* edited by W. L. Bijker, 205–24. Cambridge, MA: MIT Press.

Alberti, K. G. 1998. "Tropical Diabetes: An Elusive Concept." *Practical Diabetes International* 5 (4): 152–55.

Alcorn, Ted. 2019. "The Strange Marketplace for Diabetes Test Strips." *New York Times,* Jan. 15. https://www.nytimes.com/2019/01/14/health/diabetes -test-strips-resale.html.

Alegria, Henry, Kathy Carvalho-Knighton, and Victor Alegria. 2009. "Assessing Land-Based Sources of Pollutants to Coastal Waters of Southern Belize." National Oceanic Atmospheric Administration (NOAA). https://repository .library.noaa.gov/view/noaa/590.

Alemu, S., A. Dessie, E. Seid, E. Bard, P. T. Lee, E. R. Trimble, D. I. W. Phillips, and E. H. O. Parry. 2009. "Insulin-Requiring Diabetes in Rural Ethiopia: Should We Reopen the Case for Malnutrition-Related Diabetes?" *Diabetologia* 52 (9): 1842–45.

Ali, Marion. 2011. "2 Chinese Women Brutally Murdered." *Channel 5 News Belize,* April 4. Accessed May 5, 2011. http://edition.channel5belize.com/archives/52075.

Alruhaili, M. 2010. "Type 1 Diabetes in the Tropics: The Protective Effects of Environmental Factors." *Africa Health* 11:20–24.

Amandala. 2010. "Eyannie's Funeral Draws 4,000." September 17, 2010.

Anand, Nikhil. 2017. *Hydraulic City.* Durham, NC: Duke University Press.

Anderson, Alexander. [ca. 1798] 1983. *Alexander Anderson's Geography and History of St. Vincent, West Indies,* edited by R. A. Howard and E. S. Howard. Cambridge, MA: Arnold Arboretum.

Anderson, Mark. 2009. *Black and Indigenous: Garifuna Activism and Consumer Culture in Honduras.* Minneapolis: University of Minnesota Press.

Anderson, Roger. 2014. "Nerve Transfers Limit Pain for Amputees." *Clinical Breakthroughs, Northwestern Medicine News Center,* March 21. http:// news.feinberg.northwestern.edu/2014/03/dumanian_nerve_research/.

Anderson, Warwick. 2006. *Colonial Pathologies: American Tropical Medicine, Race, and Hygiene in the Philippines.* Durham, NC: Duke University Press.

Anderson-Fye, Eileen P. 2004. "A 'Coca-Cola' Shape: Cultural Change, Body Image, and Eating Disorders in San Andres, Belize." *Culture, Medicine, and Psychiatry* 28 (4): 561–95.

———. 2010. "Maria: Cultural Change and Posttraumatic Stress in the Life of a Belizean Adolescent Girl." In *Formative Experiences,* edited by C. Worthman et al. Cambridge: Cambridge University Press.

Anzilotti, Eillie. 2018. "This New Prosthetic Limb Transmits Sensations Directly to the Nervous System." *Fast Company,* April 17. www.fastcompany .com/40559245/this-new-prosthetic-limb-transmit-sensations.

Appiah, Kwame Anthony. 2005. *The Ethics of Identity*. Princeton, NJ: Princeton University Press.

Armstrong, David G., Andrew J.M. Boulton, and Sicco A. Bus. 2017. "Diabetic Foot Ulcers and Their Recurrence." *New England Journal of Medicine* 376 (24): 2367–75.

Armstrong, David G., Vikram A. Kanda, Lawrence A. Lavery, William Marston, Joseph L. Mills, and Andrew J.M. Boulton. 2013. "Mind the Gap: Disparity between Research Funding and Costs of Care for Diabetic Foot Ulcers." *Diabetes Care* 36 (7): 1815–17.

Armstrong, David G., L.A. Lavery, L.B. Harkless, and W.H. Van Houtum. 1997. "Amputation and Reamputation of the Diabetic Foot." *Journal of American Podiatric Medical Association* 87 (6): 255–59.

Armstrong, David G., J. Wrobel, and J.M. Robbins. 2007. "Guest Editorial: Are Diabetes-Related Wounds and Amputations Worse than Cancer?" *International Wound Journal* 4 (4): 286–87.

Arnqvist, H.J., B. Littorin, L. Nyström, B. Scherstén, J. Ostman, et al. 1993. "Difficulties in Classifying Diabetes Presentation in the Young Adult." *Diabetic Medicine* 10 (7): 606–13.

Ávila, Tomás Alberto. 2009. *Black Caribs-Garifuna: Saint Vincent's Exiled People and the Roots of the Garifuna*. Providence: Milenio Associates.

Awe, Jaime J., Candy Gonzalez, and Cruzita Ken. 2007. *Taking Stock: Belize at 25 Years of Independence*, Vol. 1. Benque Viejo del Carmen: Cubola Books.

Bailey, C.J. 2004. "Metformin: Its Botanical Background." *Practical Diabetes* 21 (3): 115–17.

Baines, Kristina. 2015. *Embodying Ecological Heritage in a Maya Community: Health, Happiness, and Identity*. Landham, MD: Rowman & Littlefield.

Balboni, Barbara, Joseph Palacio, and Jaime Awe, eds. 2007. Taking Stock: *Belize at 25 Years of Independence*, Vol. 2. Benque Viejo del Carmen, BZ: Cubola Books.

Baldwin, James. 1998. "Many Thousands Gone" and "Notes of a Native Son." In *James Baldwin: Collected Essays*, edited by Toni Morrison, 19–34 and 63–84. New York: Library of America.

———. [1964] 2011. "The Uses of the Blues." In *The Cross of Redemption: Uncollected Writings*, 70–81. New York: Vintage International.

Balsells, Montserrat, A. García-Patterson, I. Gich, and R. Corcoy. 2009. "Maternal and Fetal Outcome in Women with Type 2 versus Type 1 Diabetes Mellitus: A Systematic Review and Metaanalysis." *Journal of Clinical Endocrinology & Metabolism* 94 (11): 4284–91.

"Barbados Defense Force Hyperbaric Chamber." 2011. Video produced by InfoOnScubaDiving. *YouTube*. Accessed April 12, 2018. https://www.youtube.com/watch?v=gIvplaCvd54.

Barker, D.J.P. 2003. "The Developmental Origins of Adult Disease." *European Journal of Epidemiology* 18:733–36.

Barker, D.J.P., C.N. Hales, C.H. Fall, C. Osmond, K. Phipps, and P.M. Clark. 1993. "Type 2 (Non-insulin-dependent) Diabetes Mellitus, Hypertension and Hyperlipidaemia (Syndrome X): Relation to Reduced Fetal Growth." *Diabetologia* 36 (1): 62–7.

Barrett, Duncan, and Nuala Calvi. 2012. *The Sugar Girls.* New York: Harper-Collins.

Barrett, Ward. 1970. *The Sugar Hacienda of the Marqueses Del Valle.* Minneapolis: University of Minnesota Press.

Bartlett, Stephen. 2015. "'Our Lands Are Critical to Our Lives': Afro-Indigenous Hondurans Defend Land and Food Sovereignty." *Institute for Agriculture & Trade Policy,* October 8. Accessed April 11, 2018. https://www.iatp.org/blog/201510/our-lands-are-critical-to-our-lives-afro-indigenous-hondurans-defend-land-and-food-sover.

Bassett, Pambana, and Jeanette Charles. 2015. "In the Caribbean: What Are Reparations?" *Telesur,* October 27.

Batalis, N.I., and J.A. Prahlow. 2004. "Accidental Insulin Overdose." *Journal of Forensic Sciences* 49 (5): 1117–20.

Beard, Jo Ann. 2006. "Werner." *Tin House* 8 (1): 72–90.

Beckert, Sven. 2014. *Empire of Cotton: A Global History.* New York: Alfred A. Knopf.

Beckert, Sven, and Christine Desan, eds. 2018. *American Capitalism: New Histories.* New York: Columbia University Press.

Beckles, Hilary. 2013. *Britain's Black Debt: Reparations for Caribbean Slavery and Native Genocide.* Kingston: University of West Indies Press.

———. 2014. "Address to the British Parliament on Reparations." https://wadadlipen.wordpress.com/2014/11/21/fyi-sir-hilary-beckles-addresses-the-british-parliament-on-reparations/.

Begum, Ghazzla, Adam Stevens, Emma Smith, Kristin Connor, John Challis, F. Bloomfield, and A. White. 2012. "Epigenetic Changes in Fetal Hypothalamic Energy Regulating Pathways Are Associated with Maternal Undernutrition and Twinning." *FASEB Journal* 26 (4): 1694–703.

Behar, Ruth. 2003. *Translated Woman: Crossing the Border with Esperanza's Story.* Boston: Beacon Press.

Belcher, D.W. 1970. "Diabetes Mellitus in Northern Ethiopia." *Ethiopia Medical Journal* 8 (2): 73–74.

Beliso-De Jesús, Aisha. 2014. "Santería Copresence and the Making of African Diaspora Bodies." *Cultural Anthropology* 29 (3): 503–26.

Belize Ministry of Health. 1996. "Diagnostic Situation on the Use of DDT and the Control and Prevention of Malaria in Belize." Belize City, BZ.

———. 2014. *Belize Health Sector Strategic Plan 2014–2024.* Pan American Health Organization.

———. 2017. *Annual HIV Statistical Report.* Belmopan, BZ.

Belize Times. 2010. "Jose Cruz's Fight for Justice." *Belize Times,* March 5. www.belizetimes.bz/2010/03/05/jose-cruz%E2%80%99s-fight-for-justice/.

Bell, R., S.V. Glinianaia, P.W. Tennant, R.W. Bilous, and J. Rankin. 2012. "Peri-Conception Hyperglycaemia and Nephropathy Are Associated with Risk of Congenital Anomaly in Women with Pre-Existing Diabetes: A Population-Based Cohort Study." *Diabetologia* 55 (4): 936–47.

Benítez-Rojo, Antonio. 2001. *The Repeating Island: The Caribbean and the Postmodern Perspective.* Durham, NC: Duke University Press.

Benjamin, Ruha. 2015. "From Park Bench to Lab Bench: What Kind of Future Are We Designing?" Video. *TEDxBaltimore,* February 5. https://www .youtube.com/watch?v=_8RrX4hjCro.

Benn Torres, Jada, and Gabriel A. Torres-Colon. 2018. "Operationalizing Race within the Context of Paracommunicability: A Case Study of Uterine Fibroids among African Descended Women." Paper presented as part of Communicability in Crisis panel at American Anthropological Association Annual Meeting, November 28.

Benton, Adia. 2015. *HIV Exceptionalism: Development through Disease in Sierra Leone.* Minneapolis: University of Minnesota Press.

Benyshek, Daniel, and James Watson. 2006. "Exploring the Thrifty Genotype's Food-Shortage Assumptions: A Cross-Cultural Comparison of Ethnographic Accounts of Food Security among Foraging and Agricultural Societies." *American Journal of Physical Anthropology* 131 (1): 120–26.

Benyshek, D. C., C. S. Johnston, and J. F. Martin. 2006. "Glucose Metabolism Is Altered in the Adequately-Nourished Grand-Offspring (F3 Generation) of Rats Malnourished during Gestation and Perinatal Life." *Diabetologia* 49 (5): 1117–19.

Benyshek, D. C., J. F. Martin, and C. S. Johnston. 2001. "A Reconsideration of the Origins of the Type 2 Diabetes Epidemic among Native Americans and the Implications of Intervention Policy." *Medical Anthropology* 20(1):25–64.

Beran D., M. Ewen, and R. Laing. 2016. "Constraints and Challenges in Access to Insulin: A Global Perspective." *Lancet Diabetes Endocrinology* 4(3):275–85.

Beran, D., and J. S. Yudkin. 2006. "Diabetes Care in Sub-Saharan Africa." *Lancet* 368 (9548): 1689–95.

Berg, Jeremy, John Tymoczko, and Lubert Stryer. 2002. *Biochemistry, 5th Edition.* New York: W. H. Freeman.

Berlant, Lauren. 2007. "Slow Death (Sovereignty, Obesity, Lateral Agency)." *Critical Inquiry* 33 (4): 754–80.

———. 2008. "Thinking About Feeling Historical." *Emotion, Space and Society* 1:4–9.

Bertazzi, Pier Alberto, Dario Consonni, Silvia Bachetti, Maurizia Rubagotti, Andrea Baccarelli, Carlo Zocchetti, and Angela C. Pesatori. 2001. "Health Effects of Dioxin Exposure: A 20-Year Mortality Study." *American Journal of Epidemiology* 153 (11): 1031–44.

Bessire, Lucas. 2014. *Behold the Black Caiman: A Chronicle of Ayoreo Life.* Chicago: University of Chicago Press.

Biehl, João. 2005. *Vita: Life in a Zone of Social Abandonment.* Berkeley: University of California Press.

———. 2007. *The Will to Live: AIDS Therapies and the Politics of Survival.* Berkeley: University of California Press.

———. 2016. "Anthropology of Becomings: World on Edge, Lives, Entanglements, Stories." Friday Morning Seminar in Culture, Psychiatry, and Global Mental Health, Apr. 15. Weatherhead Center, Harvard University.

Biehl, João, and Peter Locke. 2017. *Unfinished: The Anthropology of Becoming.* Durham, NC: Duke University Press.

Biehl, João, and Adriana Petryna. 2013. *When People Come First: Critical Studies in Global Health*. Princeton, NJ: Princeton University Press.

Biruk, Crystal. 2018. *Cooking Data: Culture and Politics in an African Research World*. Durham, NC: Duke University Press.

Biswas, Atanu, Manish Bharara, Craig Hurst et al. 2010. "Use of Sugar on the Healing of Diabetic Ulcers: A Review." *Journal of Diabetes Science and Technology* 4 (5): 1139–45.

Blakeslee, Sandra. 2007. "A Small Part of the Brain, and Its Profound Effects." *New York Times,* February 6.

———. 2009. "Willem Kolff, Doctor Who Invented Kidney and Heart Machines, Dies at 97." *New York Times,* February 12.

Blanchette, Alex. 2018. "Industrial Meat Production." *Annual Review of Anthropology.* 47:185–99.

Blass, E.M., and D.J. Shide. 1994. "Some Comparisons Among the Calming and Pain-Relieving Effects of Sucrose, Glucose, Fructose and Lactose in Infant Rats." *Chem Senses* 19 (3): 239–49.

Bliss, Catherine. 2012. *Race Decoded: The Genomic Fight for Social Justice*. Palo Alto, CA: Stanford University Press.

Bliss, Michael. 1982. *The Discovery of Insulin*. Chicago: University of Chicago Press.

Bodden, Monica. 2010. "Teenager Killed by Ruthless Robbers." *7 News Belize*, August 12.

Bolland, O. Nigel. 1977. *The Formation of Colonial Society: Belize, from Conquest to Crown Colony*. Baltimore: Johns Hopkins University Press.

———. 2003. *Colonialism and Resistance in Belize: Essays in Historical Sociology*. Benque Viejo del Carmen, BZ: Cubola Books.

Bolland, Nigel, and Assad Shoman. 1977. *Land in Belize, 1765–1871*. Kingston: University of the West Indies.

Bond, David. 2013. "Governing Disaster: The Political Life of the Environment during the BP Oil Spill." *Cultural Anthropology* 28 (4): 694–715.

Boon, James. 1999. *Verging on Extra-Vagance*. Princeton, NJ: Princeton University Press.

Borges, Jorge Luis. 1995. "Blindness." In *Art of the Personal Essay,* edited by Phillip Lopate, 377–87. New York: Anchor Books.

Bourgois, Philippe. 1995. *In Search of Respect: Selling Crack in El Barrio*. Cambridge: Cambridge University Press.

———. 2009. "Recognizing Invisible Violence." In *Global Health in Times of Violence,* edited by B. Rylko-Bauer, L. Whiteford, and P. Farmer, 18–40. Santa Fe: School of Advanced Research.

Bowe, Benjamin, Yan Xie, Tingting Li, Yan Yan, Hong Xian, and Ziyad Al-Aly. 2018. "The 2016 Global and National Burden of Diabetes Mellitus Attributable to PM2-5 Air Pollution." *The Lancet: Planetary Health* 2 (7): E301–12.

Brandes, Stanley. 1997. "Sugar, Colonialism, and Death." *Comparative Studies in Society and History* 39 (2): 270–99.

Brandt, Allan M. 1997. "Behavior, Disease, and Health in the Twentieth Century United States: The Moral Valance of Individual Risk." In *Morality and Health,* edited by Allan Brandt and Paul Rozin. New York: Routledge.

Braverman, Irus. 2018. *Coral Whisperers: Scientists on the Brink*. Berkeley: University of California Press.

Briggs, Charles L. 2017. "Towards Communicative Justice in Health." *Medical Anthropology: Cross-Cultural Studies in Health and Illness* 36(4):287–304.

Briggs, Charles, and Clara Mantini-Briggs. 2016. *Tell Me Why My Children Died: Rabies, Indigenous Knowledge, and Communicative Justice*. Durham, NC: Duke University Press.

Brotherton, Sean. 2012. *Revolutionary Medicine*. Durham, NC: Duke University Press.

Brown, E. 1996. "Halfway Technologies." *Physician Executive* 22 (12): 44–45.

Brown, Norman O. 1959. *Life against Death*. Middletown, CT: Wesleyan University Press.

Brown, Vincent. 2008. "Eating the Dead: Consumption and Regeneration in the History of Sugar." *Food and Foodways* 16 (2): 117–26.

———. 2010. *The Reaper's Garden: Death and Power in the World of Atlantic Slavery*. Cambridge, MA: Harvard University Press.

Browne, Simone. 2015. *Dark Matters: On the Surveillance of Blackness*. Durham, NC: Duke University Press.

Buber, Martin. 1952. "On the Suspension of the Ethical." *The Eclipse of God: Studies in the Relation between Religion and Philosophy*, 146–56. New York: Harper and Row.

Buckley, Alex J., Anne L. Jaquiery, and Jane E. Harding. 2005. "Nutritional Programming of Adult Disease." *Cell and Tissue Research* 322 (1): 73–79.

Bukhman, Gene, Charlotte Bavuma, Crispin Gishoma, Neil Gupta, Gene F. Kwan, Richard Laing, and David Beran. 2015. "Endemic Diabetes in the World's Poorest People." *Lancet Diabetes Endocrinology* 3 (6):402–3.

Bullard, Mary Kenyon. 1973. *The Recognition of Psychiatric Disorder in British Honduras*. Oregon: University of Oregon.

Bullard, Robert, and Glenn Johnson. 2000. "Environmental Justice: Grassroots Activism and Its Impact on Public Policy Decision Making." *Journal of Social Issues* 56 (3): 555–78.

Bulwer, Bernard. 2010. "Violence and the Health of a Nation." *Guardian* (Belize), April 29.

Burdon, John, ed. 1931. *Archives of British Honduras: From the Earliest Date to A.D. 1800*. Vol. 1. London: Sifton Praed & Co.

Buyandelger, Manduhai. 2013. *Tragic Spirits: Shamanism, Memory, and Gender in Contemporary Mongolia*. Chicago: University of Chicago Press.

CABI (Centre of Agriculture and Biosciences International). 2018. Invasive Species Compendium. Accessed April 5, 2018. https://www.cabi.org/isc/datasheet/48162.

Caduff, Carlo. 2015. *The Pandemic Perhaps: Dramatic Events in a Public Culture of Danger*. Berkeley: University of California Press.

Cain, Earnest. 1933. *Cyclone: Official Record of the Hurricane and Tidal Wave Which Destroyed the City of Belize*. Devon: A. H. Stockwell.

Canguilhem, Georges. 1991. *The Normal and the Pathological*. New York: Zone Books.

CARICOM Reparations Commission. 2013. "10-Point Reparation Plan." http://caricomreparations.org/caricom/caricoms-10-point-reparation-plan/.

Castro, Jerry. 2005. "Lidani Garifuna Times Interviews Dr. Joseph Palacio." *Garinet*. https://www.garinet.com/main.php?module=gcms&node=gcms_front &action=get_content_detail&content_id=2497&category_id=202&parent _id=224.

Cavell, Stanley. 1986. "The Uncanniness of the Ordinary." Tanner Lectures on Human Values, Stanford University, April 3 and 8.

Cayetano, Isani. 2011. "One More Asian Belizean Murdered." 2011. Accessed May 20, 2016. http://edition.channel5belize.com/archives/52348.

Cayetano, Marion, and E. Roy Cayetano. 2005. "Garifuna Language, Dance and Music: A Masterpiece of the Oral and Intangible Heritage of Humanity. How Did It Happen?" In Palacio 2005a, 230–50.

Cayetano, E. Roy, ed. 1993. *The People's Garifuna Dictionary*. Dangriga, BZ: National Garifuna Council.

———. 2009. "Song and Ritual as a Key to Understanding Garifuna Personality." In *St. Vincent's Exiled People and the Origin of the Garifuna: A Historical Compilation*, edited by Tomás Alberto Ávila, 216–30. Providence: Mileno.

Chakrabarti, Pratik. 2010. *Materials and Medicine: Trade, Conquest, and Therapeutics in the Eighteenth Century*. Manchester: Manchester University Press.

Channel 5 News Belize. 2010. "Asian Community Unites against Crime on the Occasion of Hellen Yu's Funeral." August 19.

Ciego, Albert. 2012. "Popular KHMH Doctor Murdered." *Amandala*, June 19.

Clarke, S.F., and J.R. Foster. 2012. "A History of Blood Glucose Meters and Their Role in Self-Monitoring of Diabetes Mellitus." *British Journal of Biomedical Science* 69 (2): 83–93.

Clegern, Wayne. 1967. *British Honduras: Colonial Dead End, 1859–1900*. Baton Rouge: Louisiana State University Press.

Coates, Ta-Nehisi. 2014. "The Case for Reparations." *Atlantic*, June. https://www.theatlantic.com/magazine/archive/2014/06/the-case-for-reparations /361631/.

Colburn, Theo, Dianne Dumanoski, and John Peterson Myers. 1997. *Our Stolen Future*. New York: Plume.

Cole, Teju. 2017. *Blind Spot*. New York: Random House.

Collier, Stephen J., Jamie Cross, Peter Redfield, and Alice Street. 2017. "Little Development Devices/Humanitarian Goods." *Limn* 9. https://limn.it/issues /little-development-devices-humanitarian-goods/.

Corruccini, Robert, Jerome Handler, and Keith Jacobi. 1985. "Chronological Distribution of Enamel Hypoplasias and Weaning in a Caribbean Slave Population." *Human Biology* 57 (4): 699–711.

Crawford, Michael, ed. 1984. *Current Developments in Anthropological Genetics, Volume 3: Black Caribs*. New York: Plenum Press.

Crist, Carolyn. 2018. "Limb Amputation Rates for Blocked Arteries Vary by Race and Setting." *Reuters*, February 15.

Crosbie, Paul, Yvette Herrera, Myrna Manzanares, Silvana Woods, Cynthia Crosbie, and Ken Decker, eds. 2005. *Kriol-Inglish Dikshineri*. Belmopan, BZ: Belize Kriol Project.

Cuffe, Sandra. 2015. "Defender Shot in Honduras." *Intercontinental Cry*, Dec. 6. https://intercontinentalcry.org/garifuna-land-defender-shot-honduras/.

Dalí, Salvador. 1998. *The Collected Writings of Salvador Dalí*. Cambridge: Cambridge University Press.

Danticat, Edwidge. 2004. *The Dew Breaker*. New York: Vintage.

Darcel, F. C. 1954. *A History of Agriculture in the Colony of British Honduras*. British Department of Agriculture.

Das, Veena. 2015. *Affliction: Health, Disease, Poverty*. New York: Fordham University Press.

Das, Veena, and Clara Han, eds. 2015. *Living and Dying in the Contemporary World: A Compendium*. Berkeley: University of California Press.

Davita Kidney Care. 2018. "Arteriovenous (AV) Fistula—The Gold Standard Hemodialysis Access." https://www.davita.com/treatment-services/dialysis/preparing-for-dialysis/arteriovenous-av-fistula-the-gold-standard-hemodialysis-access.

Dawdy, Shannon Lee. 2008. *Building the Devil's Empire: French Colonial New Orleans*. Chicago: University of Chicago Press.

Deane, Green. 2019. "Sugar Cane on the Run." *Eat the Weeds and Other Things, Too*. http://www.eattheweeds.com/saccharum-officinarum-sweet-wild-weed-2/.

de-Graft Aikins, Ama. Forthcoming. *Sugar Disease, Bitter Medicine: Living with Diabetes in Ghana*. Cambridge: International African Institute.

de-Graft Aikins, Ama, Samuel Agyei-Mensah, and Charles Agyemang, eds. 2014. *Chronic Non-Communicable Diseases in Ghana: Multidisciplinary Perspectives*. Accra: University of Ghana Readers, African Books Collective.

de la Monte, S. M., and J. R. Wands. 2008. "Alzheimer's Disease Is Type 3 Diabetes-Evidence Reviewed." *Journal of Diabetes Science and Technology* 2 (6): 1101–13.

de las Casas, Bartolomé. [1474–1566] 1906. "Narrative of the Third Voyage of Columbus as Contained in Casas's History." In *The Northmen, Columbus and Cabot*, edited by Julius Olson and Edward Bourne, 317–66. New York: Charles Scribner's & Sons.

Desmond, Matthew. 2016. *Evicted*. New York: Broadway Books.

Diamond, Jared. 2003. "The Double Puzzle of Diabetes." *Nature* 423 (6940): 599–602.

Diaz, Natalie. 2012. *When My Brother Was an Aztec*. Port Townsend: Copper Canyon Press.

Dodu, Silas. 1967. "Diabetes in the Tropics." *British Medical Journal* 2 (5554): 747–50.

Dumit, Joseph. 2012. *Drugs for Life*. Durham, NC: Duke University Press.

Dunn, Richard. 1972. *Sugar and Slaves*. Chapel Hill: University of North Carolina Press.

Durkheim, Émile. [1912] 1995. *Elementary Forms of Religious Life*. New York: Free Press.

Durnwald, C. O., and M. B. Landon. 2011. "Insulin Analogues in the Management of Pregnancy Complicated by Diabetes Mellitus." *Current Diabetes Reports* 11 (1): 28–34.

Duster, Troy. 1990. *Backdoor to Eugenics*. New York: Routledge.

Edgell, Zee. 1982. *Beka Lamb*. Johannesburg: Heinemann.

Edwards, M. L. 2010. "Hyperbaric Oxygen Therapy. Part 1: History and Principles." *Journal Veterinary Emergency Critical Care* 20 (3): 284–88.

Elgyzri, T., J. Larsson, J. Thörne, K. F. Eriksson, and J. Apelgvist. 2013. "Outcome of Ischemic Foot Ulcer in Diabetic Patients Who Had No Invasive Vascular Intervention." *European Journal of Vascular and Endovascular Surgery* 46 (1): 110–7.

El-Haj, Nadia Abu. 2007. "The Genetic Reinscription of Race." *Annual Review of Anthropology* 36 (1): 283–300.

Elmore, Bartow. 2016. *Citizen Coke: The Making of Coca-Cola Capitalism*. New York: W. W. Norton.

Evans-Pritchard, E. E. 1937. *Witchcraft, Oracles and Magic among the Azande*. Oxford: Clarendon Press.

Eveleth, Rose. 2014. "State-of-the-Art Prosthetics Are Incredible, but Not Always Useful." *PBS: Nova Next*, March 5. www.pbs.org/wgbh/nova/next/tech/durable-prostheses/.

Fanon, Frantz. 1963. *The Wretched of the Earth*. New York: Grove Press.

Farmer, Paul. 1999. *Infections and Inequalities*. Berkeley: University of California Press.

Fassin, Didier. 2007. *When Bodies Remember: Experiences and Politics of AIDS in South Africa*. Berkeley: University of California Press.

———. 2011. *Humanitarian Reason: A Moral History of the Present*. Berkeley: University of California Press.

Fausto-Sterling, Anne. 2016. "Response to Dorothy Roberts Tanner Lecture on Human Values." November 3, Harvard University.

Fee, Margery. 2006. "Racializing Narratives: Obesity, Diabetes and the 'Aboriginal' Thrifty Genotype." *Social Science & Medicine* 62 (12): 2988–97.

Ferreira, Mariana Leal, and Gretchen Lang, eds. 2006. *Indigenous Peoples and Diabetes: Community Empowerment and Wellness*. Durham, NC: Carolina Academic Press.

Fessenden, Marissa. 2015. "It's Cheaper to Make Diabetes Test Strips Out of Silk than Paper in India." *Smithsonian Magazine*, January 9. www.smithsonianmag.com/smart-news/why-its-cheaper-make-diabetes-test-strips-out-silk-rather-paper-india-180953860/?no-ist.

Feudtner, Chris. 2003. *Bittersweet: Diabetes, Insulin, and the Transformation of Illness*. Chapel Hill: University of North Carolina Press.

Fidler, David. 2008. "A Theory of Open-Source Anarchy." *Indiana Journal of Global Legal Studies* 15 (1): 259–84.

Finkler, Kaja. 2001. "The Kin of the Gene: The Medicalization of the Family and Kinship in American Society." *Current Anthropology* 42 (2): 235–63.

———. 2003. "Illusions of Controlling the Future: Risk and Genetic Inheritance." *Anthropology and Medicine* 10 (1): 51–70.

Fischer, Michael M. J. 2013. "The Peopling of Technologies." In *When People Come First*, 347–74. Princeton, NJ: Princeton University Press.

Flavelle, Christopher. 2017. "A Coral Reef Gets an Insurance Policy of its Own." *Bloomberg*, July 20. https://www.bloomberg.com/news/articles/2017-07-20/a-coral-reef-gets-an-insurance-policy-of-its-own.

Flomenhoft, G., M. Cayetano, and C. Young. 2007. "Black Gold, White Gold and the Gentrification of Belize." *Belizean Studies* 29 (1): 4–19.

Fortun, Kim. 2001. *Advocacy after Bhopal: Environmentalism, Disaster, New Global Orders*. Chicago: University of Chicago Press.

Fortun, Kim, and Mike Fortun. 2005. "Scientific Imaginaries and Ethical Plateaus in Contemporary U.S. Toxicology." *American Anthropologist* 107 (1): 43–54.

Foster, Byron. 2005. "Heart Drum: Spirit Possession in the Garifuna Communities of Belize." In *Garifuna: A Nation Across Borders*, edited by Joseph Palacio, 159–75. Benque Viejo del Carmen, BZ: Cubola.

Foster, John Bellamy. 2000. *Marx's Ecology: Materialism and Nature*. New York: Monthly Review Press.

Foucault, Michel. 2007. *Security, Territory, Population: Lectures at the Collège de France, 1977–78*. New York: Palgrave Macmillan.

Fowler, Michael J. 2008. "Microvascular and Macrovascular Complications of Diabetes." *Clinical Diabetes* 26 (2): 77–82.

Frohlich, Xaq, Mikko Jauho, Bart Penders, and David Schleifer, eds. 2014. "Food Infrastructures." *Limn* 4. https://limn.it/issues/food-infrastructures/.

Fullwiley, Duana. 2010. "Revaluating Genetic Causation: Biology, Economy and Kinship in Dakar, Senegal." *American Ethnologist* 37 (4): 638–61.

———. 2011. *The Enculturated Gene: Sickle Cell Health Politics and Biological Difference in West Africa*. Princeton, NJ: Princeton University Press.

Fung, Jason. 2018. *The Diabetes Code*. Vancouver: Greystone Books.

Gálvez, Alyshia. 2018. *Eating NAFTA: Trade, Food Policies, and the Destruction of Mexico*. Berkeley: University of California Press.

Gann, Thomas. 1918. *The Maya Indians of Southern Yucatan and Northern British Honduras*. Washington, DC: Smithsonian Institution.

Garcia, Angela. 2010. *The Pastoral Clinic: Addiction and Dispossession along the Rio Grande*. Berkeley: University of California Press.

Gardner, Amanda. 1999. "Flatbush Diabetes." *New York Daily News*, Nov. 22. https://www.nydailynews.com/flatbush-diabetes-article-1.843164.

Garifuna Women's Project. 2009. *Umalali*. Album. Stone Tree Records, Benque Viejo del Carmen, Belize.

Gayle, Herbert. 2019. "The Failure of Suppression." Lecture at Bliss Center, Belize City. https://www.youtube.com/watch?v=C7A2pq7E1pM.

Gayle, Herbert, Nelma Mortis, Jamuna Vasquez, Raymond James Mossiah, Melvin Hewlett, and Alindy Amaya. 2010. *Report: Male Social Participation and Violence in Urban Belize*. Belize City: Belize Ministry of Education.

Geary, James. 2011. *I Is an Other: The Secret Life of Metaphor and How it Shapes the Way We See the World*. New York: Harper.

Gebel, Erika. 2013. "Making Insulin: A Behind-the-Scenes Look at Producing a Lifesaving Medication." *Diabetes Forecast*, July.

Geertz, Clifford. 2000. *Available Light*. Princeton, NJ: Princeton University Press.

Geil, Mark. 2017. "Military-Funded Prosthetic Technologies Benefit More than Just Veterans." *Conversation*, May 24. https://theconversation.com/military-funded-prosthetic-technologies-benefit-more-than-just-veterans-76891.

Geissler, P. Wenzel. 2013. "The Archipelago of Public Health." In *Making and Unmaking Public Health in Africa: Ethnographic and Historical*

Perspectives, edited by Ruth Jane Prince and Rebecca Marsland, 231–56. Athens: Ohio University Press.

Geronimus, Arline T., Margaret Hicken, Danya Keene, and John Bound. 2006. "'Weathering' and Age Patterns of Allostatic Load Scores among Blacks and Whites in the United States." *American Journal of Public Health* 96 (5): 826–33.

Gewertz, Deborah, and Frederick Errington. 2010. *Cheap Meat: Flap Food Nations in the Pacific Islands*. Berkeley: University of California Press.

Gill, G. V., J.-C. Mbanya, K. L. Ramaiya, and S. Tesfaye. 2009. "A Sub-Saharan African Perspective of Diabetes." *Diabetologia* 52 (1): 8–16.

Gill, G. V., A. Tekle, A. Reja, D. Wile, P. J. English, M. Diver, A. J. K. Williams, and S. Tesfaye. 2011. "Immunological and C-Peptide Studies of Patients with Diabetes in Northern Ethiopia: Existence of an Unusual Subgroup Possibly Related to Malnutrition." *Diabetologia* 54 (1): 51–57.

Glover, Gina, Jessica Rayner, and Geof Rayner. 2015. *The Metabolic Landscape*. London: Black Dog.

Gluckman, P. D., and M. A. Hanson, eds. 2006. *Developmental Origins of Health and Disease*. Cambridge: Cambridge University Press.

Godfrey, Keith M., and David J. P. Barker. 2000. "Fetal Nutrition and Adult Disease." *American Journal of Clinical Nutrition* 71 (5): S1344–52.

Godfrey, K. M., A. Sheppard, P. D. Gluckman, K. A. Lillycrop, G. C. Burdge et al. 2011. "Epigenetic Gene Promoter Methylation at Birth Is Associated with Child's Later Adiposity." *Diabetes* 60 (5): 1528–34.

Gomez-Marquez, Jose. 2016. "Insulinomics." *Medium,* October 26. https://medium.com/@jfgm/insulinomics-9cd1af157677.

Gonzalez, Nancie. 1988. *Sojourners of the Caribbean: Ethnogenesis and Ethnohistory of the Garifuna*. Chicago: University of Illinois Press.

Good, Mary-Jo DelVecchio, Byron Good, and Jesse Grayman. 2010. "Complex Engagements: Responding to Violence in Postconflict Aceh." In *Contemporary States of Emergency,* edited by Didier Fassin and Mariella Pandolfi, 241–68. New York: Zone Books.

Good, Mary-Jo DelVecchio, S. T. Hyde, Sarah Pinto, and Byron Good, eds. 2008. *Postcolonial Disorders*. Berkeley: University of California Press.

Gordillo, Gastón. 2014. *Rubble: The Afterlife of Destruction*. Durham, NC: Duke University Press.

Gough, Ethan, Englebert Emmanuel, Valerie Jenkins, Lorraine Thompson, Enrique Perez, Alberto Barcelo, Robert Gerzoff, and Edward Gregg. 2008. "Survey of Diabetes, Hypertension and Chronic Disease Risk Factors." Belize City: Pan American Health Organization (PAHO) and Belize Ministry of Health.

Gould, Stephen Jay. 1996. *The Mismeasure of Man*. New York: W. W. Norton.

Graham, Elizabeth. 1994. *The Highlands of the Lowlands: Environment and Archaeology in the Stann Creek District, Belize, Central America*. Madison: Prehistory Press.

Graziano, Michael. 2016. "How Phantom Limbs Explain Consciousness." *Atlantic,* Feb. 4. https://www.theatlantic.com/science/archive/2016/02/phantom-limbs-explain-consciousness/459780/.

Great Britain. 1965. *British Honduras Colonial Report.*

Green Reef. 2010. "The Peculiar Parrotfish: Reef Brief." *San Pedro Sun.* https:// ambergriscaye.com/reefbriefs/briefs91.html.

Greene, Jeremy, and Kevin Riggs. 2015. "Why Is There No Generic Insulin? Historical Origins of a Modern Problem." *New England Journal of Medicine* 372:1171–75.

Grondahl, Paul. 2012. "Growing Diabetic Population Fuels a Black Market." *Albany Times Union,* January 30. Accessed April 8, 2018.

Grove, Richard. 1995. *Green Imperialism: Colonial Expansion, Tropical Island Edens and the Origins of Environmentalism, 1600–1860.* Cambridge: Cambridge University Press.

Groves, Stephen. 2018. "Despite Historically Low Crime across New York, East Flatbush Still Plagued by Violence." *Bklyner,* Feb. 22. https://bklyner .com/east-flatbush-violence/.

Guthman, Julie. 2011. *Weighing In: Obesity, Food Justice, and the Limits of Capitalism.* Berkeley: University of California Press.

Gutierrez-Sumner, Isha. 2019. *Weiga | Let's Eat.* https://www.weigaletseat.com/.

H.T. 2013. "Eating Themselves to Death." *Economist,* April 10. Accessed April 11, 2018. https://www.economist.com/blogs/americasview/2013/04 /diabetes-mexico.

Haagsma, J. A., N. Graetz, I. Bolliger, M. Naghavi, H. Higashi et al. 2016. "The Global Burden of Injury: Incidence, Mortality, Disability-Adjusted Life Years and Time Trends from the Global Burden of Disease Study, 2013." *Injury Prevention* 22 (1): 3–18.

Hacking, Ian. 1986. "Making Up People." In *Reconstructing Individualism,* edited by T. L. Heller, M. Sosna, and D. E. Wellbery. Stanford, CA: Stanford University Press.

Hales, C. N., and D. J. Barker. 1992. "Type 2 (Non-Insulin-Dependent) Diabetes Mellitus: The Thrifty Phenotype Hypothesis." *Diabetologica* 35:595–601.

———. 2001. "The Thrifty Phenotype Hypothesis." *British Medical Bulletin* 60 (1): 5–20.

Hall, Victoria, Reimar W. Thomsen, Ole Henriksen, and Nicolai Lohse. 2011. "Diabetes in Sub Saharan Africa, 1999–2011." *BMC Public Health* 11: 564.

Hamdy, Sherine. 2008. "When the State and Your Kidneys Fail: Political Etiologies in an Egyptian Dialysis Ward." *American Ethnologist* 35 (4): 553–69.

———. 2012. *Our Bodies Belong to God.* Berkeley: University of California Press.

Han, Clara. 2012. *Life in Debt: Times of Care and Violence in Neoliberal Chile.* Berkeley: University of California Press.

Handler, Jerome. 1969. "The Amerindian Slave Population of Barbados in the Seventeenth and Early Eighteenth Centuries." *Caribbean Studies* 8 (4): 38–64.

Handler, Jerome S., and Robert S. Corruccini. 1983. "Plantation Slave Life in Barbados: A Physical Anthropological Analysis." *Journal of Interdisciplinary History* 14 (1): 65.

Handy, D. E., R. Castro, and J. Loscalzo. 2011. "Epigenetic Modifications: Basic Mechanisms and Role in Cardiovascular Disease." *Circulation* 123 (19): 2145–56.

Hanger, Inc. 2015. "Our History: Acknowledging Our Past, Innovating Our Future." Accessed May 26, 2016. http://www.hanger.com/history/Pages/default.aspx.

Hanson, M. A., and P. D. Gluckman. 2011. "Developmental Origins of Health and Disease: Moving from Biological Concepts to Interventions and Policy." *International Journal of Gynecology and Obstetrics* 115 (1): S3–5.

Haraway, Donna. 2015. "Anthropocene, Capitalocene, Plantationocene, Chthulucene: Making Kin." *Environmental Humanities* 6:159–65.

Hardin, Jessica. 2018. "Embedded Narratives: Metabolic Disorders and Pentecostal Conversion in Samoa." *Medical Anthropology Quarterly* 32 (1): 22–41.

Hartman, Saidiya. 2007. *Lose Your Mother: A Journey Along the Atlantic Slave Route.* New York: Farrar, Straus, and Giroux.

Hatch, Anthony Ryan. 2016. *Blood Sugar: Racial Pharmacology and Food Justice in Black America.* Minneapolis: University of Minnesota Press.

Hayden, Melvin, Suresh Tyagi, Michelle Kerklo, and Mark Nicolls. 2005. "Type 2 Diabetes Mellitus as a Conformational Disease." *Journal of the Pancreas* 6 (4): 287–302.

Hayes, Tyrone and Guy Raz. 2016. "How Do Common Chemicals Affect Frogs, Rats—And Maybe Us?" NPR.org. https://www.npr.org/templates/transcript/transcript.php?storyId=497844694.

Hecht, Gabrielle. 2019. "Air in the Time of Oil." *Los Angeles Review of Books,* Provocation series. https://blog.lareviewofbooks.org/provocations/air-time-oil/.

Heijmans, B., E. W. Tobi, A. D. Stein, H. Putter, G. J. Blauw, E. Susser, P. E. Slagboom, and L.H. Lumey. 2008. "Persistent Epigenetic Differences Associated with Prenatal Exposure to Famine in Humans." *Proceedings of the National Academy of Sciences* 105 (44): 17046–49.

Helmreich, Stefan. 2014. "Homo microbis: The Human Microbiome, Figural, Literal, Political." *Thresholds* 42:52–59.

———. 2016. *Sounding the Limits of Life: Essays in the Anthropology of Biology and Beyond.* Princeton, NJ: Princeton University Press.

Herbert, Christopher. 2009. *War of No Pity: The Indian Mutiny and Victorian Trauma.* Princeton, NJ: Princeton University Press.

Herr, Michael. [1977] 1991. *Dispatches.* New York: Vintage.

Hill Collins, Patricia. 2017. "On Violence, Intersectionality and Transversal Politics." *Ethnic and Racial Studies* 40 (9): 1460–73.

Hirschman, Albert O. 1970. *Exit, Voice, and Loyalty.* Cambridge, MA: Harvard University Press.

Holmes, Seth. 2013. *Fresh Fruit, Broken Bodies: Migrant Farmworkers in the United States.* Berkeley: University of California Press.

Hoover, Elizabeth. 2017. *The River Is in Us: Fighting Toxics in a Mohawk Community.* Minneapolis: University of Minnesota Press.

Hopkins, Ruth. 2011. "Epigenetics: Scientific Evidence of Intergenerational Trauma." *Indian Country Today.* Accessed December 15, 2011. https://indiancountrymedianetwork.com/news/opinions/epigenetics-scientific-evidence-of-intergenerational-trauma/.

Horton, Richard, Robert Beaglehole, Ruth Bonita, John Raeburn, Martin McKee, and Stig Wall. 2014. "From Public to Planetary Health: A Manifesto." *Lancet* 383 (9920): 847.

Howard, Richard A. 1996. "The St. Vincent Botanical Garden—The Early Years." *Harvard Papers in Botany* 8:1–6.

Hugh-Jones, P. 1955. "Diabetes in Jamaica." *Lancet* 269 (6896): 891–97.

Hurley, Dan. 2013. "Grandma's Experiences Leave a Mark on Your Genes." *Discover Magazine,* May. http://discovermagazine.com/2013/may/13 -grandmas-experiences-leave-epigenetic-mark-on-your-genes.

Hussein, Julia. 2017. "Non-Communicable Diseases during Pregnancy in Low and Middle Income Countries." *Obstetric Medicine* 10 (1): 26–29.

Ibañez, Daniel, and Nikos Katsikis. 2014. *New Geographies 06: Grounding Metabolism.* Cambridge, MA: Harvard University Press.

IDF (International Diabetes Federation). 2005. "The Role of Urine Glucose Monitoring in Diabetes: A Valuable Technology in Appropriate Settings." *IDF Position Statement.* Brussels.

———. 2010. "Foreword." https://diabetesatlas.org/resources/previous-editions .html.

———. 2015. "IDF Diabetes Atlas, 7th Edition." https://www.idf.org/our-activities/advocacy-awareness/resources-and-tools/13:diabetes-atlas -seventh-edition.html.

———. 2016. *Annual Report 2016.* https://www.idf.org/component/attachmen ts/?task=download&id=1153.

———. 2017. "IDF Diabetes Atlas, 8th Edition." https://diabetesatlas.org/IDF_ Diabetes_Atlas_8e_interactive_EN/.

Idlebrook, Craig. 2014. "Understanding Insulin Sticker-Shock." *Insulin Nation,* Dec. 22. https://insulinnation.com/treatment/medicine-drugs/understanding -insulin-sticker-shock/.

Innis, Michelle. 2016. "Climate-Related Death of Coral around World Alarms Scientists." *New York Times,* Apr. 9.

Jackson, Jean. 2005. "Stigma, Liminality, and Chronic Pain: Mind-Body Borderlands." *American Ethnologist* 32 (3): 332–53.

Jackson, Michael. 2011. *Life within Limits: Well-Being in a World of Want.* Durham, NC: Duke University Press.

Jackson, Steven. 2014. "Rethinking Repair." *Media Technologies: Essays on Communication, Materiality and Society*, edited by T. Gillespie, P. Boczkowski, and K. Foot. Cambridge, MA: MIT Press.

Jain, S. Lochlann. 1999. "The Prosthetic Imagination: Enabling and Disabling the Prosthesis Trope." *Science, Technology & Human Values* 24 (1): 31–54.

———. 2007. "Living in Prognosis: Toward an Elegiac Politics." *Representations* 98 (1): 77–92.

———. 2013. *Malignant: How Cancer Becomes Us.* Berkeley: University of California Press.

Jain, Sudhir K., and Rashmisnata Barman. 2017. "Bacteriological Profile of Diabetic Foot Ulcer with Special Reference to Drug-Resistant Strains in a Tertiary Care Center in North-East India." *Indian Journal of Endocrinology and Metabolism* 21 (5): 688–94.

James, C. L. R. [1938] 1989. *The Black Jacobins.* New York: Vintage Books.

James, Erica Caple. 2010. *Democratic Insecurities: Violence, Trauma, and Intervention in Haiti.* Berkeley: University of California Press.

Jax, Thomas W. 2010. "Metabolic Memory: A Vascular Perspective." *Cardiovascular Diabetology* 9:51.

Johns Hopkins Medicine. 2018. "Amputation." Johns Hopkins Health Library. https://www.hopkinsmedicine.org/health/treatment-tests-and-therapies/amputation.

Johnson, Carolyn. 2016. "Why Treating Diabetes Keeps Getting More Expensive." *Washington Post,* October 31.

Johnson, Melissa. 2018. *Becoming Creole: Nature and Race in Belize.* New Brunswick, NJ: Rutgers University Press.

Johnson, Paul Christopher. 2007. "On Leaving and Joining Africanness through Religion: The 'Black Caribs' across Multiple Diasporic Horizons." *Journal of Religion in Africa* 37:174–211.

Johnson, Walter. 2018. "To Remake the World: Slavery, Racial Capitalism, and Justice." *Boston Review,* Forum One. http://bostonreview.net/forum/walter-johnson-to-remake-the-world.

Jones, Andrew. 2013. "Medical Equipment Donated to Developing Nations Usually Ends Up on the Junk Heap." *Scientific American,* May 6. https://www.scientificamerican.com/article/medical-equipment-donated-developing-nations-junk-heap/.

Jung, Carl. 1989. *Memories, Dreams, Reflections,* edited by Aniela Jaffé. New York: Random House Vintage.

Jusionyte, Ieva. 2018. *Threshold: Emergency Responders on the US-Mexico Border.* Oakland: University of California Press.

Kaiser, Kristine. 2011. "Preliminary Study of Pesticide Drift into the Maya Mountain Protected Areas of Belize." *Bulletin of Environmental Contamination and Toxicology* 86 (1): 56–59.

Kane, Stephanie. 1998. *AIDS Alibis: Sex, Drugs, and Crime in the Americas.* Philadelphia: Temple University Press.

Kauanui, J. Kēhaulani. 2016. "'A Structure, Not an Event': Settler Colonialism and Enduring Indigeneity." *Lateral: Journal of the Cultural Studies Association* 5 (1) (Spring). https://doi.org/10.25158/L5.1.7.

Kelley, Trista. 2013. "U.S. Insulin Prices Rise as Sanofi, Novo Awaits Rivals." *Bloomberg,* Aug. 15. https://www.bloomberg.com/news/articles/2013-08-15/u-s-insulin-prices-rise-as-sanofi-novo-await-rivals.

Kenner, Ali. 2013. "Invisibilities: Provocation." *Cultural Anthropology Fieldnotes,* June 15. www.culanth.org/fieldsights/invisibilities-provocation.

Kerns, Virginia. 1983. *Women and the Ancestors: Black Carib Kinship and Ritual.* Chicago: University of Illinois Press.

Kew Royal Botanic Gardens. 1892. Bulletin of Miscellaneous Information, 1892, 64: 92–104.

Kew Royal Botanic Gardens. 1893. Bulletin of Miscellaneous Information, 1893, 81: 231–296.

Kim, Julie Chun. 2014. "Natural Histories of Indigenous Resistance: Alexander Anderson and the Caribs of St. Vincent." *Eighteenth Century* 55 (2–3): 217–33.

Kim, Katie. 2011. "New Mexico Doctor Brutally Murdered in Belize." KRQE News. November 12, 2011.

Ki-moon, Ban. 2009. "United Nations Secretary-General Ban Ki-moon's Concluding Remarks at Forum Global Health." United Nations Secretary-General. June 5. www.un.org/sg/STATEMENTS/index.asp?nid=3922.

Kincaid, Jamaica. 1988. *A Small Place.* New York: Farrar, Straus and Giroux.

Kinnear, T. W. G., T. A. Grillo, and B. A. Elliot. 1964. "Excerpta Med." *International Congress Series* 74 (288).

Kistenberg, Rob. 2005. "Amputation Prevention Strategies in Developing Nations: A Study of Belize." Master's thesis, University of Texas, Houston.

Kleinman, Arthur. 1997. *Writing at the Margin: Discourse Between Anthropology and Medicine.* Berkeley: University of California Press.

Kleinman, Arthur, and Rachel Hall-Clifford. 2010. "Afterword: Chronicity— Time, Space, and Culture." In *Chronic Conditions, Fluid State,* edited by Lenore Manderson and Carolyn Smith-Morris, 247–52. Piscataway, NJ: Rutgers University Press.

Klonoff, David C. 2015. "What Do Your Fingernails Say about You? Can They Indicate That You Have Diabetes?" *Journal of Diabetes Science and Technology* 9 (6): 1167–69.

Knol, M. J., J. R. Twisk, A. F. Beekman, R. J. Heine, F. J. Snoek and F. Pouwer. 2006. "Depression as a Risk Factor for the Onset of Type 2 Diabetes Mellitus. A Meta-analysis." *Diabetologia* 49 (5): 837–45.

Kolbert, Elizabeth. 2014. *The Sixth Extinction: An Unnatural History.* New York: Henry Holt & Co.

Konig, M., and A. R. Shuldiner. 2012. "The Genetic Interface between Gestational Diabetes and Type 2 Diabetes." *Journal of Maternal-Fetal & Neonatal Medicine* 25 (1): 36–40.

Krieger, Nancy. 2012. "Methods for the Scientific Study of Discrimination and Health: An Ecosocial Approach." *American Journal of Public Health* 102 (5): 936–44.

———. 2013. *Epidemiology and the People's Health.* Oxford: Oxford University Press.

Kuzawa, Christopher W., and Elizabeth Sweet. 2009. "Epigenetics and the Embodiment of Race: Developmental Origins of US Racial Disparities in Cardiovascular Health." *American Journal of Human Biology* 21 (1): 2–15.

Lakoff, Andrew. 2017. *Unprepared: Global Health in a Time of Emergency.* Berkeley: University of California Press.

Lakoff, George, and Mark Johnson. 1980. *Metaphors We Live By.* Chicago: University of Chicago Press.

Lamoreaux, Janelle. 2016. "What If the Environment Is a Person? Lineages of Epigenetic Science in a Toxic China." *Cultural Anthropology* 31 (2): 188–214.

Landecker, Hannah. 2013a. "Postindustrial Metabolism: Fat Knowledge." *Public Culture* 25, 3 (71): 495–522.

———. 2013b. "Metabolism, Reproduction, and the Aftermath of Categories." *Life (Un)ltd: Feminism, Bioscience, Race* 11 (3). http://sfonline.barnard.edu/life-un-ltd-feminism-bioscience-race/metabolism-reproduction-and-the-aftermath-of-categories/.

———. 2015. "Antibiotic Resistance and the Biology of History." *Body & Society* 22 (4): 19–52. https://doi.org/10.1177%2F1357034X14561341.

———. 2018. "The Food of Our Food: Medicated Feed and the Industrialization of Metabolism." Paper presented at Center for Science, Technology, Medicine & Society, March 21, Berkeley, CA.

Langston, Nancy. 2011. *Toxic Bodies: Hormone Disruptors and the Legacy of DES.* New Haven, CT: Yale University Press.

Laymon, Kiese. 2018. *Heavy: An American Memoir.* New York: Simon & Schuster.

Leinonen, Pekka, Vilho Hiilesmaa, Risto Kaaja, and Kari Teramo. 2001. "Maternal Mortality in Type 1 Diabetes." *Diabetes Care* 24 (8): 1501–2.

Levi, Primo. 1995. *The Periodic Table.* New York: Schocken.

Lévi-Strauss, Claude. 1966. *The Savage Mind.* New York: Free Press.

Lilienfeld, D. E. 2000. "John Snow: The First Hired Gun?" *American Journal of Epidemiology* 152 (1): 4–9.

Lim, E. L., K. G. Hollingsworth, B. S. Aribisala, M. J. Chen, J. C. Mathers, and R. Taylor. 2011. "Reversal of Type 2 Diabetes: Normalisation of Beta Cell Function in Association with Decreased Pancreas and Liver Triacylglycerol." *Diabetologia* 54 (10): 2506–14.

Litvak, Jorge. 1975. "Diabetes Mellitus: A Challenge for the Countries of the Region." *PAHO Bulletin* 9 (4): 317–24.

Livingston, Julie. 2012. *Improvising Medicine: An African Oncology Ward in an Emerging Cancer Epidemic.* Durham, NC: Duke University Press.

Llewellyn, Robin. 2013. "Rediscovering the Half-Forgotten Farms of the Garifuna." *Los Angeles Review of Books,* January 13.

Lock, Margaret. 1993. *Encounters with Aging: Mythologies of Menopause in Japan and North America.* Berkeley: University of California Press.

———. 2013. "The Epigenome and Nature/Nurture Reunification: A Challenge for Anthropology." *Medical Anthropology* 32 (4).

Lucas, B. G. 1967. "Hyperbaric Oxygen Therapy: Its History and Current Scope." *Medical and Biological Illustration* 17 (3): 174–80.

Macpherson, Anne. 2007. *From Colony to Nation: Women Activists and the Gendering of Politics in Belize, 1912–1982.* Lincoln: University of Nebraska Press.

Malinowski, Bronislaw. 1935. *Coral Gardens and Their Magic, Volume I: Soil-Tilling and Agricultural Rites in the Trobriand Islands.* New York: Routledge.

Manderson, Lenore, and Carolyn Smith-Morris, eds. 2010. *Chronic Condition, Fluid States: Chronicity and the Anthropology of Illness.* Brunswick, NJ: Rutgers University Press.

Manderson, Lenore, and Narelle Warren. 2016. "'Just One Thing after Another': Recursive Cascades and Chronic Conditions." *Medical Anthropology Quarterly* 30 (4): 479–97.

Manjapra, Kris. 2018. "Plantation Dispossessions: The Global Travel of Agricultural Racial Capitalism." In *American Capitalism: New Histories,* edited by Sven Beckert and Christine Desan, 361–88. New York: Columbia University Press.

Marcus, George, and Michael Fischer. 1996. *Anthropology as Cultural Critique, 2nd edition.* Chicago: University of Chicago Press.

Marks, Jonathan. 2007. "The Long Shadow of Linnaeus's Human Taxonomy." *Nature* 447:28. www.nature.com/articles/447028a.

Martin, Emily. 1990. "Toward an Anthropology of Immunology: The Body as Nation State." *Medical Anthropology Quarterly* 4 (4): 410–26.

Martin, J.F., C.S. Johnston, C.T. Han, and D.C. Benyshek. 2000. "Nutritional Origins of Insulin Resistance: A Rat Model for Diabetes-Prone Human Populations." *Journal of Nutrition* 130 (4): 741–44.

Marx, Leo. 1964. *The Machine in the Garden.* New York: Oxford University Press.

Masco, Joe. 2010. "Bad Weather: On Planetary Crisis." *Social Studies of Science* 40 (1): 7–40.

Mathangi, D., R. Deepa, V. Mohan, M. Govindarajan, and A. Namasivayam. 2000. "Long Term Ingestion of Cassava (Tapioca) Does Not Produce Diabetes or Pancreatitis in the Rat Model." *International Journal of Gastrointestinal Cancer* 27 (3): 203–8.

Mauss, Marcel. 1966. *The Gift.* London: Cohen and West.

Mauvais-Jarvis, Franck, E. Sobngwi, R. Porcher, J.P. Riveline, J. Kevorkian, C. Vaisse, G. Charpentier, P.J. Guillausseau, P. Vexiau, and J.F. Gautier. 2004. "Ketosis-Prone Type 2 Diabetes in Patients of Sub-Saharan African Origin." *Diabetes* 53:645–53.

Mbanya, Jean Claude, Ayesha Motala, Eugene Sobngwi, Felix Assah, and Sostanie Enoru. 2010. "Diabetes in Sub-Saharan Africa." *Lancet* 375 (9733): 2254–66.

McClaurin, Irma. 1996. *Women of Belize: Gender and Change in Central America.* New Brunswick, NJ: Rutgers University Press.

McCollum, Siobhan. 2019. "The Cultural Impacts of Sargassum Invasion." Belize NICH / Institute for Social and Cultural Research Symposia, April 4, 2019.

McCutchon, Samuel. 1874. Samuel McCutchon papers, 1832–1874. In "Records of Ante-Bellum Southern Plantations from the Revolution through the Civil War, Part I." University Publications of America Records of Antebellum Southern Plantations Series I, Part 1, Reels 5–6. LSU Libraries Special Collections.

McDermott, Robyn. 1998. "Ethics, Epidemiology and the Thrifty Gene: Biological Determinism as a Health Hazard." *Social Science and Medicine* 47 (9): 1189–95.

McKay, Ramah. 2018. *Medicine in the Meantime: The Work of Care in Mozambique.* Durham, NC: Duke University Press.

McMillan, D.E., and P.H. Geevarghese. 1979. "Dietary Cyanide and Tropical Malnutrition Diabetes." *Diabetes Care* 2 (2): 202–8.

McMullin, Juliet. 2010. *The Healthy Ancestor: Embodied Inequality and the Revitalization of Native Hawai'ian Health.* Walnut Creek, CA: Left Coast Press.

Mendenhall, Emily, Brandon Kohrt, Shane Norris, David Ndetei and Dorairaj Prabhakaran. 2017. "Non-communicable disease syndemics: poverty, depression, and diabetes among low-income populations." *Lancet* 389(10072): 951–963.

Mendenhall, Emily, and Merrill Singer. 2019. "Comment on 'The Global Syndemic of Obesity, Undernutrition, and Climate Change.'" *Lancet* 393 (10173): 741.

Mendenhall, Emily, and Shane A. Norris. 2015. "When HIV Is Ordinary and Diabetes New: Remaking Suffering in a South African Township." *Global Public Health* 10 (4): 449–62.

Mendosa, David. 2000. "Meter Memories." *Diabetes Wellness Letter,* 1–6.

Mesnage, Robin, George Renney, Gilles-Eric Séralini, Malcolm Ward, and Michael N. Antoniou. 2017. "Multiomics Reveal Non-Alcoholic Fatty Liver Disease in Rats Following Chronic Exposure to an Ultra-Low Dose of Roundup Herbicide." *Nature, Scientific Reports* 7 (39328). doi:10.1038/srep39328.

Metropolitan Museum of Art. 2013. *Search for the Unicorn: An Exhibition in Honor of The Cloisters' 75th Anniversary,* May 15–Aug 18.

Meyers, Allan. 2012. *Outside the Hacienda Walls: The Archaeology of Plantation Peonage in Nineteenth-Century Yucatán.* Tucson: University of Arizona Press.

Michaels, Anne. 1998. *Fugitive Pieces.* New York: Vintage.

Mika, Marissa. 2015. "Research Is Our Resource: Surviving Experiments and Politics at an African Cancer Institute, 1950-Present." PhD diss., University of Pennsylvania. https://repository.upenn.edu/edissertations/1898.

Mintz, Sidney. 1974. *Worker in the Cane: A Puerto Rican Life History.* New York: W. W. Norton.

———. 1985. *Sweetness and Power: The Place of Sugar in Modern History.* New York: Penguin.

Mitaishvili, Ramaz. 2010. *Dialysis.* Los Angeles: RM Global Health.

Mitchell, Timothy. 2011. *Carbon Democracy: Political Power in the Age of Oil.* New York: Verso.

Moberg, Mark. 1997. *Myths of Ethnicity and Nation: Immigrants, Work and Identity in the Belize Banana Industry.* Knoxville: University of Tennessee Press.

Mobile Equine Hyperbaric Oxygen Therapy. 2019. "Hyperbaric Oxygen Therapy: A Simple Concept." http://www.mehotcenters.com/overview/simple -concept/.

Mohan, V., R. Mohan, L. Susheela, C. Snehalatha, G. Bharani, V. K. Mahajan, A. Ramachandran, M. Viswanathan, and E. M. Kohner. 1985. "Tropical Pancreatic Diabetes in South India: Heterogeneity in Clinical and Biochemical Profile." *Diabetologia* 28 (4): 229–32.

Mol, Annemarie. 2002. *The Body Multiple: Ontology in Medical Practice.* Durham, NC: Duke University Press.

———. 2008. *The Logic of Care: Health and the Problem of Patient Choice.* New York: Routledge.

———. 2009. "Living with Diabetes: Care beyond Choice and Control." *Lancet* 373 (9677): 1756–57.

Montoya, Michael. 2011. *Making the Mexican Diabetic: Race, Science, and the Genetics of Inequality.* Berkeley: University of California Press.

———. 2014. "Healthy Dissent: Urban Ecologies and the Art of Metabolic Politics." Paper presented as part of Metabolizing Environment panel at American Anthropological Association Annual Meeting, Dec. 3.

Moore, Jason W. 2000. "Sugar and the Expansion of the Early Modern World-Economy." *Fernand Braudel Center Review* 23 (3): 409–33.

Moran-Thomas, Amy. 2010a. "In Search of the 'Philanthropic Plum': Diabetes Research, Hookworm Interventions, and Comparative Philanthropy in Historical Perspective." Rockefeller Archives Center Research Reports. http://www.rockarch.org/publications/resrep/moranthomas.php.

———. 2010b. "The Paradox of Non-Communicable Epidemic." *West African Research Association News,* Spring, 8.

———. 2016. "Breakthroughs for Whom? Global Diabetes Care and Equitable Design." *New England Journal of Medicine* 375:2317–19.

———. 2017. "Glucometer Foils." *Limn* 9. https://limn.it/articles/glucometer-foils/.

Morrison, Errol, and Dalip Ragoobirsingh. 1992. "J-Type Diabetes Revisited." *Journal of the National Medical Association* 84 (7): 603–8.

Morrison, Toni. 1987. *Beloved.* New York: Vintage.

———. 2008. *What Moves at the Margin.* Jackson: University Press of Mississippi.

Morton, Timothy. 2000. "Blood Sugar." In *The Poetics of Spice: Romantic Consumerism,* 174–206. Cambridge: Cambridge University Press.

Moss, Michael. 2014. *Salt Sugar Fat.* New York: Penguin Random House.

Moss, Nancy, Michael C. Stone, and J. Smith. 1992. "Child Health Outcomes among Central American Refugees and Immigrants in Belize." *Social Science and Medicine* 36 (3): 203–17.

Mueller, Lucas. 2019. "Toxic Relationships: Health and the Politics of Science and Trade in the Postcolonial World." PhD diss., MIT HASTS.

Murphy, Michelle. 2013. "Distributed Reproduction, Chemical Violence, and Latency." *Life(UN)LTD: Feminism, Bioscience, Race* 11 (3): 1–2. http://sfonline.barnard.edu/life-un-ltd-feminism-bioscience-race/distributed-reproduction-chemical-violence-and-latency/o/.

———. 2017. "Alterlife and Decolonial Chemical Relations." *Cultural Anthropology* 32 (4): 494–503.

Nading, Alex. 2016. "Local Biologies, Leaky Things, and the Chemical Infrastructure of Global Health." *Medical Anthropology: Cross-Cultural Studies in Health and Illness* 36 (2): 141–56.

Nash, Linda. 2007. *Inescapable Ecologies: A History of Environment, Disease, and Knowledge.* Berkeley: University of California Press.

National Garifuna Council of Belize. [1998] 2015. "The Garifuna Agenda." http://www.ngcbelize.org/content/view/47/176.

Neel, B. A., and R. M. Sargis. 2011. "The Paradox of Progress: Environmental Disruption of Metabolism and the Diabetes Epidemic." *Diabetes* 60 (7): 1838–48.

Neel, James. 1962. "Diabetes Mellitus: A "Thrifty" Genotype Rendered Detrimental by "Progress"?" *American Journal of Human Genetics* 14 (4): 353–62.

Neil, M.J.E. 2015. "Pain after Amputation." *British Journal of Anaesthesia Education* 16 (3): 107–12.

Nelson, Alondra. 2016. *The Social Life of DNA: Race, Reparations, and Reconciliation After the Genome.* Boston: Beacon Press.

Nelson, Diane. 2015. *Who Counts? : The Mathematics of Life and Death after Genocide*. Durham, NC: Duke University Press.

Nerlich, Andreas, Albert Zink, Ulrike Szeimies, and Hjalmar Hagedorn. 2000. "Ancient Egyptian Prosthesis of the Big Toe." *Lancet* 356(9248): 2176–9.

Nestle, Marion. 2015. "Coca-Cola Says Its Drinks Don't Cause Obesity. Science Says Otherwise." *Guardian,* August 11.

Nguyen, Vihn-Kim. 2010. *The Republic of Therapy: Triage and Sovereignty in West Africa's Time of AIDS*. Durham, NC: Duke University Press.

Niewöhner, Jörg, and Margaret Lock. 2018. "Situating Local Biologies: Anthropological Perspectives on Environment/Human Entanglement." *BioSocieties* 13(4): 681–97.

Nixon, Rob. 2011. *Slow Violence and the Environmentalism of the Poor*. Cambridge, MA: Harvard University Press.

Nobel Women's Initiative. 2015. "Meet Miriam Miranda, Honduras." Dec. 9. https://nobelwomensinitiative.org/meet-miriam-miranda-honduras/.

Nolan, Christopher, Peter Damm, and Marc Prentki. 2011. "Type 2 Diabetes across Generations: From Pathophysiology to Prevention and Management." *Lancet* 378 (9786): 169–81.

Nwokolo, Chukuedu. 1986. "Tropical Diabetes." *Lancet* 328 (8509): 755.

Ofra, Danielle. 2019. "The Insulin Wars." *New York Times,* Jan. 18. https://www.nytimes.com/2019/01/18/opinion/cost-insurance-diabetes-insulin.html.

Oldenziel, R. 2011. "Islands: The United States as Networked Empire." In *Entangled Geographies: Empire and Technopolitics in the Global Cold War,* edited by G. Hecht, 13–42. Cambridge: MIT Press.

Oreskes, Naomi, and Erik Conway. 2011. *Merchants of Doubt: How a Handful of Scientists Obscured the Truth on Issues from Tobacco Smoke to Global Warming*. New York: Bloomsbury Press.

O'Rourke, Megan. 2014. "What's Wrong With Me? The Mysteries of Chronic Illness." Fellows Presentation, Radcliffe Institute for Advanced Study, Harvard University, December 10.

Osgood, N.D., R.F. Dyck, and W.K. Grassmann. 2011. "Inter- and Intragenerational Impact of Gestational Diabetes on the Epidemic of Type 2 Diabetes." *American Journal of Public Health* 101(1): 173–79.

Osseo-Asare, Abena Dove. 2008. "Bioprospecting and Resistance: Transforming Poisoned Arrows into Strophantin Pills in Colonial Gold Coast." *Social History of Medicine* 21 (2): 269–90.

Packard, Randall M. 2016. *A History of Global Health: Interventions into the Lives of Other Peoples*. Baltimore: Johns Hopkins University Press.

PAHO (Pan American Health Organization). 2002. "Belize." In *Health in the Americas,* 64–75. Washington, DC: Pan American Health Organization.

Palacio, I. Myrtle. 2011. *Adugurahani: A Walk Through Garifuna Spiritualism*. Belize City: Gleesima Research and Services.

Palacio, Joseph. 1982. "Food and Social Relations in a Garifuna Village." PhD diss., University of California, Berkeley.

———. 1983. "Food and Body in Garifuna Belief Systems." *Cajanus* 16 (3): 149–60.

————, ed. 2005a. *The Garifuna: A Nation across Borders—Essays in Social Anthropology.* Benque Viejo del Carmen, BZ: Cubola Books.

————. 2005b. "The Multifaceted Garifuna: Juggling Cultural Spaces in the 21st Century." In Palacio 2005a.

————, ed. 2005c. "Reconstructing Garifuna Oral History-Techniques and Methods in the History of a Caribbean People." In Palacio 2005a.

————. 2007. "How Did the Garifuna Become an Indigenous People? Reconstructing the Cultural Persona of an African-Native American People in Central America." *Revista Pueblos y Fronteras Digital* 2 (4). https://doi.org/10.22201/cimsur.18704115e.2007.4.226.

Palacio, Joseph O., Carlson Tuttle, and Judith Rae Lumb. 2011. *Garifuna Continuity in Land: Barranco Settlement and Land Use 1862 to 2000.* Caye Caulker, BZ: Producciones de la Hamaca.

Paradies, Y. C., M. J. Montoya, and S. M. Fullerton. 2007. "Racialized Genetics and the Study of Complex Diseases: The Thrifty Genotype Revisited." *Perspectives in Biology and Medicine* 50 (2): 203–27.

Parreñas, Juno Salazar. 2018. *Decolonizing Extinction: The Work of Care in Orangutan Rehabilitation.* Durham, NC: Duke University Press.

Patel, Raj. 2012. *Stuffed and Starved: The Hidden Battle for the World Food System.* New York: Melville House.

Patient Safety Authority. 2010. "Medication Errors with the Dosing of Insulin: Problems across the Continuum." *PA Patient Safety Advisory* 7 (1): 9–17.

Paxson, Heather. 2013. *The Life of Cheese: Crafting Food and Value in America.* Berkeley: University of California Press.

Pecoraro, Roger E., Gayle E. Reiber, and Ernest M. Burgess. 1990. "Pathways to Diabetic Limb Amputation: Basis for Prevention." *Diabetes Care* 13 (5): 513–21.

People v Latham. 2012. Court of Appeal, Fourth District, Division 1, California. Apr. 18.

Pepper, Christopher B., Thomas R. Rainwater, Steven G. Platt, Jennifer A. Dever, and Todd A. Anderson. 2004. "Organochlorine Pesticides in Chorioallantoic Membranes of Morelet's Crocodile Eggs from Belize." *Journal of Wildlife Diseases* 40 (3): 493–500.

Persson, Martina, Mikael Norman, and Ulf Hanson. 2009. "Obstetric and Perinatal Outcomes in Type 1 Diabetic Pregnancies." *Diabetes Care* 32 (11): 2005–9.

PETA (People for the Ethical Treatment of Animals). 2019. "Are Animal Ingredients Included in White Sugar?" *PETA FAQs.* www.peta.org/about-peta/faq/are-animal-ingredients-included-in-white-sugar/.

Peterson, Kristin. 2014. *Speculative Markets: Drug Circuits and Derivative Life in Nigeria.* Durham, NC: Duke University Press.

Petryna, Adriana. 2018. "Wildfires at the Edges of Science: Horizoning Work amid Runaway Change." *Cultural Anthropology* 33 (4): 570–95.

Pfeiffer, James, and Rachel Chapman. 2010. "Anthropological Perspectives on Structural Adjustment and Public Health." *Annual Review of Anthropology* 39 (1): 149–65.

Phillips, D. I., D. J. P. Barker, C. N. Hales, S. Hirst, and C. Osmond. 1994. "Thinness at Birth and Insulin Resistance in Adult Life." *Diabetologia* 37 (2): 150–54.

Pinto, Sarah. 2008. *Where There is No Midwife: Birth and Loss in Rural India.* New York: Berghahn Books.

Plumer, Brad. 2018. "How More Carbon Dioxide Can Make Food Less Nutritious." *New York Times,* May 23.

Pollin, T. I. 2011. "Epigenetics and Diabetes Risk: Not Just for Imprinting Anymore?" *Diabetes* 60 (7): 1859–60.

Pomet, Pierre. [1694] 1712. *A Compleat History of Druggs Divided into Three Classes, Vegetable, Animal and Mineral; With Their Use in Physick, Chymistry, Pharmacy, and Several Other Arts.* London: Printed for R. Bonwicke et al.

Porter, Michael, and Elizabeth Teisberg. 2006. *Redefining Healthcare: Creating Value-Based Competition on Results.* Boston: Harvard Business School Press.

Poudrier, Jennifer. 2008. "The Geneticization of Aboriginal Diabetes and Obesity: Adding Another Scene to the Story of the Thrifty Gene." *Canadian Review of Sociology* 44 (2): 237–61.

Pringle, Heather. 2010. "Sugar Masters in a New World." *Smithsonian.com,* January 12. Accessed April 10, 2018. https://www.smithsonianmag.com /history/sugar-masters-in-a-new-world-5212993/.

Prosthetic Hope International. 2011. "Project Hope Belize: How It all Began." http://www.prosthetichope.org/projects/belize/.

Puar, Jasbir. 2017. *The Right to Maim: Debility, Capacity, Disability.* Durham, NC: Duke University Press.

Quammen, David. 2018. *The Tangled Tree: A Radical New History of Life.* New York: Simon & Schuster.

Rabinow, Paul. 1995. *French Modern: Norms and Forms of the Social Environment.* Chicago: University of Chicago Press.

———. 1999. "Artificiality and Enlightenment: From Sociobiology to Biosociality." In *Essays on the Anthropology of Reason,* 91–111. Princeton, NJ: Princeton University Press.

Radin, Joanna. 2017. *Life on Ice: A History of New Uses for Cold Blood.* Chicago: University of Chicago Press.

Ralph, Laurence. 2012. "What Wounds Enable: The Politics of Disability and Violence in Chicago." *Disability Studies Quarterly* 32 (3). http://dsq-sds.org /article/view/3270/3099.

———. 2014. *Renegade Dreams: Living through Injury in Gangland Chicago.* Chicago: University of Chicago Press.

Ramos, Adele. 2009. "Dialysis Patients, Kidney Association Cry for Help." *Amandala,* December 15.

———. 2010. "R. I. P. Jose Cruz, Dialysis Advocate—Dead at 41." *Amandala,* December 14.

———. 2017. "Graveyard in Monkey River Menaced by Erosion." *Amandala,* May 10.

Rankine, Claudia. 2014. *Citizen: An American Lyric.* Minneapolis, MN: Graywolf Press.

Rao, R.H. 1988. "Diabetes in the Undernourished: Coincidence or Consequence." *Endocrinology Review* 9 (1): 67–87.

Rapp, Rayna. 1999. *Testing Women, Testing the Fetus: The Social Impact of Amniocentesis in America.* New York: Routledge.

Redfield, Peter. 2012. "Bioexpectations: Life Technologies as Humanitarian Goods." *Public Culture* 24 (166): 157–84.

———. 2013. *Life in Crisis: The Ethical Journey of Doctors without Borders.* Berkeley: University of California Press.

Reid, Basil, Peter Siegel, Nicholas Dunning, Corinne Hofman, Stéphen Rostain, Victor Thompson, and Scott Fitzpatrick. 2018. "Caribbean and Circum-Caribbean Farmers." In *The Archaeology of Caribbean and Circum-Caribbean Farmers 6000 BC-AD 1500*, 1–32. New York: Routledge.

Rettig, Richard. 2011. "Special Treatment: The Story of Medicare's ESRD Entitlement." *New England Journal of Medicine* 364:596–98.

Reynolds, Cuyler, ed. 1911. *Hudson-Mohawk Genealogical and Family Memoirs.* Vol. 1. New York: Lewis Historical, 61–65.

Reynolds Whyte, Susan, ed. 2014a. *Second Chances: Surviving AIDS in Uganda.* Durham, NC: Duke University Press.

———. 2014b. "The Publics of the New Public Health: Life Conditions and 'Lifestyle Diseases' in Uganda." In *Making and Unmaking Public Health in Africa*, edited by Ruth Prince and Rebecca Marsland, 187–207. Athens: Ohio University Press.

Rhodes-Pitts, Sharifa. 2013. *Harlem Is Nowhere.* New York: Little Brown / Back Bay Books.

Rich, Adrienne. [1971] 2016. "The Burning of Paper Instead of Children." In *Collected Poems*, edited by Claudia Rankine. 299–306. New York: W. W. Norton.

Richardson, Robert. 2009. "Belize and Climate Change: The Costs of Inaction." Belmopan, BZ: U.N. Development Program.

Ringholm, L., U. Pedersen-Bjergaard, B. Thorsteinsson, P. Damm, and E.R. Mathiesen. 2012. "Hypoglycaemia during Pregnancy in Women with Type 1 Diabetes." *Diabetic Medicine* 29 (5): 558–66.

Roberts, Dorothy. 2012. *Fatal Invention: How Science, Politics, and Big Business Re-create Race in the Twenty-first Century.* New York: New Press.

———. 2016. "The Old Biosocial and the Legacy of Unethical Science." Tanner Lectures on Human Values, Harvard University, November 2–3.

Roberts, Elizabeth. 2015. "Bio-Ethnography." *Somatosphere,* February 26, http://somatosphere.net/2015/02/bio-ethnography.html.

———. 2017. "What Gets Inside: Violent Entanglements and Toxic Boundaries in Mexico City." *Cultural Anthropology* 32 (4): 592–619.

Robinson, Cedric. 1983. *Black Marxism: The Making of the Black Racial Tradition.* Chapel Hill: University of North Carolina Press.

Rock, Melanie. 2003. "Sweet Blood and Social Suffering: Rethinking Cause-Effect Relationships in Diabetes, Distress, and Duress." *Medical Anthropology Quarterly* 22 (2): 131–74.

———. 2005a. "Classifying Diabetes; or, Commensurating Bodies of Unequal Experience." *Public Culture* 17 (3): 467–86.

————. 2005b. "Figuring Out Type 2 Diabetes through Genetic Research: Reckoning Kinship and the Origins of Sickness." *Anthropology and Medicine* 12 (2): 115–27.

Rodriguez, Richard. 2007. "Disappointment." In *Best American Essays*, edited by David Foster Wallace, 221–33. Boston: Houghton Mifflin.

Rodriguez, Tori. 2015. "Descendants of Holocaust Survivors Have Altered Stress Hormones." *Scientific American*, March 1. https://www.scientificamerican .com/article/descendants-of-holocaust-survivors-have-altered-stress -hormones/.

Rogers, Lee C., Robert G. Frykberg, David G. Armstrong, Andrew Boulton, Michael Edmonds et al. 2011. "The Charcot Foot in Diabetes." *Diabetes Care* 34 (9): 2123–29.

Rosaldo, Renato. 2004. "Grief and a Headhunter's Rage." In *Violence in War and Peace: An Anthology*, edited by N. Scheper-Hughes and P. Bourgois, 150–56. Hoboken, NJ: Blackwell.

Rosenberg, Charles. 1992. *Explaining Epidemics and Other Studies in the History of Medicine*. Cambridge: Cambridge University Press.

Rouse, Carolyn. 2009. *Uncertain Suffering: Racial Health Care Disparities and Sickle Cell Disease*. Berkeley: University of California Press.

Rugnetta, Michael. 2018. "Phantom Limb Syndrome." *Encyclopaedia Britannica, Inc.* https://www.britannica.com/science/phantom-limb-syndrome.

Russell, Andrew, and Lee Vinsel. 2018. "After Innovation, Turn to Maintenance." *Technology and Culture* 59(1): 1–25.

Russell, Kristin, Jonathan Stevens, and Theodore Stern. 2009. "Insulin Overdose among Patients with Diabetes: A Readily Available Means of Suicide." *Journal of Clinical Psychiatry* 11 (5): 258–62.

Saguy, Abigail, and Rene Almeling. 2005. "Fat Panic! The Obesity Epidemic as Moral Panic." Paper presented at the annual meeting of the American Sociological Association, Philadelphia, PA, Aug. 12.

Samal, K.C., A. Kanungo, and C.B. Sanjeevi. 2002. "Clinicoepidemiological and Biochemical Profile of Malnutrition-Modulated Diabetes Mellitus." *Annals of the New York Academy of Sciences* 958:131–37.

Sangaramoorthy, Thurka, and Adia Benton. 2012. "Enumeration, Identity, and Health." *Medical Anthropology* 31 (4):287–91.

Schaffer, Amanda. 2019. "Living with Type 1 Diabetes When you Can't Afford Insulin." *New Yorker*, Feb. 22. https://www.newyorker.com/news/as-told-to /living-with-type-1-diabetes-when-you-cant-afford-insulin.

Scheffler, Robin Wolfe. 2019. *A Contagious Cause: The American Hunt for Cancer Viruses and the Rise of Molecular Medicine*. Chicago: University of Chicago Press.

Scheper-Hughes, Nancy. 1993. *Death without Weeping: The Violence of Everyday Life in Brazil*. Berkeley: University of California Press.

————. 1995. "The Primacy of the Ethical: Propositions for a Militant Anthropology." *Current Anthropology* 36:3.

Schnell, M., M.E. Carvajal, and B. Anchustegui. 1993. "Effect of Cassava Bread Supplementation on Energy Intake of Rats." *Archeology of Latin American Nutrition* 43 (3): 217–20.

Schroeder, William, and Helmut Huebert. 1996. *Mennonite Historical Atlas*. Winnipeg, Canada: Springfield.

Schuler, Monica. 1989. "Review of *The Black Saturnalia*." *The Americas* 46 (2): 248–50.

Schulz, Laura C. 2010. "The Dutch Hunger Winter and the Developmental Origins of Health and Disease." *Proceedings of the National Academy of the Sciences* 107 (39): 16757–58.

Schwartz, Claire. 2016. "An Interview with Claudia Rankine." *TriQuarterly*, July 15. http://www.triquarterly.org/issues/issue-150/interview-claudia-rankine.

Scott, Julius S. 2018. *The Common Wind: Afro-American Currents in the Age of the Haitian Revolution*. New York: Verso.

Sebald, W. G. 1998. *Rings of Saturn*. New York: New Directions.

Seeberg, Jens, and Lotte Meinert. 2015. "Can Epidemics Be Noncommunicable? Reflections on the Spread of 'Noncommunicable' Diseases" *Medicine Anthropology Theory* 2:54–71.

Selin, Noelle Eckley, and Sae Yun Kwon. 2018. "Another Problem with China's Coal: Mercury in Rice." *The Conversation*. https://theconversation.com/another-problem-with-chinas-coal-mercury-in-rice-92974.

Sen, D. K., and G. S. Sarin. 1980. "Tear Glucose Levels in Normal People and in Diabetic Patients." *British Journal of Ophthalmology* 64 (9): 693–95.

Sepa, A., A. Frodi, and J. Ludvigsson. 2005. "Mother's Experiences of Serious Life Events Increase Risk of Diabetes-Related Autoimmunity in Their Children." *Diabetes Care* 28 (10): 2394–99.

Shakespeare, William. [1610] 2016. *The Tempest*. Washington, DC: New Folger Shakespeare Library.

Shaper, A. G. 1964. "Aetiology of Chronic Pancreatic Fibrosis with Calcification Seen in Uganda." *British Medical Journal*, June, 1607–9.

Shapiro, Nicholas. 2015. "Attuning to the Chemosphere: Domestic Formaldehyde, Bodily Reasoning, and the Chemical Sublime." *Cultural Anthropology* 30 (3): 368–93.

Sharp, Lesley. 2013. *The Transplant Imaginary: Mechanical Hearts, Animal Parts, and Moral Thinking in Highly Experimental Science*. Berkeley: University of California Press.

Sharpe, Christina. 2016. *In the Wake: On Blackness and Being*. Durham, NC: Duke University Press.

———. 2017. "'What Does It Mean to Be Black and Look at This?' A Scholar Reflects on the Dana Schutz Controversy." *Hyperallergic*, March 24, with interviewer S. Mitter. https://hyperallergic.com/368012/what-does-it-mean-to-be-black-and-look-at-this-a-scholar-reflects-on-the-dana-schutz-controversy/.

Shobhana, R., P. Rama Rao, A. Lavanya, R. Williams, C. Padma, V. Vijay, and A. Ramachandran. 2002. "Cost Incurred by Families Having Type 1 Diabetes in a Developing Country: A Study from Southern India." *Diabetic Research and Clinical Practice* 55 (1): 45–48.

Shoman, Assad. 1994. *Thirteen Chapters of a History of Belize*. Belize City: Angelus Press.

Simmons, Donald. 2001. *Confederate Settlements in British Honduras*. Jefferson, NC: McFarland.

Simmons, Kristen. 2017. "Settler Atmospherics." *Cultural Anthropology,* November 20. https://culanth.org/fieldsights/1221-settler-atmospherics.

Simpson, Audra. 2014. *Mohawk Interruptus: Political Life across the Borders of Settler States.* Durham, NC: Duke University Press.

Singerman, David Roth. 2015. "Inventing Purity in the Atlantic Sugar World, 1860–1930." *Enterprise & Society* 16 (4): 780–91.

Singh, Bhrigupati. 2015. *Poverty and the Quest for Life: Spiritual and Material Striving in Rural India.* Chicago: University of Chicago Press.

Smith-Morris, Carolyn. 2006. *Diabetes among the Pima: Stories of Survival.* Tucson: University of Arizona Press.

Solomon, Harris. 2016. *Metabolic Living: Food, Fat, and the Absorption of Illness in India.* Durham, NC: Duke University Press.

Song, Rhan-Ju. 2004. "Reconstructing Infant Diet and Weaning Behavior of Ancient Maya from Lamanai, Belize." PhD diss, University of Massachusetts at Amherst.

Sontag, Susan. 1988. *Illness as Metaphor and AIDS and Its Metaphors.* New York: Picador.

Sovik, O, and H. Thordarson. 1999. "Dead-in-Bed Syndrome in Young Diabetic Patients." *Diabetes Care* 22 (s2): B40–42.

Staiano, Kathryn. 1986. *Interpreting Signs of Illness: A Case Study in Medical Semiotics.* New York: Mouton de Gruyter.

Statistical Institute of Belize. 2011. "Belize Population and Housing Census: 2010 Country Report." Belmopan, Belize.

Stapleton, Sahael, Yanik Bababekov, Numa Perez, Zhi Ven Fong, and Daniel Hashimoto et al. 2018. "Variation in Amputation Risk for Black Patients: Uncovering Potential Sources of Bias and Opportunities for Intervention." *Journal of the American College of Surgeons* 226 (4): 641–9.

Star, Susan Leigh. 1999. "The Ethnography of Infrastructure." *American Behavioral Scientist* 43:377–91.

Stevens, Carl, David L. Schriger, Brian Raffetto, Anna Davis, David Zingmond, and Dylan Roby. 2014. "Geographic Clustering of Diabetic Lower Extremity Amputations in Low Income Regions of California." *Health Affairs* 33 (8): 1383–90.

Stevenson, Lisa. 2014. *Life Beside Itself: Imagining Care in the Canadian Arctic.* Berkeley: University of California Press.

Stewart, Kathleen. 2013. "Studying Unformed Objects: The Provocation of a Compositional Mode." *Fieldsights,* June 30. https://culanth.org/fieldsights/studying-unformed-objects-the-provocation-of-a-compositional-mode.

Stocker, Claire, Jonathan Arch, and Michael Cawthorne. 2005. "Fetal Origins of Insulin Resistance and Obesity." *Proceedings of the Nutrition Society* 64 (2): 143–51.

Stoler, Ann Laura, ed. 2013. Imperial Debris: On Ruins and Ruination. Durham: Duke University Press.

Stone, Michael C. 1994. "Caribbean Nation, Central American State: Ethnicity, Race, and National Formation in Belize, 1798–1990." PhD diss., University of Texas at Austin.

Strebel, Ignaz, Alain Bovet, and Philippe Sormani, eds. 2019. *Repair Work Ethnographies.* Singapore: Palgrave Macmillan.

Street, Alice. 2014. *Biomedicine in an Unstable Place: Infrastructure and Personhood in a Papua New Guinean Hospital*. Durham, NC: Duke University Press.

———. 2017. "Deep Diagnostics." "Little Development Devices/Humanitarian Goods." *Limn* 9.

Subramanian, Ajantha. 2009. *Shorelines: Space and Rights in South India*. Stanford, CA: Stanford University Press.

Sutherland, Anne. 1998. *The Making of Belize: Globalization in the Margins*. Westport, CT: Bergin & Garvey.

Sweeney, James. 2007. "Caribs, Maroons, Jacobins, Brigands, and Sugar Barons: The Last Stand of the Black Caribs on St. Vincent." *African Diaspora Archaeology* 10 (1): 1–38.

Sweeny, Robert. 2005. "Para-Sights: Multiplied Perspectives on Surveillance Research in Art Educational Spaces." *Surveillance & Society* 3(2–3): 240–50.

Sweitz, Sam. 2012. *On the Periphery of the Periphery: Household Archaeology at Hacienda San Juan Bautista Tabi, Yucatán, Mexico*. New York: Springer.

TallBear, Kim. 2013. *Native American DNA: Tribal Belonging and the False Promise of Genetic Science*. Minneapolis: University of Minnesota Press.

———. 2011. "Why Interspecies Thinking Needs Indigenous Standpoints." *Cultural Anthropology*, April 18. https://culanth.org/fieldsights/260-why-interspecies-thinking-needs-indigenous-standpoints.

Taussig, Michael. 1989. "History as Commodity." *Critique of Anthropology* 9 (1): 7–23.

Taylor, Christopher. 2012. *The Black Carib Wars: Freedom, Survival, and the Making of the Garifuna*. Jackson: University of Mississippi Press.

Taylor, Douglas. 1951. *The Black Carib of British Honduras*. New York: Wenner-Gren Foundation.

Thayer, Zaneta M, and Amy L. Non. 2015. "Anthropology Meets Epigenetics: Current and Future Directions." *American Ethnologist,* Nov 2. https://doi.org/10.1111/aman.12351.

Thiong'o, Ngugi wa. 2009. *Something Torn and New*. Philadelphia: BasicCivitas Books.

Thomas, Deborah. 2011. *Exceptional Violence: Embodied Citizenship in Transnational Jamaica*. Durham, NC: Duke University Press.

———. 2016. "Time and the Otherwise: Plantations, Garrisons and Being Human in the Caribbean." *Anthropological Theory* 16 (2–3): 177–200.

Todd, Zoe. 2017. "Fish, Kin and Hope: Tending to Water Violations in *amiskwaciwâskahikan* and Treaty Six Territory." *Afterall* 43:102–7.

Toomer, Jean. [1923] 2019. *Cane*. New York: Penguin Classics.

Torlone, Elisabetta, Graziano Di Cianni, Domenico Mannino, and Annunziata Lapolla. 2009. "Insulin Analogs and Pregnancy: An Update." *Acta Diabetologica* 46 (3): 163–72.

Trapp, Adele. 2011. "Sugar and Bullets—Belize's Leading Killers." *Amandala*, November 17. http://amandala.com.bz/news/sugar-and-bullets-belizes-leading-killers/.

Trethewey, Natasha. 2010. *Beyond Katrina: A Meditation on the Mississippi Gulf Coast*. Athens: University of Georgia Press.

Tripathy, B. B., and K. C. Samal. 1993. "Protein Deficient Diabetes Mellitus (PDDM) in India." *International Journal of Diabetes in Developing Countries* 13:3–13.

———. 1997. "Overview and Consensus Statement on Diabetes in Tropical Areas." *Diabetes Metabolic Review* 13 (1): 63–76.

Trouillot, Michel-Rolph. [1995] 2015. *Silencing the Past: Power and the Production of History*. Boston: Beacon Press.

Trujillo, Angelina. 2007. "Insulin Analogs and Pregnancy." *Diabetes Spectrum* 20 (2): 94–101.

Tsing, Anna Lowenhaupt. 1993. *In the Realm of the Diamond Queen: Marginality in an Out-of-the-Way Place*. Princeton, NJ: Princeton University Press.

———. 2015. *The Mushroom at the End of the World: On the Possibility of Life in Capitalist Ruins*. Princeton, NJ: Princeton University Press.

Tuchman, Arleen M. 2011. "Diabetes and Race: A Historical Perspective." *American Journal of Public Health* 101(1):24–33.

Tuck, Eve. 2009. "Suspending Damage: A Letter to Communities." *Harvard Educational Review* 79 (3): 409–28.

Tulloch, J. A., and D. MacIntosh. 1961. "J-type Diabetes." *Lancet* 2:119–21.

Turkle, Sherry. 2007. *Evocative Objects: Things We Think With*. Cambridge: MIT Press.

Turner, Victor. 1967. *The Forest of Symbols*. Ithaca, NY: Cornell University Press.

———. 1974. *Dramas, Fields and Metaphors: Symbolic Action in Human Society*. Ithaca, NY: Cornell University Press.

Ukpc, I. S. 1996. "Managing Tropical Diabetes Mellitus in Pemba, Mozambique: Which Way Out." *Tropical Doctor* 26 (1): 8–9.

Ulrich, Kate. 2017. "Some Chemical and More-Than-Human Transformations of Sugar/Energy." *Environment and Society*, June 21.

United Nations. 2014. "Global Study on Homicide." Vienna: United Nations Office on Drugs and Crime.

U.S. Environmental Protection Agency. 2008. "Cruise Ship Discharge Assessment Report." EPA Report # 842-R-07-005. Washington, DC.

U.S. National Kidney Foundation. 2018. "Global Facts." www.kidney.org/kidneydisease/global-facts-about-kidney-disease#_ENREF_3.

Valentine, Jerris. 2002. *Garifuna Understanding of Death*. Belmopan, BZ: National Garifuna Council of Belize.

van Braght, Thieleman J. Thieleman. [1660] 1950. *The Bloody Theater: Or Martyrs Mirror of the Defenseless Christians*. Scottsdale, PA: Mennonite Publishing House.

van Crevel, Reinout, Steven van de Vijver, and David A. J. Moore. 2017. "The Global Diabetes Epidemic: What Does It Mean for Infectious Diseases in Tropical Countries?" *Lancet* 5 (6): 457–68.

van der Donck, Adriaen. 1655. "Description of the New Netherlands." Collections of the New-York Historical Society. New-York: Printed for the Society, 1841. Second Series, v. 1, 125–42.

Vannier, Christian. 2011. "The Influence of Medical Tourism on Health Belief Systems in Rural Belize." Paper presented at the American Anthropological Association 110th Annual Meeting, Montreal.

Vas, Prashant, Michael Edmonds, and Nikolaos Papanas. 2017. "Nutritional Supplementation for Diabetic Foot Ulcers: The Big Challenge." *International Journal of Lower Extremity Wounds* 16 (4): 226–29.

Vasquez, Jules. 2011. "Chinese Community Holds Funeral for Three Murder Victims." 7 News Belize. April 11, 2011. www.7newsbelize.com/sstory .php?nid=19425.

Vaughan, Megan. 2018. "Conceptualising Metabolic Disorder in Southern Africa: Biology, History and Global Health." *BioSocieties* 14 (1): 123–42.

Vaughn, Sarah. 2017. "Disappearing Mangroves: The Epistemic Politics of Climate Adaptation in Guyana." *Cultural Anthropology* 32 (2): 242–68.

Velmurugan, G., T. Ramprasath, K. Swaminathan et al. 2017. "Gut Microbial Degradation of Organophosphate Insecticides-Induces Glucose Intolerance via Gluconeogenesis." *Genome Biology* 18 (1): 8.

Vizenor, Gerald. 1999. *Manifest Manners: Narratives on Postindian Survivance.* Lincoln: University of Nebraska Press.

Vogel, Sarah A. 2009. "The Politics of Plastics: The Making and Unmaking of Bisphenol A 'Safety.'" *American Journal of Public Health* 99 (S3): S559–66.

Voltaire, Jean Francois. [1759] 1918. *Candide.* New York: Modern Library.

Wailoo, Keith, Alondra Nelson, and Catherine Lee. 2012. *Genetics and the Unsettled Past: The Collision of DNA, Race, and History.* Piscataway, NJ: Rutgers University Press.

Walcott, Derek. 1992. "The Antilles: Fragments of Epic Memory." Nobel Lecture, December 7. In *Nobel Lectures, Literature 1991–1995,* edited by Sture Allén. Singapore: World Scientific.

Wald, Priscilla. 2008. *Contagious: Contagious: Cultures, Carriers, and the Outbreak Narrative.* Durham, NC: Duke University Press.

Walker, Kara. 2014. "A Subtlety, or the Marvelous Sugar Baby." *Art 21.* https:// art21.org/watch/extended-play/kara-walker-a-subtlety-or-the-marvelous -sugar-baby-short/.

Walley, Christine. 2013. *Exit Zero: Family and Class in Postindustrial Chicago.* Chicago: University of Chicago Press.

Walvin, James. 2018. *Sugar: The World Corrupted, From Slavery to Obesity.* New York: Pegasus Books.

Wang, Shu-Li, Jeng-Min Chiou, Chien-Jen Chen, Chin-Hsiao Tzeng, Wei-Ling Chou et al. 2003. "Prevalence of Non-insulin-dependent Diabetes Mellitus and Related Vascular Diseases in Southwestern Arseniasis-Endemic and Nonendemic Areas in Taiwan." *Environmental Health Perspectives* 111 (2): 155–59.

Wardian, Jana. 2018. "The Smell of Diabetes." *Clinical Diabetes* 36(3): 257–58.

Weaver, Mary Jo. 2019. *Sugar and Tension: Diabetes and Gender in Modern India.* New Brunswick, NJ: Rutgers University Press.

Weisz, George, and Etienne Vignola-Gagné. 2015. "The World Health Organization and the Globalization of Chronic Noncommunicable Disease." *Population and Development Review* 41 (3): 507–32.

Wells, J.C. 2007. "The Thrifty Phenotype as an Adaptive Maternal Effect." *Biological Review of the Cambridge Philosophical Society* 82 (1): 143–72.

Wendland, Claire. 2010. *A Heart for the Work: Journeys Through an African Medical School.* Chicago: University of Chicago Press.

Wendt, Diane. 2013. "Two Tons of Pig Parts: Making Insulin in the 1920s." *American History / Smithsonian Institute,* November 1. http://american history.si.edu/blog/2013/11/two-tons-of-pig-parts-making-insulin-in-the-19 20s.html.

Weston, Kath. 2017. *Animate Planet: Making Visceral Sense of Living in a High-Tech Ecologically Damaged World.* Durham, NC: Duke University Press.

Wetsman, Nicole. 2019. "23andMe Now Claims Its DNA Tests Can Predict Your Risk of Diabetes." *Popular Science,* March 12. https://www.popsci .com/23andme-prediabetes-test-survey-useful.

Whaley, Arthur. 2003. "Ethnicity/Race, Ethics, Epidemiology." *Journal of the National Medical Association* 95 (8): 736–42.

Whipps, Heather. 2008. "How Sugar Changed the World." *Live Science,* June 2.

Whitmarsh, Ian. 2008. *Biomedical Ambiguity: Race, Asthma, and the Contested Meaning of Genetic Research in the Caribbean.* Ithaca, NY: Cornell University Press.

———. 2011. "American Genomics in Barbados: Race, Illness, and Pleasure in the Science of Personalized Medicine." *Body & Society* 17 (2–3): 159–81.

———. 2013a. "Troubling 'Environments': Postgenomics, Bajan Wheezing, and Lévi-Strauss." *Medical Anthropology Quarterly* 27 (4): 489–509.

———. 2013b. "The Ascetic Subject of Compliance: The Turn to Chronic Diseases in Global Health." In *When People Come First: Evidence, Actuality and Theory in Global Health,* edited by João Biehl and Adriana Petryna, 302–24. Princeton: Princeton University Press.

Whitmarsh, Ian, and David S. Jones, eds. 2010. *What's the Use of Race? Modern Governance and the Biology of Difference.* Cambridge, MA: MIT Press.

Whitmarsh, Ian, and Elizabeth F.S. Roberts. 2016. "Nonsecular Medical Anthropology." *Medical Anthropology: Cross-Cultural Studies in Health and Illness* 35 (3): 203–8.

WHO (World Health Organization). 2016. *Global Report on Diabetes.* http:// apps.who.int/iris/bitstream/handle/10665/204871/9789241565257_eng.pdf ;jsessionid=1A92569A44430A5469766FDDD25DCFF6?sequence=1.

Wiedman, Dennis, and G.C. Lang. 2005. "Striving for Healthy Lifestyles: Contributions of Anthropologists to the Challenge of Diabetes in Indigenous Communities." In *Indigenous Peoples and Diabetes: Community Empowerment and Wellness.* Durham, NC: Carolina Academic Press.

Wilk, Richard. 2006a. *Fast Food/Slow Food: The Cultural Economy of the Global Food System.* Lanham, MD: AltaMira Press.

———. 2006b. *Home Cooking in the Global Village: Caribbean Food from Buccaneers to Ecotourists.* Oxford: Berg.

———. 2007. "The Extractive Economy: An Early Phase of the Globalization of Diet, and Its Environmental Consequences." In *Rethinking Environmental History,* edited by Alf Hornborg, J.R. McNeill, Joan Martinez-Alier, 179–98. Lanham: AltaMira Press.

Wilkinson, D., I.M. Chapman, and L.K. Heilbronn. 2012. "Hyperbaric Oxygen Therapy Improves Peripheral Insulin Sensitivity in Humans." *Diabetic Medicine* 29 (8): 986–89.

Williams, Eric. [1944] 2005. *Capitalism and Slavery*. Chapel Hill: University of North Carolina Press.

Wilson, William Julius. 1990. *The Truly Disadvantaged: The Inner City, the Underclass, and Public Policy*. Chicago: University of Chicago Press.

Wirtz, Veronika. 2019. "Introduction to MIT Seminar: Meeting the Challenge of Ensuring Global Access to Insulin." Keynote speaker, MIT Center for Biomedical Innovation, February 19.

Wolfe, Patrick. 2006. "Settler Colonialism and the Elimination of the Native." *Journal of Genocide Research* 8 (4): 387–409.

Woods, Jacqueline. 2003. "First Dialysis Centre Opens in Belize." Channel 5 News Belize. March 12, 2003. http://edition.channel5belize.com/archives /15509.

Wool, Zoë H. 2015. *After War: The Weight of Life at Walter Reed*. Durham, NC: Duke University Press.

World Bank. 2018. GDP per capita (US$). https://data.worldbank.org/indicator /NY.GDP.PCAP.CD?locations=ZJ-CL.

Wright, Uldine K. 2017. "Diabetic Foot: A Preliminary Study." *Belize Journal of Medicine* 6 (2): 24–27.

Yaghi, K., Y. Yaghi, A. A. McDonald, G. Yadegarfar, E. Cecil, J. Seidl, E. Dubois, S. Rawaf, and A. Majeed. 2012. "Diabetes or War? Incidence of and Indications for Limb Amputation in Lebanon, 2007." *Eastern Mediterranean Health Journal* 18 (12): 1178–86.

Yajnik, C. S. 2004. "Early Life Origins of Insulin Resistance and Type 2 Diabetes in India and Other Asian Countries." *Journal of Nutrition* 134 (1): 205–10.

Yates-Doerr, Emily. 2015. *The Weight of Obesity: Hunger and Global Health in Postwar Guatemala*. Berkeley: University of California Press.

———. 2017. "Where is the Local?: Partial Biologies, Ethnographic Sitings." *HAU* 7 (2): 377–401.

Young, Colin. 2008. "Belize's Ecosystems: Threats and Challenges to Conservation in Belize." *Tropical Conservation Science* 1 (1): 18–33.

Young, Colville, and Michael Phillips. 2007. "Sugar." In *Snapshots of Belize*, 95–104. Belize: Cubola.

Zhao, Yuxing, Heather L. Wieman, Sarah R. Jacobs, and Jeffrey C. Rathmell. 2008. "Mechanisms and Methods in Glucose Metabolism and Cell Death." *Methods in Enzymology* 442:439–57.

Zuberi, Tukufu. 2001. *Thicker than Blood: How Racial Statistics Lie*. Minneapolis: University of Minnesota Press.

Zuidema, P. J. 1955. "Calcification and Cirrhosis of the Pancreas in Patients with Deficient Nutrition." *Doumenta de Medicina Geographica et Tropica* 7 (3): 229–51.

Index